# TREATMENT OF RETINOPATHY OF PREMATURITY

# Treatment of Retinopathy of Prematurity

**Joseph W. Eichenbaum, M.D.**
Clinical Instructor of Ophthalmology
Mount Sinai Medical School
Assistant Attending
Manhattan Eye, Ear and Throat Hospital
New York, New York

**Alfred E. Mamelok, A.B., M.D.**
Clinical Associate Professor of Ophthalmology
Cornell Medical College
Attending Surgeon and Director of Uveitis Clinic
Manhattan Eye, Ear and Throat Hospital
New York, New York

**Rainer N. Mittl, M.D.**
Assistant Professor of Ophthalmology
College of Physicians and Surgeons
Assistant Attending
Columbia-Presbyterian Medical Center
New York, New York

**Juan Orellana, M.D.**
Assistant Clinical Professor of Ophthalmology
Mount Sinai Medical School
New York, New York

**YEAR BOOK MEDICAL PUBLISHERS, INC.**
CHICAGO • LONDON • BOCA RATON • LITTLETON, MASS.

**Library of Congress Cataloging-in-Publication Data**
Treatment of retinopathy of prematurity / [edited by]
Joseph W. Eichenbaum.
p. cm.
Includes bibliographical references.
ISBN 0-8151-3049-X
1. Retrolental fibroplasia—Treatment. I. Eichenbaum, Joseph W.
[DNLM: 1. Retinopathy of Prematurity—therapy. WW 270 T784]
RJ313.T74 1990
618.92'09773—dc20 89-70655
DNLM/DLC CIP
for Library of Congress



1 2 3 4 5 6 7 8 9 0 YR 94 93 92 91 90

Sponsoring Editor: David K. Marshall
Assistant Managing Editor, Text and Reference: Jan Gardner
Production Project Coordinator: Karen Halm
Proofroom Supervisor: Barbara M. Kelly

# CONTRIBUTORS

**Albert L. Ackerman, M.D.**
*Associate Clinical Professor of Ophthalmology*
*Albert Einstein College of Medicine*
*Adjunct Attending*
*Montefiore Hospital*
*Bronx, New York*

**Joseph W. Eichenbaum, M.D.**
*Clinical Instructor of Ophthalmology*
*Mount Sinai Medical School*
*Assistant Attending*
*Manhattan Eye, Ear and Throat Hospital*
*New York, New York*

**John T. Flynn, M.D.**
*Professor, Bascom Palmer Eye Institute*
*University of Miami*
*Miami, Florida*

**Alfred E. Mamelok, A.B., M.D.**
*Clinical Associate Professor of Ophthalmology*
*Cornell Medical College*
*Attending Surgeon and*
*Director of Uveitis Clinic*
*Manhattan Eye, Ear and Throat Hospital*
*New York, New York*

**Rainer N. Mittl, M.D.**
*Assistant Professor of Ophthalmology*
*College of Physicians and Surgeons*
*Assistant Attending*
*Columbia-Presbyterian Medical Center*
*New York, New York*

**Juan Orellana, M.D.**
*Assistant Clinical Professor of Ophthalmology*
*Mount Sinai Medical School*
*New York, New York*

**Arnall Patz, M.D.**
*Professor of Ophthalmology*
*and Director, Emeritus*
*The Wilmer Institute*
*The Johns Hopkins Medical Institutions*
*Baltimore, Maryland*

**Rand Spencer, M.D.**
*Clinical Assistant Professor of Ophthalmology*
*University of Texas*
*Southwestern Medical School*
*Attending Staff*
*Baylor University Medical Center*
*Dallas, Texas*

**Harvey W. Topilow, M.D.**
*Associate Clinical Professor of Ophthalmology*
*Albert Einstein College of Medicine*
*Attending Surgeon Retina Service*
*Montefiore Hospital*
*Bronx, New York*

# INTRODUCTION

Over the last 44 years a plethora of literature has emerged on retrolental fibroplasia (RLF) and retinopathy of prematurity (ROP). There appears to have been an "oxygen epidemic" from the late 1940s through the mid 1950s. During this period ROP was the leading cause of blindness in neonates. This resulted in the mid 1950s in three prospective, controlled studies and one large retrospective review of the use of oxygen in nurseries. Although the percentage of arterial oxygen delivered per se could not be incriminated, the duration of oxygen administration was found to be of significance. However, most centers developed guidelines in neonatal oxygen therapy that differed from the conclusions of the large multicenter, cooperative controlled studies.

Over the next 25 years a number of factors, including phototoxicity, ischemia, elevated oxygen levels, low oxygen levels, adrenocortical deficiency, elevated and low carbon dioxide levels, vitamin E or A deficiency, iron deficiency, maternal factors, multiple gestation, poor nutrition, cyanotic congenital heart disease, anencephaly, exchange and replacement transfusion, complications of pregnancy, congenital anomalies, intraventricular hemorrhage, septicemia, and prematurity itself, were advanced as possible causes of the disease. Despite meticulous attention to oxygen use, however, the disease is increasingly prevalent at this writing; in fact, it has occurred in term infants who have never been given supplemental oxygen as well as in the hypoxic infant.

Court awards, mostly based on excessive oxygen therapy, have run into the millions of dollars. However, the disease of fibrovascular proliferation in the neonatal retina, or ROP, remains an enigma.

**Joseph W. Eichenbaum, M.D.**

# FOREWORD

In the epidemic of Retinopathy of Prematurity (ROP) in the early 1950s, overuse of oxygen was identified as the major cause of the disorder. It is significant that during the epidemic, very low birth weight infants, those with markedly immature retinal vessels and hence greater susceptibility to ROP, rarely survived. With modern neonatal intensive care, including arterial blood-gas monitoring and other sophisticated measures, a significant population of these infants with very immature retinas and high risk for ROP are surviving. ROP is occurring in this new population of high risk, small premature infants in spite of the most meticulous monitoring of oxygen.

Recognizing that a significant number of new cases of ROP are developing, the authors present a useful update on treatment and address several key aspects of ROP. These include a historical overview by Dr. Joseph Eichenbaum and a special chapter on medicolegal aspects by Dr. Alfred Mamelok.

Dr. John Flynn, who has contributed so greatly to the modern understanding of ROP, has written a chapter on the clinical overview of the disorder. Current concepts on the natural history, suggested pathogenesis, and the new international classification are included.

Drs. Harvey Topilow and Albert Ackerman have provided chapters on the rationale for cryotherapy and present their experiences in the use of cryotherapy for advanced stage 3 ROP.

For the first time since Terry's original identification of ROP in the early 1940s, a successful form of treatment has been conclusively documented. The multicenter national clinical trial on cryotherapy provided the large sample size necessary to confirm the studies of several individual investigators who reported on this method of treatment. Cryotherapy reduced the incidence of adverse outcome from severe ROP by approximately 50% in the collaborative study. Dr. Rand Spencer, a principal investigator in the study, has summarized the findings and recommendations from this collaborative effort.

Dr. Rainer Mittl has provided an update on vitrectomy surgery, which permits the treatment of the more advanced stages of ROP. Dr. Juan Orellana has presented chapters describing scleral buckling for stages 4 and 5 ROP and the "open-sky" vitrectomy technique for stage 5 disease.

The authors are to be congratulated on this useful contribution to the contemporary management of ROP.

**Arnall Patz, M.D.**
*Professor of Ophthalmology*
*and Director, Emeritus*
*The Wilmer Institute*
*The Johns Hopkins Medical Institutions*
*Baltimore, Maryland*

# PREFACE

Retinopathy of prematurity (ROP), or retrolental fibroplasia as it was originally named, has had a most curious life span as a twentieth century disease. The enigmatic findings of the disease, with scar tissue behind the neonate lens associated with retinal detachment, have been responsible for the two largest "epidemics" of blindness in neonates in modern times. These outbreaks of the disease occurred approximately 25 years apart, in the mid 1950s and late 1970s. Initially, excessive oxygen use in the newborn nurseries was implicated as the cause of the disease. However, just as the directives against hyperoxic therapy were known to have been enforced, a new ROP epidemic in the late 1970s surfaced. Restricting oxygen in neonates was also shown to result in increased brain damage in infants. Neonatologists, pediatricians, obstetricians, and ophthalmologists have recently attempted to view the disease as a problem of prematurity itself. Nonetheless, the literature is replete with exceptions. Many reports cite ROP in full-term infants. Certain studies suggest the efficacy of vitamin E in treating the disease; others deny any statistically significant role of the vitamin. Retinal buckling, drainage of subretinal fluid, and cryotherapy seem to offer hope. Their application, timing and relationship to the mechanisms of the disease, however, remain controversial. Thus in the last 45 years, although much has been written about the cause and therapy of ROP, little is actually understood.

Despite this woefully puzzling predicament over the state of our medical knowledge, malpractice suits relative to administration of oxygen in infants over the last 25 years have been legion, with awards into the millions of dollars. Cases are still being brought to trial regarding optimal therapy. Yet many of our newer concepts of understanding, managing, and treating ROP have barely achieved clinical recognition and acceptance.

It was with the concept of our uncertainty as clinicians and the lack of clear understanding of the cause and management of ROP that the editors met to discuss the contents of this text. The medical as well as the legal literature was reviewed to highlight what has been learned from medical research and what telescoped into the courtroom. Experts in vitrectomy, retinal buckling, and cryotherapy were asked to write on their experiences and strategies in ROP. *Therapy of Retinopathy of Prematurity* presents the history of ROP, the frustrating medicolegal implications, and the controversial management of this disabling disease, along with hope of providing a stepping stone to further understanding.

**Joseph W. Eichenbaum, M.D.**

*I wish to acknowledge my gratitude to Ms. Belinda Daniel for her typing of many portions of the text and for her careful and considerate suggestions, perseverance, and devotion.*

*Many thanks to my wife, Dr. Annette Eichenbaum, for her understanding, patience, and support as well as timely review of statistical material.*

*Many thanks to my co-editors, Drs. Mamelok, Mittl, and Orellana, whose insights and judgments made this text possible.*

*I wish to express my sincere gratitude to Dr. Arnall Patz for reviewing large portions of this manuscript and for providing additional historical information as well as suggestions on various chapters of the text. I thank Dr. Richard Green for providing didactic photomicrographs from his work on ROP. Special thanks to Dr. Steven Podos for reviewing the entire manuscript.*

*Last, but not least, I would like to express my appreciation to my children, Kenny and Gary, whose simple but loving and gentle support of the project helped make it all worthwhile.*

**Joseph W. Eichenbaum, M.D.**

# CONTENTS

# Color Plates

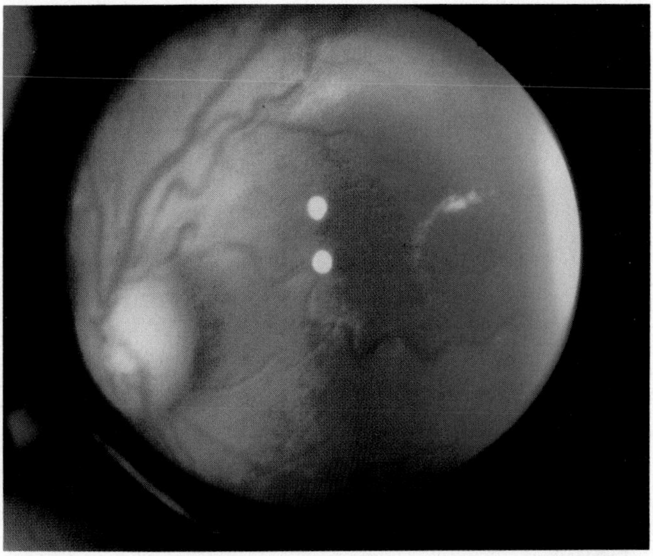

**PLATE 1.**
Plus disease, with tortuous arterioles and dilated venules. Note bright red arteriolized blood in venules as a result of high flow rate through the peripheral AV shunt. (From Topilow HW, Ackerman AL, Wang FM: *Ophthalmology* 1985; 92:379–387. Used by permission.)

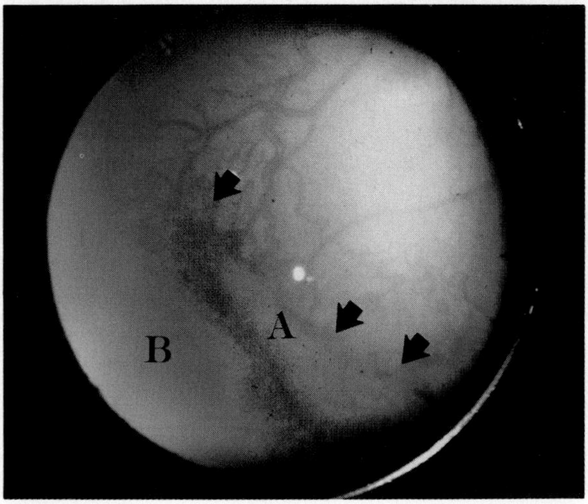


**PLATE 2.**
Stage 3+ ROP. Retinal vessels terminate in abnormal vascular arcades in an elevated thickened AV shunt *(A)* with a wide zone of avascular retina *(B)* anteriorly. Ragged confluent growth of preretinal neovascularization is noted along the posterior border of the AV shunt *(arrows)*.

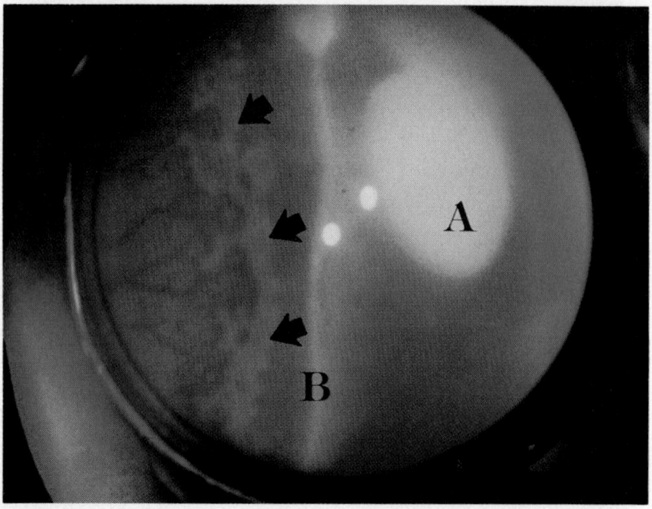


**PLATE 3.**
Cryotherapy *(A)* is applied to the wide avascular zone anterior to the AV shunt *(B)*. Confluent preretinal neovascularization *(arrows)* is noted posterior to the AV shunt. (From Topilow HW, Ackerman AL, Wang FM: *Ophthalmology* 1985; 92:379–387. Used by permission.)

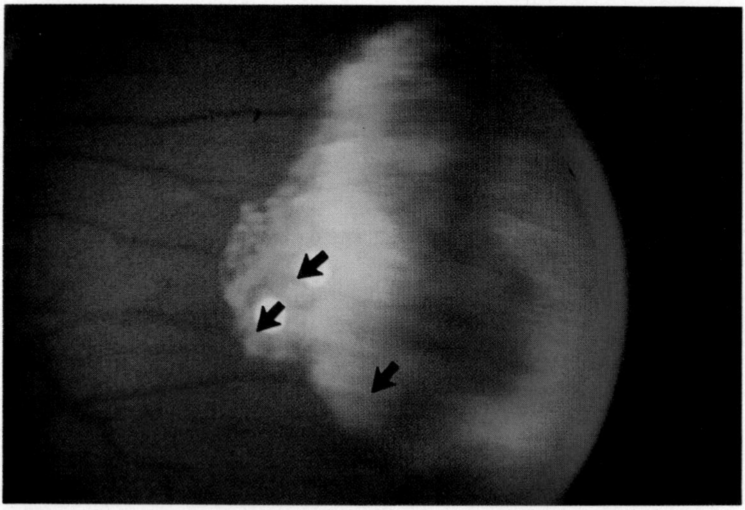

**PLATE 4.**
Cryotherapy reaction 3 weeks after treatment, with complete resolution of the AV shunt and preretinal neovascularization previously located posterior to the area of treatment. Retinal vessels *(arrows)* now extend anteriorly into the zone of treatment, which had been avascular. (From Topilow HW, Ackerman AL, Wang FM: *Ophthalmology* 1985; 92:379–387. Used by permission.)

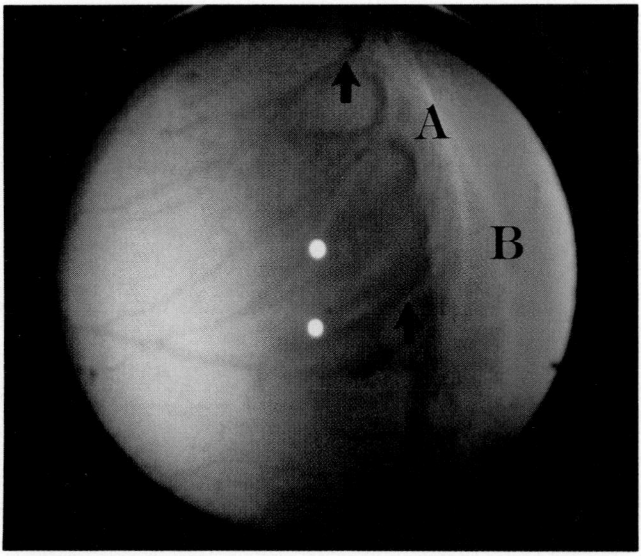


**PLATE 5.**
Confluent preretinal neovascularization *(A)* covers the AV shunt. Wide zone of avascular retina *(B)* is presently anteriorly. Vitreous traction causes elevation of preretinal neovascularization and retinal vessels *(arrows)*, which terminate in the underlying AV shunt.

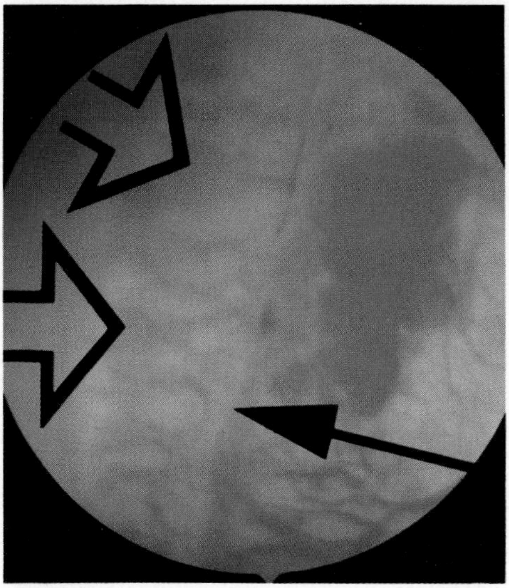

**PLATE 6.**
Relatively early growth of new vessels *(open arrows)* beyond previous peripheral shunt *(solid arrow)*.

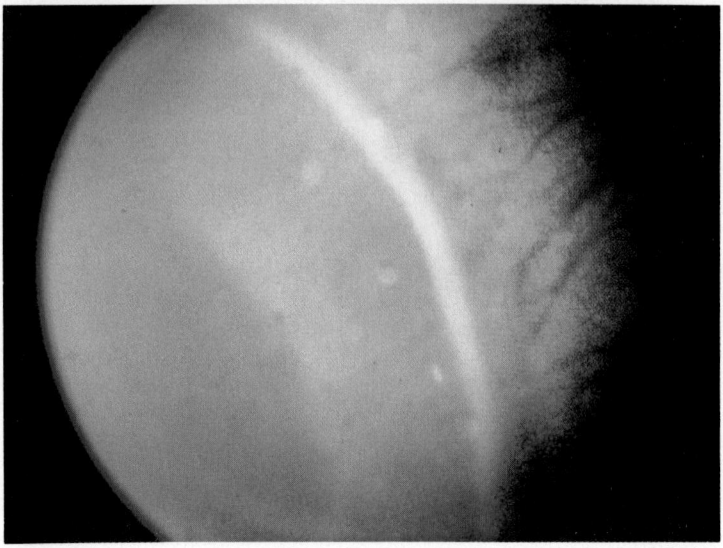

**PLATE 7.**
Last stage of regressing ROP with white fribrosis of "old" peripheral shunt and generalized attenuation of vessel caliber.

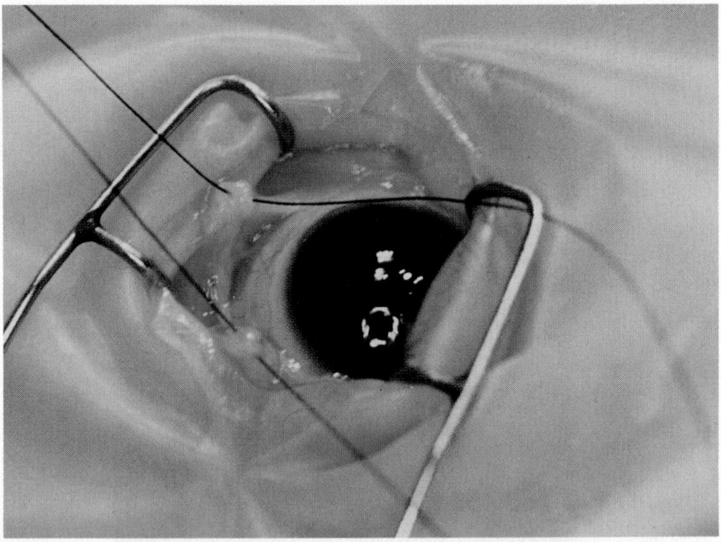

**PLATE 8.**
Relaxing incisions are made in the conjunctiva in oblique quadrants, and the edges are tagged with black silk to facilitate reapposition at the end of the procedure.

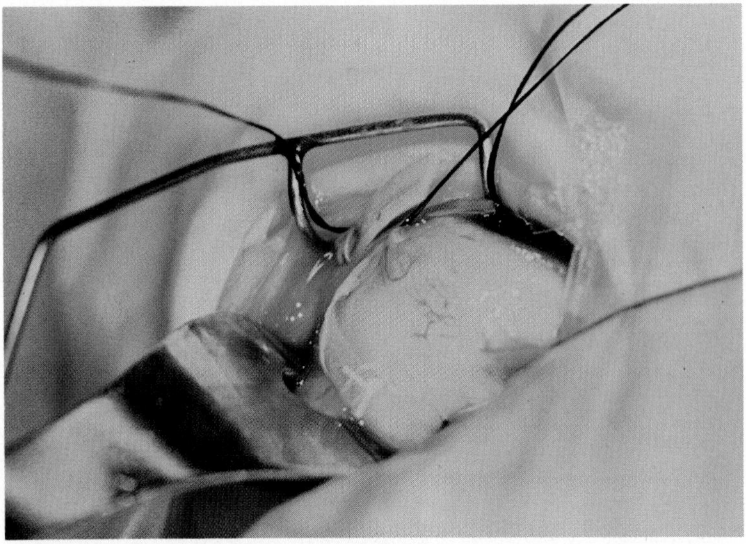

**PLATE 9.**
The band is in position and the excessive strip of solid silicone has been trimmed. The buckle will support areas of vitreoretinal traction.

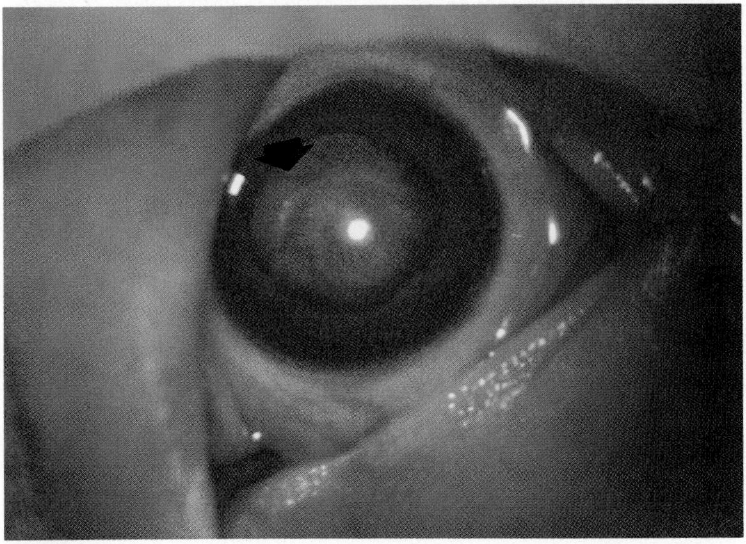

**PLATE 10.**
Prominent retinal vessels in the detached retina *(arrow)* are easily seen through the clear crystalline lens. The center of this funnel has a moderately transparent membrane bridging the funnel opening.

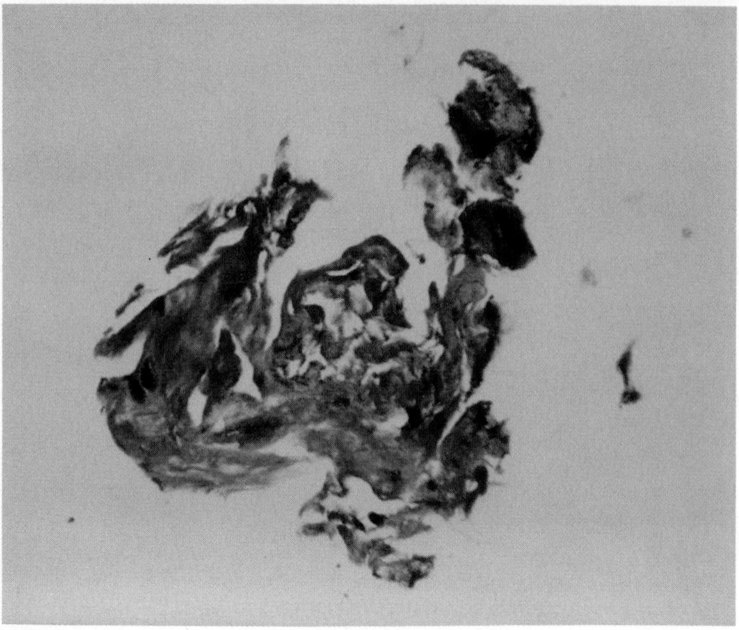

**PLATE 11.**
Specimen taken from a 2-year-old child. The tissue, which was located behind the lens and bridging the funnel, demonstrates a large amount of minimally vascularized connective tissue. (Masson-trichrome; ×60.)

Chapter 1

# Medicolegal Aspects of Retinopathy of Prematurity

Alfred E. Mamelok, M.D.

Since the mid-1950s, there has been an explosion of malpractice actions against physicians who treat retinopathy of prematurity (ROP). In many cases, similar actions have been taken against hospitals and manufacturers of appliances, including devices that supply oxygen and control humidity in incubators.

Most of these cases were based on the findings of the National Cooperative Study of 1953–1954. Studies during that era demonstrated a generally increased risk of retrolental fibroplasia (RLF) among infants treated in a high-oxygen group, compared with infants given limited oxygen. This fact was given much play in the medical and lay press and other media, alerting a good percentage of the victims of this disease or their parents to the possibility of litigation. As will be shown below, most of the cases cited "improper administration of oxygen" to the claimant. That analysis of the data also repeatedly showed that some babies in the low-oxygen groups went on to develop RLF, whereas many in the high-oxygen group had no signs of the disease, which is almost never mentioned when these malpractice cases are reviewed. Nor has it been mentioned, as one study showed, that there is no single arterial oxygen tension level at which premature infants will uniformly show changes of ROP; this implies that there is no uniform level at which this disease will develop. Why certain premature infants are more susceptible to the disease than others remains one of many questions still unanswered.

Lucey and Dangman reviewed the subject in the latter part of 1983[1] in a comprehensive article that concluded that RLF should not be considered an avoidable iatrogenic disease in very low birth weight infants, and that its cause in these infants is not known. They postulated that it is probably incorrect to make the assumption that "excessive" use of oxygen in treating prematurely born infants is the cause of this disease. They cited three prospective controlled studies and one large retrospective review as demonstration of their position. They pointed out that when the experiences of the four original studies were combined, 37% (51/137) of the high-oxygen group of infants did not develop RLF, while 22% (89/407) of the low-oxygen group of infants did develop the disease. Further, they located 95 infants of low birth weight who never received oxygen but nevertheless developed ROP. They pointed to one study which produced evidence suggesting that lack of oxygen, rather than excess oxygen, might be the cause.

Another study showed increased risk for the disease among infants who received exchange transfusions. One study analyzed several cases of unilateral RLF or marked discrepancies in the severity of the disease between the two eyes in human infants, which is inconsistent with a simple, generalized, toxic (hyperoxic) etiology.

Other questions such as the role of vitamin E have received much attention in the medical literature and much controversy still surrounds this aspect of the problem. As the results of studies and research proliferate, the work of plaintiff malpractice attorneys will become more difficult, if not impossible, until a true breakthrough occurs in prevention.

Because the number of premature infants saved at lower and lower birth weights continually increases, we can expect the problem to remain with us for a long time.

Attorneys need established facts, statutes, and precedents in order to successfully argue their cases before judges and juries. Perdue, an attorney writing in the textbook, *Retinopathy of Prematurity* by McPherson, Hittner, and Kretzer[2] states:

> If qualified medical experts are willing to present the necessary scientific knowledge, a medical standard may be established to the law's satisfaction. In the area of retinopathy of prematurity, this could involve claims for damages arising from improper oxygen therapy; withholding vitamin E prophylaxis; for death or hepatic failure as a result of using vitamin E, not F.D.A approved; for late retinal screening, so that cryotherapy could not be properly applied; and for withholding cryotherapy.

In malpractice litigation involving cases of retinopathy of prematurity, this would be the plaintiff lawyer's dream, but as is obvious from the above, from a general review of the literature, and in other parts of this book, the necessary scientific knowledge is nowhere near being established, and such a medical standard cannot be established to the law's satisfaction.

Nevertheless, in the arena of malpractice litigation, high awards have been granted where even the defendant admitted negligence by "prolonged exposure to relatively high concentrations of oxygen." This is illustrated in *Penetrante v United States*[3] (Table 1–1, case 14), in which awards of $2,292,123 to one twin and $900,000 to the second twin were made by the United States District Court in a nonjury retrial. How relatively high the concentration of oxygen was and the details of the monitoring were not mentioned. Interestingly, one twin was extremely bright intellectually, while the other, who was totally blind and who received the larger award, was severely mentally retarded. No mention was made about whether the mental retardation was the result of lack of sufficient oxygen. Is there a trade-off between cerebral damage and eye damage, especially when we cannot prove the eye damage is simply caused by "excess oxygen"? In the legal analysis of these cases, the traditional medical concept of risk vs. benefit becomes the issue. A fascinating aspect of this case is that the defendant admitted negligence and presented no evidence in his defense, despite the many articles in the literature and the research studies that questioned the role of oxygen as a sole etiology of ROP. This gave the plaintiff attorneys an opportunity to produce expert medical testimony by an ophthalmologist, a neurologist, and a clinical psychologist. The ophthalmologist testified that the second infant, who was blind in the right eye, had vision of 20/50 in the left eye when his head was turned to a degree when he attempted to read the eye chart, and that he was more likely by 20% to have a retinal detachment in the left eye in his later years. If this did occur, the best result would be a failure of the retina to reattach, such that no vision in the left eye could exist. The ophthalmologist further testified that the second twin was directed to avoid all contact sports and other activities which could cause jarring of the head, that he would be unable to obtain a driver's license or a license to drive for hire, and that his range of future employment possibilities would be limited accordingly. The neurologist testified that the second infant was not well-coordinated, and had difficulty doing chores his peers might perform. While his intelligence was judged normal, if not superior, serious psychological problems were anticipated according to the results of psychological tests. On appeal, the apellate court held that "the award for damages was not excessive nor shocking."

In the case of *Burton v Brooklyn Doctor's Hospital*[4] (Table 1–1, case 18), the allegation was that a baby who was five to six weeks premature developed RLF as a result of being exposed to a "high oxygen state" for 28 days in an incubator, causing irreversible blindness. Except for faint light perception in his left eye, the plaintiff was totally blind. His attorneys alleged that he suffered daily pain and irritation which had worsened in recent years. An opinion was rendered that because his eyes were shrinking, they would have to be enucleated and replaced with plastic eyes. At the trial, the jury found for the plaintiff, awarding him $2,887,000 in damages. This amount was

**TABLE 1–1.**
Cases Involving Administration of Oxygen to Premature Infants

| Case | Dates | Issues | Outcome |
|---|---|---|---|
| 1. *Toth v Community Hospital at Glen Cove* 22 NY 2d 255 (NY App) | July 6, 1965: NY Supreme Ct, Trial Term, Nassau Co.<br>July 10, 1967: App Div 2d Depart.<br>July 5, 1967: Court of Appeals. | RLF and blindness allegedly caused by improper oxygen administration by ophthalmologist, pediatrician, and hospital. | 1. Complaints dismissed. Jury verdict in favor of pediatrician and ophthalmologist.<br>2. Divided court in appellate division.<br>3. New trial against hospital and pediatrician but not ophthalmologist ordered by court of appeals. |
| 2. *Swank v Halivopoulos* 108 NJ Super 120 (NJ Super Ct App Div) | Argued November 24, 1969: NJ Super Ct.<br>Decided December 29, 1969, by App Div. | Administration of excess oxygen to plaintiff, allegedly causing RLF (less than 40% administered and only for 5 days). | Verdict for the defendant.<br>Affirmed on appeal. |
| 3. *Huie v Newcomb Hospital* 112 NJ Super 429 (NJ Super Ct App Div) | Argued November 23, 1970.<br>Decided December 7, 1970 (Super Ct, Law Div). | Order requiring defendant physician to produce and submit for examination by plaintiff's attorney an article previously prepared for publication by physician. Physician appealed. Original action against physician and hospital for injury and disability sustained by infant by reason of allegedly negligent administration of oxygen. | Superior court entered order requiring physician to produce article. Order affirmed by appellate division. |
| 4. *Siirila v Barrios* 66 WI 2d 394 (WI Supreme Ct) | February 4, 1975. | Loss by parents of child's aid, comfort, society, and companionship as a result of injuries sustained allegedly by administration of excess oxygen causing RLF. | Circuit court, Milwaukee County, ruled for defendant.<br>Reversed by Supreme Court. |

| | | | |
|---|---|---|---|
| 5. *Kanon v Brookdale Medical Center* 87 Misc 2d 816 (Supreme Ct Special Term Kings County, Part I) | November 5, 1975. | Amendment by plaintiffs of their complaint of medical malpractice in cases of RLF in premature infants born between 1953 and 1975 to include class action allegations and to add additional party defendants. | Motion denied. |
| 6. *Poulin v Zartman* Nos. 2120, 2127 (AK Supreme Ct) | November 12, 1975. | Titration technique of oxygen administration. Proper treatment of jaundice and brain damage. Respiratory distress syndrome. Lack of prenatal care. Background of father. Informed consent. Proof of insurance. Violation of duty by certain jurors. Supervision. | Superior court entered judgment on verdict against plaintiff. Supreme court affirmed in part and reversed in part, remanding new trial regarding issue of proper supervision. ("Issue of methodology and informed consent may not be retried."). |
| 7. *Siirila v Barrios* 398 MI 576 No. 11 (MI Supreme Ct) | December 21, 1976. | Continued exposure to oxygen of premature infant in an Isolette as cause for RLF and permanent blindness. | Judgment for defendants, a general practitioner and a hospital, upheld by court of appeals, 58 MI App 725, 228 N.W. 2d 801, and affirmed by Supreme Court. |
| 8. *Quick v Aetna Casualty & Surety Co.* No 13251 (LA App 2d Cir) | May 23, 1977. En Banc rehearing denied June 22, 1977. | Improper administration of oxygen to child while in incubator. | Plaintiff denied by expiration of statute of limitations by first judicial Court. Affirmed by court of appeals. |
| 9. *Greenberg v Bishop Clarkson Memorial Hospital* 201 Neb. 215 No. 41477 (NE Supreme Ct) | June 21, 1978. | Proper use of oxygen in case of respiratory distress developing RLF. Inadequate number of nurses in special nursery. | District court entered judgment for defendants. Supreme Court affirmed in part regarding nurses and instruction of jury summarizing allegations in one instruction but reversed and remanded on instruction that testimony of disa- |

(*continued*)

**TABLE 1–1** (*cont.*).
Cases Involving Administration of Oxygen to Premature Infants

| Case | Dates | Issues | Outcome |
|---|---|---|---|
| | | | greement by other doctors of equal skill and learning as to what treatment should have been does not establish negligence was prejudicial error to the plaintiff's cause. |
| 10. *Comley v Emmanuel Lutheran Charity Board* 35 or App. 465 No. 417–542; CA 8489 (OR App) | Argued and submitted December 19, 1977. Decided August 1, 1978. | "Negligent prescription, administration, and supervision of oxygen therapy caused her to sustain RLF." Concealment of this fact from plaintiff. | Circuit court, Multuomah County, granted summary judgment in favor of Board and the two doctors. Affirmed in part and reversed in part and remanded regarding second doctor, as his actions fell outside of immunity given to governmental employment for discretionary acts. |
| 11. *Hill v Boles* No. 60788 (MO Supreme Ct En Banc) | July 27, 1979. | Negligent administration of oxygen causing RLF. | Circuit court, City of St. Louis, granted summary judgment for the hospital and judgment on a jury verdict for the physician. Reversed and remanded by Supreme Court because defense council, over objection, was allowed to argue failure of plaintiff to produce surgeon as a witness in view of evidence as to the relationship between defendant treating physician and surgeon. Also, on remand, plaintiff could show that the hospital's negli- |

| | | | |
|---|---|---|---|
| | | | gence contained beyond the date of abolishment of the doctrine of charitable immunity, then he would have a valid cause of action against the hospital. |
| 12. *Ohler v Tacoma General Hospital and Air Shields, Inc.* 92 WA 2d 507 No. 45247 (WA Supreme Ct En Banc) | August 16, 1979. | Excessive concentrations of oxygen and administration of oxygen in the first few days of the infant's life, causing RLF. | Superior Court, Pierce County, entered summary judgment in favor of defendants on ground that woman's claims were barred by statute of limitations. Supreme Court reversed and remanded, based on the use of the discovery rule for medical malpractice cases governed by the three-year limitation period (RLW 4.16.010 and 4.16.080 [2]). |
| 13. *Air Shields, Inc. and Southern Hospital and Clinic, Inc. v Spears* No. 6026 (TX Civil App Waco) | October 18, 1979. Rehearing denied November 29, 1979. | Warnings allegedly not given by manufacturer of incubators regarding danger of oxygen to premature infants. | Award of $100,000 for past mental suffering and physical disfigurement; $900,000 for future mental suffering and physical disfigurement; $500,000 for loss of future earnings; $10,000 for loss of past ability to care for himself; $250,000 for loss of future ability to care for himself; modified and affirmed by Court of Appeals. Hospital was entitled to recover indemnity against the manufacturer for damages recovered by minor plaintiff. |

(*continued*)

**TABLE 1–1** (*cont.*).
Cases Involving Administration of Oxygen to Premature Infants

| Case | Dates | Issues | Outcome |
|---|---|---|---|
| 14. *Penetrante v United States* 21.60 604 F 2d 1248 (ND [cal] 1979) | 1979. | Prolonged exposure of twins to relatively high concentrations of oxygen. | US district court award entering judgment against defendant of $2,292,123 to one twin and $900,000 to second twin. Judgment not reduced in appeal. |
| 15. *May v Wm. Dafoe, Providence Hospital, Air Shields, Inc.* 25 WA App 575 No. 6987–0–1 (WA App Div 1.) | March 17, 1980. Reconsideration denied April 17, 1980. | Liability of manufacturer of incubator in which infant plaintiff was placed, permitting infant's exposure to excessive amount of oxygen. | Superior court, King County, granted manufacturer's motion for a directed verdict. Affirmed by court of appeals: injuries received must be the result of the functioning of the product itself for the manufacturer to be held strictly liable for injuries. |
| 16. *Zimmerman v Nassau Hospital* 76 A.D. 2d. 92, (NY Supreme Ct, 2d Depart) | June 30, 1980. | Motion by defendant to compel plaintiffs to provide them with authorization to obtain certain medical records. | Denied by Supreme Court, Nassau County. Reversed by Supreme Court, appellate division. |
| 17. *Jones v New Hanover Memorial Hospital* No. 815 SC 440 (NC App) | February 2, 1982. | Failure of hospital to have established a policy prohibiting administration of oxygen in concentrations exceeding 40% fraction of inspired air to premature newborns, allegedly resulting in blindness of the plaintiff. | Summary judgment granted by the superior court, New Hanover County, in favor of hospital in action by former patient for alleged negligence. Affirmed by court of appeals. Plaintiff's claim barred by doctrine of charitable immunity. |
| 18. *Burton v Brooklyn Doctors Hospital* 452 NYS 2d 875 (App Div 1982) | 1982. | Prolonged liberal administration of oxygen to premature infant placed in incubator, allegedly resulting in RLF. | Jury found for plaintiff in NY Supreme Court; award of $2,887,000 for damages judged excessive by appellate division; reduced to $1,500,000. |

| | | | |
|---|---|---|---|
| 19. *Wilsher v Essex AHA*, Queens Bench Division, England | December 21, 1984. | Catheter to measure oxygen inserted in vein instead of artery; whether above contributed to or increased risk of RLF; whether with subsequent treatment with oxygen the arterial tension rose five times to a level and length of times that were dangerous, whether defendants were negligent in permitting this and caused or contributed to RLF. Etiology of optic atrophy, right eye. | Judgment in favor of plaintiff of £109,500 (pounds): "Defendants were negligent in failure to check the monitor sufficiently frequently at later periods of blood-gas readings." |
| 20. *Flores v Flushing Hospital and Medical Center and Dr. James G. Lione* 109 A.D. 2d 198 (Supreme Ct, App Div 1st Depart) | June 25, 1985. | Blindness allegedly caused by administration of excessive amounts of oxygen. Lack of informed consent. | Verdict rejecting both theories of recovery by Supreme Court, Bronx County. Reversed in part by appellate division because jury was instructed to determine whether lack of informed consent proximately resulted in injury to the infant instead of whether in fact injury resulted from treatment; otherwise affirmed. |
| 21. *Duffy v Fear* (Supreme Ct, App Div 1st Depart) | July 24, 1986. | Administration of oxygen to premature infant. Failure to remove previously inserted IUD and to inform mother of danger of IUD causing premature birth at the time she learned of pregnancy. | Verdict in favor of plaintiff by Supreme Court, Bronx County, of $1,740,000. Reversed and remanded for new trial by appellate division. |
| 22. *Kuncio v Millard Fillmore Hospital* Supreme Ct, App Div 4th Depart | February 21, 1986. | Administration to twins of high concentrations of oxygen, and failure to obtain informed consent from parents before high concentration of supplemental oxygen was administered. | Jury verdict of no cause of action in favor of hospital by Supreme Court, Erie County. Judge granted motion to set aside verdict. Latter reversed and denied by appellate division. |

held by the Supreme Court appellate division to be excessive because it exceeded $1,500,000. On the other hand, the Court also held that the plaintiff's proof clearly established that the prolonged liberal administration of oxygen to which he had been subjected had caused his blindness. To date, no conclusive evidence for such a proof exists.

After the publication of the Cooperative Study, the upper "safe" limit of oxygen concentration was accepted to be 40%. The duration of exposure was also considered to be important because it could be controlled fairly well. However, other controls were found to be necessary. One of the most important was $PO_2$ measurement (arterial oxygen tension). In the late 1970s, transcutaneous monitoring was introduced and offered the opportunity for noninvasive measurements of $PO_2$. Thus far, unfortunately, ROP cannot be prevented by routine transcutaneous $PO_2$ monitoring.[5] The reason for this was explained by Flynn, in his work with 300 premature infants during the past two years who has used this modality at the Bascom-Palmer Eye Institute. The blood levels of these infants fluctuate violently and very frequently during any 24-hour period.[6] The technology for controlling these levels has not become available to date. It is perhaps for this reason that this subject has not been brought up at malpractice trials, for it might make both the judge and the jury realize how difficult it is to prevent ROP and how many perverse etiologies are ascribed to this condition.

As stated above, most action for damages has been based on the excessive use of oxygen. In the case of *Toth v Community Hospital at Glen Cove*[7] (Table 1–1, case 1), such action was brought against the pediatrician, the ophthalmologist and the hospital by lawyers for prematurely born babies blinded or partially blinded by RLF allegedly caused by administration of 6 L of oxygen per minute (50% to 60% oxygen), instead of 4 L/min (30% to 40% oxygen concentration), as ordered by the pediatrician. The Supreme Court trial term, Nassau County, entertained judgment on July 6, 1965, dismissing the complaint to the hospital at the end of the entire case in favor of the pediatrician and ophthalmologist on a jury verdict. The Supreme Court apellate division, second judicial department, entered an order on July 10, 1967, affirming, by a divided court, the judgment of the trial term, and the lawyers for the babies appealed. The court of appeals (Judge Keating) held that evidence required submission to the jury of the issue of whether the pediatrician was negligent in failing to discover that nurses were administering 6 L of oxygen per minute instead of 4 L/min, and that the lawyers for the babies made out a prima facie case against the hospital when they introduced substantial evidence to establish that the nurses had not conformed to the pediatrician's orders. The order of the appellate division was modified to order a new trial against the hospital and the pediatrician and otherwise to affirm. It is interesting to note in the opinion of Judge Keating that he quotes the Cooperative Study, stating, "While the use of oxygen might mitigate brain damage, it did not reduce mortality rate at all and did cause RLF, resulting in blindness in many infants. This was the result here." The judge himself, on appeal, and without a jury, made this decision on his own, being convinced of a simplistic etiology of the disease in question.

The case against the ophthalmologist held that first, he should have discovered the retrolental fibroplasia during his examination of the babies on July 17, 1967, and that second, regardless of whether RLF had manifested itself by that date, he should have made a recommendation about the advisability of continuing the oxygen treatment. The trial court dismissed the complaint against the hospital on the grounds that the evidence did not show that 6 L/min had been continuously given, and that the alleged deviation from the physician's orders was a proximate cause of the children's loss of sight. (Proximate cause refers to a cause that directly or with no mediating agency produces an effect, or, specifically, a cause that arises out of a wrongdoer's negligence or conduct, with the result that the wrongdoer can be held liable for the particular harm that in fact resulted therefrom, as distinguished from a remote cause or any superventing or concurring cause for which the wrongdoer is not deemed chargeable under those rules.) The jury returned a verdict in favor of the doctors. On appeal, the appellate division affirmed, with one justice dissenting, for the hospital and the pediatrician. The appellate division stated that there was ample evidence to support the jury's finding that the defendant pediatrician, who viewed the oxygen treatment as a necessary, calculated risk, had acted in accordance with acceptable medical practice. The appellate division stated that at no time had the hospital claimed that authorization had been given, either by the pediatrician or the standing orders of the premature nursery, to give 6 L of oxygen continuously. It follows that the case against the hospital should not have been dismissed. With respect to the ophthalmologist, the appellate division stated that although this doctor had been aware of the retrolental fibroplasia controversy, there was no evidence to indicate that he thought that the four liters of oxygen the children were then scheduled to receive, were particularly dangerous. The order of the appellate division was modified to order a new trial against the defendants, Community Hospital at Glen Cove, and the pediatrician in the case.

In a dissenting opinion by Judge Bergan, the question of the pediatrician's vulnerability was discussed. Judge Bergan conceded that oxygen had caused the injury, but stated that this did not make the pediatrician liable. The judge felt that the pediatrician had practiced with the same skill and knowledge that would have been practiced by other pediatricians of his time, in his specialty area, and under similar circumstances. He stated that the prime purpose of the procedure had been to save the lives of the children.

That later knowledge showed that serious side effects might have been avoided should not spell out a liability under this record. Judge Bergan did not feel that the "second theory" of negligence regarding the administration of oxygen was enough to remand the case for a new trial, especially because the plaintiff's lawyers did not describe this second theory to the jury in enough detail to establish it.

From the above, it can be seen that the ophthalmologist and the pediatrician were both vulnerable to charges of malpractice, but that there was adequate defense for both of their positions. In *Duffy v Fear*[8] (Table 1–1, case 21), a medical malpractice action was brought against a physician by parents on behalf of their child to recover damages for blindness the child incurred following premature birth. The Supreme Court of Bronx County (Judge Difed) entered a judgment on the jury verdict in favor of the child in the sum of $1,740,000, and the physician appealed.

In this case, the mother of the plaintiff child had an intrauterine device (IUD) within her uterus during her pregnancy. The physician was sued, accused of deviating from accepted medical standard by not removing the IUD, and because the pregnancy was unwanted and thus unjustified. He was also accused of not informing the mother that the presence of the IUD increased the risk of premature delivery — the cause of the ROP — and that if she had been so informed, she would have had an abortion.

The Supreme Court, appellate division, disagreed, stating that the first claim was not justified and the second claim was improper. The plaintiff's expert explicitly disclaimed the contention that not removing the IUD was a departure from the medical standards of 1970. Regarding abortion, the appellate division stated that the record disclosed no evidence whatever to support the finding that the plaintiff's mother, if she had been informed of the risks described by the expert on her behalf, would have had an abortion. The appellate division further invoked the explicit disapproval by the court of appeals of what has come to be known as a "wrongful life" claim as a principle of liability. They consequently faulted the lower court's instruction to the jury permitting them to return a verdict for the plaintiff on such a claim. Finally, the trial court was faulted because it failed to submit to the jury the issue of proximate cause of the IUD as the cause of the premature birth, an issue squarely disputed by defense testimony. As a result, the lower court's decision was reversed and remanded for a new trial. This is one of the few cases where hyperoxygenation was not an issue, and where prematurity was deemed to be the cause of ROP.

In recent years, new and more sophisticated points of law have entered into malpractice trials. In *Flores v Flushing Hospital and Medical Center and Dr. James G. Lione*[9] (Table 1–1, case 20), lawyers for the patient, whose blindness was allegedly caused by the administration of excessive amounts of oxygen after a premature birth, brought suit against the hospital and physician for alleged malpractice and lack of informed consent. The Supreme Court, Bronx County (Judge Orlando), entered judgment on the verdict, rejecting both theories of recovery, and the patient appealed.

The Supreme Court, appellate division (Judge Carro), held that instruction on proximate cause in an action against a physician, based on lack of informed consent regarding the possibility of blindness if an infant is administered an excess amount of oxygen at birth, was erroneous and required a new trial. Instead of requiring the jury to determine whether treatment would have occurred except for a failure to inform the parents, and whether injury in fact resulted from treatment, instructions required the jury to determine whether the lack of informed consent proximately resulted in injury to the infant. The decision was reversed in part and otherwise affirmed. The proof at trial showed that the plaintiff was subjected to concentrations of oxygen between 31% and 40% over a 13-day period. The jury found no departure from accepted medical or hospital practice as it existed in May 1970 by either the hospital or Dr. Lione, the attending physician. Further testimony showed that Dr. Lione never informed the plaintiff's parents about the risks of oxygen use, or, specifically, about the possibility of blindness. Accordingly, neither was there any discussion of the range of percentage-volume or the duration of oxygen therapy. Given the complexity of factors and outcomes in treating a grossly underweight, premature infant, the issue of lack of informed consent was clearly not reducible to whether, if so informed, the parents would have been forced to choose between death and blindness. On this issue, the jury was directed "to consider whether the infant's parents were adequately and reasonably informed and based on that, did they give their consent to the procedure and treatment undertaken by Dr. Lione?" The jury answered no to this question. The appellate division concluded that the court's charge on proximate cause may have confused the jury. They vacated the judgment of action in Dr. Lione's favor, remanding the matter for a new trial on that cause, alleging lack of informed consent.

In *Kuncio v Millard Fillmore Hospital*[10] (Table 1–1, case 22), lawyers for twins who were blinded and suffered extremely impaired eyesight as a result of developing RLF caused by their exposure to high concentrations of oxygen after they were born prematurely brought action against the hospital, alleging medical malpractice in the failure to obtain informed consent from the parents before a high concentration of supplemental oxygen was administered. After the jury returned the verdict of no cause of action in favor of the hospital, the lawyers for the twins moved to set aside the verdict for a new trial. The Supreme Court, Erie County (Judge Kuszynski), granted the motion and the hospital appealed. The Supreme Court, appellate division, held that (1) credible evidence supported the finding that exposure of premature babies to oxygen was not a deviation from accepted standards of practice (this was a marked change in attitude from previous cases, in which exposure to oxygen was presumed to be a proximate cause of damage in these infants); (2) there was sufficient credible evidence to support the finding that the parents' consent to the use of oxygen therapy was not obtained because of differing opinions about the safety of therapy, balanced against the perceived risks of brain damage or death, and that an informed, reasonably prudent person would have consented to treatment despite the risks, or that it was not the hospital's responsibility to procure informed consent from the parents; and (3) there was insufficient basis to justify setting aside the verdict on the grounds that it was influenced by extrinsic factors relating principally to jurors' dissatisfaction with the length of the trial. The Supreme Court's ruling was reversed, the motion was denied, and the jury verdict was reinstated. Nevertheless, even in this trial, experts for both parties agreed that it was deliberate exposure to oxygen that had caused the twins' blindness and that much of the trial centered on the state of the art of medicine as it was in March 1953.

Nevertheless, plaintiff's claims regarding improper use of oxygen in cases of ROP have not always been successful. In *Sirila v Barrios*[10] (Table 1–1, case 4), a father brought a medical malpractice action for his son against a general practitioner in a hospital, claiming that the baby's RLF and consequent total and permanent blindness had been caused by his continued exposure to oxygen while he was in the incubator after birth. The Circuit Court, Houghton County (Judge Condon), rendered judgment for the defendants, and the court of appeals affirmed. On further appeal, the Supreme Court (Judge Williams) held that a specialist may testify as to the standard of the general practitioner. The judgment for the defendants was affirmed. It is interesting to note that in this case, the dosage rate of oxygen was approximately 36% to 38% on November 26, 1967, and 27% to 31% between December 7 and 12, 1967. This was well below the 40% maximum, the standard of the time. Dr. Barrios, the general practitioner, testified that he knew the oxygen concentration should have been no more than 40% in the incubator, but did not know that prolonged exposure to oxygen could produce the added risk of retrolental fibroplasia. Whether oxygen exposure was prolonged in this case was in question, but Dr. Barrios stated that he had prescribed the oxygen to keep the baby alive and to prevent brain and cardiorespiratory damage.

In *Swank v Halivopoulos*[11] (Table 1–1, case 2), the question of oxygen again was raised. In this case, the orders were for oxygen below 40%, which was administered to the child continuously from September 20 to 24, 1964; the infant had been blind since September 19, 1964. On September 25, the defendant ordered oxygen to be administered as necessary and it was gradually discontinued on that day. None was given on September 26 or thereafter. The defendant testified that even though he recognized that retrolental fibroplasia was one of the known, possible dangers resulting from the use of oxygen for premature babies, he nevertheless ordered its administration in the specified amount and time because he felt that "the baby could not survive without it" and that "oxygen was a mandatory thing for this particular baby." The Superior Court, law division, entered a verdict for the defendant, and this was affirmed on appeal.

In certain cases, issues in addition to ROP have entered into consideration. In *Zartman v Poulin*[12] (Table 1–1, case 6), medical malpractice action was brought on the basis that the defendant physician improperly administered oxygen to the premature infant, thereby causing her to become totally blind, and that the physician's failure to properly treat jaundice during this period caused severe brain damage. Judgment was entered on a verdict against the plaintiff, and the plaintiff appealed. The issue of informed consent also entered into the case. The plaintiff's lawyers contended that the defendant administered treatment to the plaintiff without informed consent of either of the plaintiff's parents. This case is particularly interesting because the premature plaintiff had a definite diagnosis of respiratory distress syndrome (RDS) requiring oxygen therapy for survival, and also RLF, which was claimed to have been caused by the administered oxygen. The oxygen was given for only 1 week in 1968, in Anchorage, Alaska. Precise gauges for monitoring the amount of oxygen in the blood were not available. The patient's mental deficiency, coupled with cyanosis, raised the question of too little oxygen, yet the latter was implicated as having caused the RLF. Did the infant get too much oxygen, or too little? Other complicating issues were the patient's jaundice, and also the alleged lack of prenatal care. Concerning informed consent, the Supreme Court overruled the appellant's claim, stating that there was no evidence that the plaintiff's parents would have declined the procedure had it been adequately explained. Finally, a new trial was ordered over the issue of proper supervision. As we can see, many, many issues come to trial in addition to the actual technicalities and scientific facts regarding the disease and its management.

In many malpractice cases, there are marked differences in opinion regarding the treatment rendered by the defendant. In *Greenberg v Bishop Clarkson Memorial Hospital*[13] (Table 1–1, case 9), medical malpractice action was brought by lawyers for the infant, through her father, against the hospital where she had been born, and against the doctor who attended her after her birth, alleging that the defendant's malpractice caused the plaintiff's permanent blindness. The court held that (1) the trial court properly exercised its discretion in concluding that the facts did not justify amendment of the petition, after the parties had rested their case, to allege that the hospital had been negligent in not maintaining an adequate number of nurses in the special nursery; (2) the trial court did not err in failing to instruct the jury about each specific active negligence charge against the hospital and the doctor, but instead properly summarized those allegations in one instruction; and (3) instruction to the jury that testimony of other physicians that they would have followed different courses of treatment from that followed by defendant was prejudicial. Disagreement among doctors of equal skill and learning about what the treatment should have been did not establish negligence. It was prejudicial error to the plaintiff's cause of action against the doctor, when the plaintiff's evidence of negligence was based largely on the testimony of doctors who stated that they would have acted differently than the defendant doctor, or that treatment by the defendant doctor should have been performed differently. The verdict was affirmed in refusing to amend the petition about an inadequate number of nurses in the nursery and to summarize allegations in one instruction, but reversed in part and remanded on testimony of the various doctors.

The plaintiff, Stephanie Greenberg, was born approximately 3 months prematurely on May 15, 1972, with a birth weight of 1 lb 13 oz. On multiple occasions, her breathing stopped because of respiratory distress. The medical testimony was in conflict about when oxygen should have been used, the length of time for which it should have been necessary, the method by which oxygen levels in the baby's blood should have been measured, and the exact cause-and-effect relationship between administration of high levels of oxygen for various periods of time and the occurrence of RLF. The plaintiff's expert witness testified that the treatment given by the defendant doctor had not been in accordance with generally accepted standards of medical practice in Omaha or similar communities. The defendant's expert witnesses testified that the administration of supplemental oxygen was essential to save the baby's life, that the amounts of oxygen administered, the methods of monitoring and testing the blood levels in the blood, and the treatment were all in accordance with accepted standards of practice in the community. In this case, it is interesting that definite "authoritative" testimony was given by both sides. To this day, we know that we are still far from having the final answers to these questions. As a further detail in this case, after the parties had rested their cases, the plaintiff alleged that the defendant hospital had been negligent in not maintaining an adequate number of nurses in the special nursery. The district court had refused to allow the plaintiff to amend the petition in this manner. This was denied on appeal. The instruction to the jury, that the testimony of other physicians that they would have followed a course of treatment different from that followed by the defendant, Dr. James Wax (or a disagreement of doctors of equal skill and learning about what the treatment should have been) did not establish negligence, was deemed erroneous. As a result, the judgment in favor of the hospital was affirmed but the judgment for the defendant, James I. Wax, was reversed and the case was remanded for further proceedings.

## OTHER ISSUES OF LIABILITY

In *Comley v Emmanuel Lutheran Charity Board*[14] (Table 1–1, case 10), there were multiple issues of liability. The usual issue of oxygen administration was introduced, but in addition, the plaintiff alleged that the defendants had fraudulently and deceitfully concealed this fact from the plaintiff. The defendant, Dr. Johnson, stated in his affidavit that while under his care the plaintiff did not receive oxygen, nor did he administer oxygen or order that she be administered oxygen or oxygen incubation. The plaintiff did not file responsive affidavits. Further complicating the case was a movement for the same rejudgment by the Board and Drs. Nunon and Johnson made on the grounds that plaintiff's claim against them was barred under the doctor sovereign immunity and immunity of state officers and employees. The alleged false statements were deemed not to be a part of the cause of action because if there had been no liability initially, or concealment of liability, actionable facts could not have created liability when none existed. The state employee, Dr. Nunon, was deemed not immune because a plaintiff's complaint charges that conduct that falls outside of a discretionary act is an exception. No governmental discretion had been involved, and Dr. Nunon was subject to criticism for the same balance of risk against benefit which every physician must undertake when treating patients. Therefore, judgment for Dr. Nunon was reversed and remanded for retrial. Regarding the Board and Dr. Johnson, however, the judgment regarding them was affirmed because their actions had occurred prior to the effective date of exposure or liability under the Tort Claims Act.

Charitable immunity is defined as immunity to liability given to a hospital under a specific law of the state by virtue of the hospital's rendering services for no charge to patients unable to pay. This issue came up in *Jones v New Hanover Memorial Hospital*[15] (Table 1–1, case 17, and *Hill v Boles*[16] (Table 1–1, case 11). In the former case, even though there had been an allegation of the use of more than 40% oxygen, the court entered an order granting the hospital's motion for the same rejudgment, stating that the plaintiff's claim against the defendant hospital was barred by the doctrine of charitable immunity as a matter of law. In the latter case, the circuit court granted the same rejudgment for the hospital, and judgment on a jury verdict for the physician. On appeal, the above was reversed and remanded because the defense counsel was allowed, over objection, to argue the failure of the plaintiff to produce the surgeon as a witness. Regarding the hospital, in this case the circuit court stated that on remand the plaintiff could show that if the hospital's negligence had been contained beyond the date that the doctrine of charitable immunity had been abolished, then the plaintiff would have valid cause of action against the hospital.

Other legal technicalities have also been brought to court. For example, in *Quick v Aetna Casualty and Surety Company*[17] (Table 1–1, case 8), the parents of a premature baby brought a medical malpractice suit against a hospital, its various doctors and nurses, and their insurer for the baby's blindness allegedly caused by improper administration of oxygen to the child while she was in an incubator in the hospital. The case was denied because the complaint was brought after the statute of limitations had expired, and this was affirmed by the court of appeals.

A rash of lawsuits involving oxygen administration and ROP against the manufacturer of incubators occurred near the end of the 1970s and three are sited here.[18–20] In *Ohler v Tacoma General Hospital and Air Shields, Inc.* (Table 1–1, case 12), a 22-year-old woman brought personal injury action against a hospital which had treated her as an infant, on the theory of medical malpractice, and against the manufacturer of the incubator in which she had been placed at that time, on the theory of products liability. She alleged that the defendants caused her blindness. She had been placed in the incubator for 16 days and given oxygen. The incubator had been manufactured by Air Shields, Inc. The claimant stated that in the fall of 1974, when she was 21 years old, she heard through the news media that a school friend, who also suffered from RLF, had initiated a lawsuit alleging that her blindness had been caused by the wrongful conduct of a hospital and an incubator manufacturer, Air Shields, Inc. Within a week, she contacted her friend's attorney and in her affidavit said that she "discovered for the first time that it was possible that she did not need as much, if any, oxygen as was actually administered to her in her infancy and that her sightlessness might have been prevented." In March 1975, shortly after her 22d birthday, the claimant began her lawsuit. The superior court of Pierce County entered a summary judgment in favor of the defendant on the grounds that the patient's claims were barred by statutes of limitations. On appeal, the Supreme Court held that (1) the patient's medical malpractice claim against the hospital did not accrue until she discovered or reasonably should have discovered all of the essential elements of her possible cause of action, i.e., duty, breach, causation, and damages; (2) the material issue of fact that one patient discovered that her blindness may have been caused by a hospital's wrongful act precluded summary judgment on the grounds of the statue of limitations in medical malpractice action; (3) the plaintiff's claim against the manufacturer of the incubator in which she was placed as an infant did not accrue until after she had discovered, or reasonably should have discovered, all the essential elements of her possible products liability cause of action against the manufacturer for allegedly causing her blindness; and (4) the material issue of fact that whether the plaintiff discovered all of the elements of her possible causes of action against the incubator manufacturer more than three years before she filed suit precluded some rejudgment in the product liability action. The summary judgment in favor of Tacoma General Hospital and Air Shields, Inc.,[18] was reversed and the case was remanded for trial.

In *Air Shields, Inc., v. Spears*[19] (Table 1–1, case 13), the mother brought action against the manufacturer of the incubator, the hospital, and Drs. Rothenberg and Doncaster, for her minor son, to recover damages arising from his permanent blindness. The District Court entered judgments for the plaintiff, and the defendants appealed. The court of civil appeals held that (1) evidence sustained the finding that the manufacturer had been negligent in failing to furnish with its incubators warnings relative to the risks of giving supplemental oxygen to premature infants, and that such negligence was a proximate cause of the minor's blindness; (2) the evidence sustained an award of $100,000 for past mental suffering and physical disfigurement, $900,000 for future mental suffering and physical disfigurement, $500,000 for loss of future earnings, $10,000 for loss of past ability to care for and manage his own affairs, and $250,000 for future loss of ability to care for and manage his own affairs; (3) the evidence sustained the finding that the hospital had been negligent in its policies and procedures regarding the administration of supplemental oxygen to premature infants and that such negligence constituted a proximate cause of the minor plaintiff's blindness; and (4) because the manufacturer of the incubator owed a duty to the hospital as purchaser of the incubator, to warn of dangers in the use of machine, the hospital was entitled to recover indemnity against the manufacturer for damages recovered by the minor plaintiff. The original judgment was modified and affirmed. It is interesting that at birth the plaintiff weighed 2 lb 3 oz and that oxygen had been administered in the range of 32% to 40% on a continuous basis between April 27 and May 6, 1970. They stated that it was formally believed that oxygen was safe if kept below 40%, but that research in 1967 and 1968 determined that there was no safe percentage. The jury also rendered a finding of negligence against Dr. Rothenberg in his diagnosis and medical care and treatment of the claimant. Air Shields filed the third part of the action against Drs. Rothenberg and Doncaster, alleging that the doctors had been well aware of the risks and benefits of administration of oxygen in various concentrations for various amounts of time to premature infants, and that their negligence had caused the minor plaintiff's blindness and damage. It is interesting that all of the defendants agreed with the assumption that in the management of this patient, negligence was taken for granted because oxygen had been used. This was substantiated by Dr. Silverman, a pediatrician, who testified for the plaintiff that the claimant was permanently and completely blind because he had been exposed to oxygen levels higher than room concentration. Similarly, Dr. Doncaster, a defendant, testified that the claimant's blindness had been caused by oxygen administered during the first days of his life. Another point of interest was that in 1972 the minor plaintiff, through his father, filed suit against Drs. Rothenberg and Doncaster, asserting negligence in adminstering oxygen after the claimant's birth, causing his blindness. This suit was compromised and settled for $100,000. The agreement was that the plaintiff would give the doctors a complete release for the $100,000 for liability insurance available, but would maintain all causes of action against anyone else.

In the third case involving incubators, *May v Estate of Robert A. Maves, M.D. and Air Shields, Inc.* (Table 1–1, case 15), action based on strict liability was brought against the manufacturer of the incubator by the plaintiff, who claimed that he suffered from RLF because as an infant he had been placed in an incubator, permitting his exposure to an excessive amount of oxygen. The superior court granted the manufacturer's motion for a directed verdict and the plaintiff appealed. The court of appeals held that the manufacturer was not strictly liable, despite the plaintiff's contention that the manufacturer's letter to the hospital failed to provide an adequate warning, and that duration, not concentration, of oxygen was the critical factor in reducing the possibility of RLF. Although the manufacturer did have a duty to warn physicians about the state of current medical research with respect to retrolental fibroplasia, the plaintiff's injury was not the result of any dangerous propensity of the incubator itself, but was solely the direct and proximate result of a medical decision to administer oxygen. The motion of the superior court was affirmed. The court, in this case, came to the more logical conclusion that the doctrine of strict liability does not impose legal responsibility on a manufacturer simply because harm results from the use of a product.[21] The court did state, however, that a manufacturer may be held strictly liable for injury sustained by the use of a product which is free from defect in either design or manufacture if adequate warning about potentially dangerous propensities is not given to a user. The injury received, however, must be the result of the functioning of the product itself. In this case, the injury the claimant received was not the result of any dangerous propensity of the incubator itself. It was solely a direct and proximate result of a medical decision to administer oxygen. The court concluded that equipment manufacturers need not be trained in medical science, and for them to render advice in medical treatment would be suspect and dangerous. Their duty to warn should relate only to design, engineering, and functional dangers. The court further concluded that the analogy between a drug manufacturer and an incubator maker is not apt.

In attempts to attain recovery for plaintiffs, there have been other trials and actions regarding even more technical matters. For example, in *Huie v Newcomb Hospital*[22] (Table 1–1, case 3), the plaintiff brought actions against the hospital and physician for injury and disability sustained by the infant by reason of the allegedly negligent administration of oxygen. The superior court, law division, entered an order requiring the physician to submit for examination by the plaintiff's attorney an article previously prepared for publication by the physician, and the physician appealed. The superior court, appellate division, held that where the article on retrolental fibroplasia prepared for publication by the defendant physician concerned the relation between the use of oxygen and retrolental fibroplasia, and that inspection of the paper might lead to discovery of work which the physician viewed as authoritative at the time the paper was prepared, the plaintiffs were entitled to produce the paper for examination. Although the paper was not published, the order by the Supreme Court was affirmed.

In another case, *Zimmerman v Nassau Hospital*[23] (Table 1–1, case 16), the Supreme Court, Nassau County, denied the defendants' motion to compel plaintiffs to provide them with authorization to obtain the medical records of Dr. Gerald Kara, who had conducted two examinations on the plaintiff 12 years before litigation had commenced. Both examinations had been conducted in the presence of the attorney. The Supreme Court, appellate division, held that medical records related to examination, diagnosis, and treatment of the infant plaintiff constituted neither the attorney's work product nor material prepared for litigation, and so had to be exempt from discovery, and reversed the denial of the defendant's motion by the Supreme Court.

In *Kanon v The Brookdale Hospital Medical Center*[24] (Table 1–1, case 5), the plaintiffs, in medical malpractice action, moved for leave to amend their complaint to include class action allegations and to add additional party defendants. This motion was denied by the Supreme Court. Judge Ruben held that charges of medical malpractice allegedly resulting in the development of RLF in various classes of proposed plaintiffs, where in each matter individual plaintiffs were involved, varied in degree from plaintiff to plaintiff, and therefore a judgment about any one of the proposed plaintiffs could not bind any other involved plaintiff. Additionally, class action suit is not justified, and therefore was denied. This important decision prevented escalation of lawsuits involving ROP.

Another example of how claims can escalate in these lawsuits is illustrated by *Shockley v Thomas A. Prier, M.D.*[25] In this case, action was brought by the parents of a minor child against two doctors and their insurer for injury sustained by the child, allegedly caused by the doctors' negligence, and for loss to the parents of the child's aid, comfort, society, and companionship as a result of such injuries. The circuit court, Milwaukee County

(Judge Roller), sustained the defendants' objection to that part of the complaint seeking damages for loss of the child's aid, comfort, society, and companionship and the parents appealed. The Supreme Court (Judge Day) held that, for instant case and causes of action arising thereafter, parents may maintain action for loss of aid, comfort, society, and companionship of the injured minor child against the negligent tort feasor, provided and on condition that the parents' cause of action is combined with that of the child for the child's personal injuries. They reversed the ruling of the circuit court. Again, the case involved ROP where it was alleged that the claimant had been given excessive amounts of oxygen which caused RLF resulting in total and permanent blindness and disfigurement. This court concluded that the law should recognize the right of parents to recover for loss of aid, comfort, society, and companionship of a child during minority when such loss is caused by the negligence of another. The defendants pointed out that several states have declined to create a cause of action for loss of a child's society and companionship. These states include Alabama, New York, North Dakota, Pennsylvania, Mississippi, Rhode Island, and New Jersey.

In the final case to be referred to,[26] *Wilsher v Essex AHA, England* (Table 1–1, case 19), the plaintiff was born in 1978 at 28 weeks gestation, weighing 1,200 g. He had RDS and difficulty in breathing, for which he was given oxygen for the first 81 days of his life. In addition, he had an intraventricular hemorrhage, which led to hydrocephalus, for which operative treatment became necessary. He survived as an intelligent child but developed RLF that resulted in blindness of his left eye and very little sight in the right eye. In his opinion, Mr. Justice Peter Pain stated, "It does seem a great pity that in the process, the doctors get little credit for what they did right, and the whole basis of my inquiry is to see whether they did wrong." The issues involved the following: (1) Whether the failure of the defendant to appreciate initially that a catheter had been inserted into a vein and not into an artery amounted to negligence; (2) If so, whether this negligence caused, contributed materially to, or increased materially the risk of RLF; (3) Whether the subsequent treatment caused the oxygen arterial tension to rise on some provocations to a level and for a length of time that were dangerous; (4) If so, whether the defendants were negligent in causing or permitting this to happen; (5) If yes for (2), (3), and (4), whether this negligence caused or contributed to the RLF; and (6) Whether the partial loss of sight in the plaintiff's right eye could be attributed wholly to retrolental fibroplasia, or whether it was in part caused by optic atrophy, for which the defendants had not been responsible. After much research, and after three experts for the plaintiff and four experts for the defendants were heard, the court appreciated that the danger lay not in the concentration of oxygen used but in excessive arterial oxygen tension. The court stated that methods of measurement were now improved and that a monitor had been developed to check oxygen tension minute by minute. The court did not mention the wild, frequent fluctuations of the oxygen tension of these infants. They admitted that at the time, medical evidence led to the opinion that high arterial oxygen tension was not the sole cause of retrolental fibroplasia, but that it must be carefully controlled. They mentioned other factors such as intraventricular hemorrhage, apnea, RDS, acidosis, carbon dioxide poisoning, and hypoxia, which all may be associated with retrolental fibroplasia. They did admit that in 1978, monitors were not altogether reliable, and that it was necessary to check the monitor frequently against analysis by a blood-gas machine and, if necessary, to recalibrate the monitor.

The judge did find that the hospital had fallen below the requisite standard of care and that the doctors had failed to realize that they had inserted the catheter into a vein instead of an artery and had misread a clear x-ray from which it should have been apparent to any competent doctor that the catheter was not in an artery. He rejected the defendant's submission that a lower standard should have been expected from the house physician because he was inexperienced. The judge held that although there was no certain answer to the question of whether the RLF was caused by the defendant's negligence, on balance of probabilities, it was. The onus shifted to the defendants to prove that their breach of duty had not caused RLF and to show that the first and third periods of overexposure did not do damage. The judge stated that, indeed, the probability was that they did do damage. The problem was with the periods of overexposure, and that the increased arterial tension was assumed to be the cause of the RLF. He awarded a total of over £109,500. This occurred on December 21, 1984, although as previously stated, it has never been proved that RLF is an iatrogenic disease caused by the "excessive" use of oxygen in treating premature infants. There is certainly evidence[1] that the assumption is probably incorrect.

In conclusion, it is obvious from the above that many legal decisions and the litigation of malpractice cases involving ROP are based on facts assumed to be already proved and correct. As is obvious from the literature, these assumptions are far from valid. The legal issues involving vitamin E and the surgical management of ROP are not clear at this time, and there have been no important decisions involving either of these subjects. For this reason, the retina surgeon does not have a greater liability if surgery is or is not performed. Nor does a poor outcome necessarily mean a disastrous legal future. Nevertheless, it is obvious that ophthalmologists dealing with these children should be heavily insured in this current litigious environment. As is the case with all malpractice actions, detailed documentation of everything must be made. This includes informed consent, which is now routinely included in most bills of particulars in these cases. It is certainly a good idea for neonatologists and ophthalmologists to have in the chart parents' statements in writing that they "understand the risks, benefits, and alternatives to therapy with oxygen and/or surgery." Such a statement on the record would be of legal help to the defendant. The locality rule, the reasonable and prudent physician rule, or the custom rule would be no more helpful or harmful to defendants than they would be in any case of malpractice.

Because there are so many differences of opinion about the therapy of ROP, their relevance may be questionable in many cases. The main areas of ROP that may increase liability for the neonatologist and the ophthalmologist are the control of arterial oxygen and the balance of the oxygen level against the risk of death of the patient or cerebral damage to the patient. If the public, particularly juries, are convinced of the difficulties involved in these decisions, the liability will be decreased. Certainly, attention to every detail of each case is most important. The training physician must not rely on a covering physician to assume the care of the patient unless he is fully confident that the covering physician will supervise every detail and be knowledgeable of all the risks. In addition, the treating physician must double and triple check the nursing care and the nurses' notes. As more research is being done and as clinical statistics are collected and analyzed, it is apparent that the assumption that ROP can be eliminated solely by control of arterial oxygen tension is inappropriate. The medical profession has a difficult battle in overcoming the prejudice of legal precedents that may have been wrongfully and unscientifically established. The battle is not over yet. It is hoped that with future scientific clarification of the subject, justice will win out.

## ACKNOWLEDGEMENT

Acknowledgement is made to Brian Bandler who has been most helpful in assembling the legal cases cited.

## REFERENCES

1. Lucey JF, Dangman B: A reexamination of the role of oxygen in retrolental fibroplasia. *Pediatrics* 1984; 73:82–95.
2. McPherson AR, Hittner HM and Kretzer FL: *Retinopathy of Prematurity* Toronto: B.C. Decker Inc, 1986, p 74.
3. *Penetrante v United States* 604 F2d 1248 (ND [Cal] 1979).
4. *Burton v Brooklyn Doctors Hospital,* 452, NYS. 2 875 (App Div 1982).
5. Yu UYH, Hoodman DM, Nave JRM: Retrolental fibroplasia: Controlled study of 4 years experience in an intensive care unit. *Arch Dis Child* 1982: 57:247–252.

6. Personal Communication.
7. *Community Hospital at Glen Cove* 22 NY 2d 255 NY Ct of App June 5, 1968.
8. *Duffy v Fear*, Supreme Court, App Div, 1st Depart, Bronx, NY July 24, 1986.
9. 109 A.D. 2d 198 *Flores v Flushing Hospital and Medical Center and Dr. James G. Lione,* Supreme Court, App Div, 1st Depart, June 25, 1985.
10. *Siirrila v Barrios* 398 Mich 576 No 11 Supreme Court of Michigan Dec. 21, 1976.
11. *Swank v Halivopoulos* 108 NJ Super. 120 Super Ct App Div Argued Nov. 24, 1969. Decided Dec. 29, 1969.
12. Poulin v Zartman Nos 2120, 2127 AK Supreme Court Nov. 12, 1975.
13. *Greenberg v Bishop Clarkson Memorial Hospital* No 41477 NE Supreme Court June 21, 1978.
14. *Comley v Emmanuel Lutheran Charity Board and State Board of Higher Education of the State of Oregon.*
15. *Jones v New Hanover Memorial Hospital* No. 815 SC 440 NC Court of Appeals Feb. 2, 1982.
16. *Hatl v Boles* No 60788 MO Supreme Court En Banc June 27, 1979.
17. *Quick v Aetna Casualty & Surety Company* No. 13251 LA 2d Circuit May 23, 1977. En Banc. Rehearing denied June 22, 1977.
18. *Ohler v Tacoma General Hospital and Air Shields* No. 45247 WA Supreme Ct En Banc, Aug. 16, 1979.
19. *Air Shields, Inc. and Southmore Hospital and Clinic, Inc. v Spears* No. 6026 TX Civil App Ct (Waco). Oct. 18, 1979. Rehearing Denied Nov. 29, 1979.
20. May v Dafoe and Provident Hospital WA Court of Appeals Div I. March 17, 1980. Reconsideration denied Apr. 17, 1980.
21. *Seattle First National Bank v Talbert,* 86 WA 2d 145, 542 P. 2d 774. (1976).
22. *Huie v Newcomb Hospital* NJ Super Ct App Div. Argued Nov. 23, 1970. Decided Dec. 7, 1970.
23. *Zimmerman v Nassau Hospital,* Supreme Court 76 A.D. 2d 921, June 30, 1980.
24. *Kanon v The Brookdale Hospital Medical Center,* Supreme Court Special Term Kings County, Part I. Nov. 5, 1975.
25. *Shockley v Prier,* 66 WI 2d 394, NO 310 WI Supreme Court, Feb. 4, 1975.
26. *Wilsher v Essex AHA,* Queen's Bench Division, Dec. 21, 1984. (Printed in the *Lancet* March 9, 1985 p 589–590.)

Chapter 2

# Retrolental Fibroplasia: Early Years

Joseph W. Eichenbaum, M.D.

In Boston in February of 1941, two premature infants, each approximately 1 kg in weight, were born with nystagmus, almost flat anterior chambers, grayish red reflexes, and gray membranes with blood vessels on the back surface of both lenses. No systemic anomalies were noted. These infants were at the forefront of a blindness epidemic that extended over the next 15 years (Table 2–1).[1] This became known as the retrolental fibroplasia (RLF) epidemic, in reference to the scar tissue that developed behind the lens.

From 1942 through 1945, Terry[2–8] followed infants with RLF and reported on 117 who had the new disease. The term RLF, according to Silverman[1] originated in 1944 with Dr. Harry Messenger, a Boston ophthalmologist who was also a scholar of Latin and Greek. Terry theorized that the problem derived from the persistence and overgrowth of components of the embryonic hyaloid vascular system. He indicated, however, that some RLF victims had normal eye examinations shortly after delivery. It was he who first raised the possibility of extreme prematurity itself as being responsible for the malady.

In the cases of the two above-mentioned premature Boston infants, Silverman[1] excerpted the orders from the hospital records. Both sets of orders prescribed "constant oxygen" therapy.

In 1946, Reese and Payne[9] observed RLF in both premature and full-term infants. Persistent primary vitreous, vitreous hemorrhage causing secondary changes including a ruptured lens capsule, and glaucoma were reported. Also, an association was made between RLF and skin hemangiomas. Both were felt to derive from angioblastic mesoderm in early skin and primary vitreous. Howard,[10] in an earlier paper, had reported that hemangiomas occurred more frequently in premature infants.

**TABLE 2–1.**
The Four Most Frequent Causes of Blindness in Preschool Children in Four States (1947)*

| Causes of Blindness | Illinois | New Jersey | New York | Wisconsin |
|---|---|---|---|---|
| Retrolental Fibroplasia | 20 | 28 | 20 | 8 |
| Cataract | 9 | 18 | 15 | 14 |
| Optic atrophy | — | 21 | 9 | 5 |
| Glaucoma | 3 | 10 | 11 | — |
| Total | 48 | 96 | 93 | 38 |

*From Silverman WA: Retrolental Fibroplasia: A Modern Parable, New York, Grune & Stratton, 1980, p 55. (Used by permission.)

In 1946, Kraus[11] presented the cases of 18 children with retinal atrophy, gliosis, and retinal detachment. The aggregate of several summating congenital defects and malformations was postulated as the cause of RLF in the context of retinal and cerebral hypoplasia and hyperplasia.

In 1948 and 1949, Owens and Owens[12–14] examined over 200 premature infants at birth with a direct ophthalmoscope. None had RLF. Half of the infants were examined again at monthly intervals until age six months; 4% developed RLF. They first described RLF in serial stages of (1) dilated and tortuous retinal blood vessels, (2) retinal elevation more peripherally, (3) further elevated retina with a membrane at the edge of the field, and (4) complete retrolental membrane with blood vessels over the totally detached retina. Owens and Owens[12–14] stated that RLF was a postnatal vascular retinopathy with neovascularization and its secondary complications.

Reese[15] in 1949 noted an RLF-like condition (described by Collins in 1925) with "an opaque membrane behind the lens." Between 1925 and 1937, probable RLF facsimile cases were cited in the ophthalmologic literature with the descriptives "metastatic retinitis," "extrauterine endophthalmitis and iridocyclitis," "congenital falciform fold," "shrunken fibrous tissue cataract," "congenital connective tissue formation in the vitreous chamber," and "fibrous tissue cataract."[15] In 1948, Unsworth[16] cited an old description of apparent RLF dating back to 1820.

## REFERENCES

1. Silverman WA: *Retrolental Fibroplasia: A Modern Parable.* Grune & Stratton Inc., 1980; pp 4–66.
2. Terry TL: Extreme prematurity and fibroplastic overgrowth of persistent vascular sheath behind each crystalline lens. Preliminary report. *Am J Ophthalmol* 1942; 25:203–204.
3. Terry TL: Fibroplastic overgrowth of persistent tunica vasculosa lentis in in-

fants born prematurely. Studies in development and regression of hyaloid artery and tunica vasculosa lentis. *Am J Ophthalmol* 1942; 25:1409–1423.
4. Terry TL: Fibroplastic overgrowth of persistent tunica vasculosa lentis in premature infants. Report of cases—clinical aspects. *Arch Ophthalmol* 1943; 29:36–53.
5. Terry TL: Fibroplastic overgrowth of persistent tunica vasculosa lentis in premature infants. Etiologic factors. *Arch Ophthalmol* 1943; 29:54–68.
6. Terry TL: Retrolental fibroplasia in premature infants. Further studies on fibroplastic overgrowth of persistent tunica vasculosa lentis. *Arch Ophthalmol* 1945; 33:203–208.
7. Terry TL: Ocular maldevelopment in extremely premature infants: Retrolental fibroplasia. General considerations. *JAMA* 1945; 128:582–585.
8. Terry TL: Retrolental fibroplasia, in Levine SZ, et al. (eds): *Advances in Pediatrics,* vol 3, New York, Interscience Publishers, 1948.
9. Reese AB, Payne J: Persistence and hyperplasia of the primary vitreous: Tunica vasculosa lentis or retrolental fibroplasia. *Am J Ophthalmol* 1946; 29:1–24.
10. Howard H: A case showing multiple congenital abnormalities of the eye: The origin of the vitreous indicated by one of them. *Trans Am Ophthalmol Soc* 1917; 15:244–301.
11. Kraus AC: Congenital encephala-ophthalmic dysplasia. *Arch Ophthalmol* 1946; 36:387–144.
12. Owens WC, Owens EU: Retrolental fibroplasia in premature infants. *Tr Am Acad Ophth Otol* 1948; 53:18–41.
13. Owens WC, Owens EU: Retrolental fibroplasia in premature infants. *Am J Ophthalmol* 1949; 32:1–21.
14. Owens WC, Owens EU: Retrolental fibroplasia in premature infants: Studies on the prophylaxis of the disease. *Am J Ophthalmol* 1949; 32:1631–1637.
15. Reese AB: Persistence and hyperplasia of primary vitreous: Two entities. *Arch Ophthalmol* 1949; 41:527–549.
16. Unsworth AC: Retrolental fibroplasia. A preliminary report. *Arch Ophthalmol* 1948; 40:341–346.

Chapter 3

# The "Oxygen Era"

Joseph W. Eichenbaum, M.D.

## HUMAN INVESTIGATIONS

Several papers in the early 1950s, including those by Campbell,[1] Reese and Blodi,[2] Gyllensten and Hellstrom (from animal work),[3] Jefferson,[4] Huggert,[5] and Szewczyk,[6] strongly suggested the association of oxygen therapy and retrolental fibroplasia (RLF). In 1952 Crosse and Evans[7] in England suggested that freely used oxygen was responsible for RLF.

Patz et al.[8] and Patz,[9–12] in the first of the controlled studies in 1952, alternately assigned infants weighing less than 1,600 gm ($3^1/_2$ lb) at birth to receive either "high oxygen" (65% to 70% oxygen for 4 to 7 weeks) or "low oxygen" (<40% oxygen for 24 hours to 2 weeks). After 1 year, 60% of the surviving infants in the high oxygen group had RLF, compared with 6% in the low oxygen group. In the second year, 12 (20%) of 60 infants in the high oxygen group had RLF, compared with one (<1%) of 60 receiving low oxygen.[12] Thus discrimination was made for duration and concentration of oxygen used (Table 3–1).

Patz had indicated, even at this early date, that even if high oxygen levels were correlated with RLF, other factors could play a basic role in mild RLF where low oxygen levels were used.

In April of 1954, the Pediatric Advisory Committee to the cooperative study of oxygen recommended that the infants receive oxygen only as needed, and then in concentrations not to exceed 40%.

Reliable statistics on the number of RLF epidemic infants blinded between 1943 and 1953 are difficult to obtain. However, Silverman[13] estimated the number at 10,000 in the world. According to Heath,[14] by 1949 ROP was

**TABLE 3–1.**
Controlled Study of Retrolental Fibroplasia Outcome According to Treatment Group*

| | Outcome | | | | | |
|---|---|---|---|---|---|---|
| | | RLF Grade† | | | | |
| Treatment Group | Normal Eyes | I | II | III | IV | Total Patients |
| High oxygen | 11 | 3 | 7 | 2 | 5 | 28 |
| Low oxygen | 31 | 4 | 2 | 0 | 0 | 37 |

**From Patz A, Hoeck LE, DeLaCruz E: Studies on the effect of high oxygen administration in retrolental fibroplasia. Am J Ophthalmol 1952; 35:1248–1252. (Used by permission.)*
*†Owens and Owens classification.*

responsible for 30% of blindness in preschool children in the United States.

From 1953 to 1955 a controlled multicenter nursery cooperative study of oxygen levels in premature neonates was undertaken.[15, 16] The cooperative study did not find that the extent of RLF correlated with the percentage of oxygen supplementation per se. Kinsey did note, however, a strong relationship between the duration of oxygen therapy over several weeks and RLF. In a cooperative oxygen study there were 35 cases of cicatricial RLF among infants in the oxygen-curtailed group, compared with 12 infants in the routine (50% oxygen for 8 days) group (Tables 3–2 to 3–5). In addition, several unexpected findings were disclosed: cicatricial RLF occurred three times more frequently in twins and multiple birth infants than in singletons. Singletons, however, on average, received oxygen for longer periods and had lower gestational age than multiple birth infants did. The oxygen concentration (above that of room air) was not associated with the risk of developing RLF. Contrary to the findings of Bedrossian,[17] the rate of oxygen withdrawal did not appear to play a primary role in the vascular changes of RLF.

In May 1954 a second prospective controlled clinical trial appeared, comparing the effects of low and high oxygen therapy among premature infants at Bellevue Hospital.[18] Infants weighing 1,000 to 1,850 gm were randomly assigned to receive either high oxygen (mean 69% for a minimum of 2 weeks or until reaching 1,500 gm weight) or low oxygen (oxygen used only as clinically necessary to treat cyanosis, with a mean concentration of 38%). Two (1.4%) of 28 in the low oxygen group developed RLF, compared with 22 (61%) of 36 in the high oxygen group. However, this study did not mention the cooperative oxygen study, despite the fact that Bellevue Hospital was one of 18 hospitals in the national study (Table 3–6). Many observers believed the independent Bellevue study to be inadequate because of the paucity of cases cited and the reliance on some uncontrolled, 10-year retrospective data.[19]

In a personal communication (1989) Dr. Patz indicated that he was skeptical regarding the interpretations of RLF staging in the early 1950s. Since all observations were made with the direct ophthalmoscope, comprehensive conclusions regarding all stages of the disease were limited.

Bedrossian,[17] in a 1954 controlled trial, condemned the excessive use of oxygen and its rapid withdrawal. Oxygen, in a sense, was used as therapy for RLF.[13, 17]

In 1954 Gordon et al.[20] reported retrospectively on their experience in

**TABLE 3–2.**
Active Stages and Cicatricial Grades of Retrolental Fibroplasia in Infants of Single and Multiple Births, by Hospital*

| | Single Births, No. of Infants | | | Multiple Births, No. of Infants | | |
|---|---|---|---|---|---|---|
| Hospital | Active Stages | Cicatricial Grades | Total of Single Birth | Active Stages | Cicatricial Grades | Total of Multiple Births |
| Abington Memorial Hospital | 0 | 0 | 3 | 0 | 0 | 0 |
| Baltimore City Hospital | 6 | 3 | 22 | 0 | 0 | 3 |
| Boston Lying-In Hospital | 6 | 0 | 9 | 1 | 0 | 2 |
| Cincinnati General Hospital | 7 | 3 | 32 | 1 | 1 | 3 |
| Children's (and affiliated) Hospital (Columbus) | 3 | 0 | 27 | 3 | 2 | 4 |
| Babies' and Children's Hospital (University Hospitals of Cleveland) | 4 | 2 | 25 | 3 | 0 | 10 |
| Cooper Hospital | 1 | 0 | 4 | 0 | 0 | 3 |
| Chicago Lying-In Hospital | 7 | 3 | 12 | 0 | 0 | 2 |
| Michael Reese Hospital | 14 | 2 | 55 | 1 | 0 | 11 |
| Charity Hospital of Louisiana | 60 | 4 | 127 | 21 | 8 | 24 |
| Babies' Hospital (New York) | 9 | 2 | 58 | 0 | 0 | 8 |
| Bellevue Hospital | 0 | 0 | 31 | 1 | 1 | 4 |
| New York Hospital | 21 | 6 | 25 | 10 | 3 | 12 |
| Hospital of the University of Pennsylvania | 0 | 0 | 7 | 2 | 1 | 4 |
| Pennsylvania Hospital | 2 | 0 | 11 | 0 | 0 | 0 |
| Temple University Hospital | 5 | 1 | 16 | 3 | 1 | 5 |
| Elisabeth Steel Magee Hospital | 12 | 2 | 17 | 3 | 1 | 5 |
| Walter Reed Army Hospital | 0 | 0 | 2 | 1 | 1 | 2 |
| Total | 164 | 28 | 472 | 50 | 19 | 114† |

*From Kinsey VE, Hemphill FM: *Etiology of retrolental fibroplasia and preliminary report of the Cooperative Study of retrolental fibroplasia.* Trans Am Acad Ophthalmol *1955; 59:15–24. (Used by permission.)*
†NOTE: *Total as in original table.*

**TABLE 3–3.**
Incidence of Active Retrolental Fibroplasia*
According to Stay in Oxygen Before† Admission to the Study

| Stay in Oxygen (hr) | Incidence of Active RLF‡ n | % |
|---|---|---|
| 0 | — | — |
| 1–12 | 2/17 | 12 |
| 13–24 | 1/10 | 10 |
| 25–48 | 3/25 | 12 |

**From Kinsey VE, Hemphill FM: Etiology of retrolental fibroplasia and preliminary report of the Cooperative Study of retrolental fibroplasia.* Trans Am Acad Ophthalmol *1955; 59:15–24. (Used by permission.)*
*†Infants received no added oxygen after admission at age 48 hours.*
*‡One infant developed active Stages 3 and 4 and finally cicatricial Grade A. All others developed active RLF Stage 2 or less in poorer eye.*

Denver from 1947 to 1953. They compared the incidence of RLF among infants of birth weight of less than 1,500 gm during four periods: (1) "unscrutinized, moderate oxygen": 1947–1950, when infants were nursed in incubators with lids; (2) "unscrutinized high oxygen": 1950, when incubators with portholes were used; (3) "transition period": 3 months in 1950 when "lower oxygen" was used; (4) "scrutinized low oxygen": 1951–1953 (Table 3–7).

A lower incidence of RLF was prevalent during periods of lower oxygen use. However, during the low-oxygen period, eight of 97 infants developed the early stigmata of RLF, and two subsequently developed retrolental membranes. Three of the infants in the low-oxygen group were in oxygen for 3 days or less. Gordon et al.[20] stated that "the obvious importance of high oxygen should not exclude consideration of other etiologic factors both in the host and environment which may be interrelated." Recently Patz (personal communication, 1989) echoed this sentiment. Although the role of oxygen in RLF should certainly be downplayed, it would be incorrect to totally dismiss its adjunctive role.

Lucey and Dangerman[19] pointed out that when the experience of the four original studies (Patz, Lanman, Gordon, and Kinsey and their coworkers) were combined, only 37% of the infants in the high oxygen group had normal eyes (Table 3–8); however, 22% of those in the low oxygen group had RLF.

**TABLE 3–4.**
First Cooperative Study of Retrolental Fibroplasia*

| | No. of Patients Followed | Ophthalmologic Outcome | | | | | |
|---|---|---|---|---|---|---|---|
| | | | RLF Active Stage | | | | |
| | | Normal | I | II | III | IV | V |
| Routine $O_2$ | 53 | 15 (28%) | 13 (25%) | 12 (23%) | 7 (13%) | 5 (9%) | 1 (2%) |
| Curtailed $O_2$ | 245 | 172 (70%) | 37 (15%) | 20 (8%) | 13 (5.5%) | 2 (1%) | 1 (0.5%) |

*From: *Kinsey VE, Hemphill FM: Etiology of retrolental fibroplasia and preliminary report of the Cooperative Study of retrolental fibroplasia.* Tr Am Acad Ophthalmol *1955; 59:15–24. (Used by permission.)*

**TABLE 3–5.**
Additional Data from First Cooperative Study of Retrolental Fibroplasia*

| | No. of Patients Followed | Ophthalmologic Outcome | | | | | |
|---|---|---|---|---|---|---|---|
| | | | Cicatricial RLF Grade | | | | |
| | | Normal | I | II | III | IV | V |
| Routine $O_2$ | 53 | 40 (75.6%) | 3 (5.7%) | 2 (3.8%) | 2 (3.8%) | 2 (3.8%) | 4 (7.5%) |
| Curtailed $O_2$ | 245 | 230 (93.8%) | 4 (1.6%) | 4 (1.6%) | 2 (0.8%) | 4 (1.6%) | 1 (0.4%) |

*From *Kinsey VE, Hemphill FM: Etiology of retrolental fibroplasia and preliminary report of the Cooperative Study of retrolental fibroplasia.* Tr Am Acad Ophthalmol *1955; 59:15–24. (Used by permission.)*

**TABLE 3–6.**
Second Controlled Trial of Retrolental Fibroplasia Outcome According to Treatment Group*

| | Outcome | | | |
|---|---|---|---|---|
| | | RLF | | |
| Treatment Group | Normal Eyes | Vascular Stage | Cicatricial | Total Surviving Patients |
| High oxygen | 14 | 14 | 8 | 36 |
| Low oxygen | 26 | 2 | 0 | 28 |

*From Lanman JT, et al: Retrolental fibroplasia and oxygen therapy. JAMA 1954; 155:223–225. (Used by permission.)*

**TABLE 3–7.**
Incidence of All Residual Lesions and Retrolental Membranes*

| | Period | | | |
|---|---|---|---|---|
| | I Moderate Oxygen | II High Oxygen | III Transition | IV Low Oxygen |
| All residua | 12/80 (15%) | 9/20 (45%) | 4/14 (29%) | 8/97 (8%) |
| Retrolental membranes | 8/80 (10%) | 7/20 (35%) | 3/14 (21%) | 2/97 (2%) |

*From Gordon HH, Lucchenko L, Hix I: Observations on the etiology of retrolental fibroplasia.* Bulletin Johns Hopkins Hospital *1954; 94:34–41. (Used by permission.)*

Also, Lucey and Dangerman[19] cited reports of 159 infants (Tables 3–9 and 3–10) who had not received oxygen therapy and still developed RLF: "The validity of this observation can no longer be questioned; 64 of the infants with nonhyperoxic RLF have been reported in full-term infants born without other anomalies. These nonhyperoxic cases challenge the dogma that RLF is a unique response of the premature infant's retina to excess oxygen." It has been suggested that perhaps some full-term infants are born

**TABLE 3–8.**
Combined Results of Four Original Studies of Retrolental Fibroplasia*

| Study | High Oxygen Group (Normal Eyes/Total) | Low-Oxygen Group (RLF/Total) |
|---|---|---|
| Patz et al (<1,590 g) | 11/28 | 6/37 |
| Lanman et al (1,000–1,850 g) | 14/36 | 2/28 |
| Gordon et al (≤1,500 g) | 11/20 | 8/97 |
| Kinsey and Hemphill (<1,500 g) | 15/53 | 73/245 |
| Total | 51/137 (37%) | 89/407 (22%) |

**From Lucey JF, Dangerman B: A reexamination of this role of oxygen in retrolental fibroplasia.* Pediatrics *1984; 73:1. (Used by permission.)*

**TABLE 3–9.**
Data on 64 Full-Term (FT) Infants With Retrolental Fibroplasia (RLF)*

| Reference | Year | No. | Description | Oxygen |
|---|---|---|---|---|
| Adamkin et al | 1977 | 1 | 2,848-g infant needing exchange transfusion | None |
| Alfano | 1970 | 3 | FT | Yes |
| Brockhurst and Chishti | 1975 | 3 | Birth weight >2,950 g ($6^1/_2$ lb) | None |
| Dixon and Paul | 1951 | 1 | Eyes enucleated for suspected retinoblastoma | |
| Foris and Brockhurst | 1969 | 1 | FT | |
| Harris | 1976 | 3 | FT | None |
| Johnson et al | 1978 | 2 | Siblings, both FT | None |
| Kranshar et al | 1975 | 1 | FT, 3,800 g | Briefly in DR and $1^1/_2$ h of 100% at age 24 h |
| Oshima et al | 1971 | 10 | FT | None |
| Reese and Stepanik | 1954 | 20 | Birth weight 2,270-3,630 g (5–8 lb) | |
| Schulman et al | 1980 | 1 | 40 wk, 2,948 g | None |
| Stefani and Ehalt | 1974 | 15 | Eyes enucleated at 3-24 mo | None |
| Svedbergh and Lindstedt | 1973 | 1 | 39 wk SGA (2,120 g) | Few min |
| Unsworth | 1949 | 2 | FT | None |

**From: Lucey JF, Dangerman B, A reexamination of this role of oxygen in retrolental fibroplasia.* Pediatrics *1984; 73:1. (Used by permission.)*
*SGA = small for gestational age; DR = delivery room.*

**TABLE 3–10.**
Data on 95 Preterm Infants Not Given Oxygen With Development of Retrolental Fibroplasia*

| Reference | Year | No. | Description |
|---|---|---|---|
| Bembridge et al | 1952 | 1 | |
| Brockhurst and Chishti | 1975 | 3 | Birth weight 1,400–1,600 g (3–3½ lb), born before oxygen available |
| Coxon | 1951 | 2 | Birth weight <1,400 g (3 lb) |
| Flynn et al | 1980 | 7 | All <1,500 g |
| Huggert | 1954 | 4 | |
| Johnson et al | 1978 | 11 | Birth weight <1,750 g |
| Messer et al | 1979 | 2 | Birth weight 1,000 gm in 1, and 1,200 g in 1 who was in 25% oxygen for 1 h only |
| Nishimura et al | 1975 | 1 | |
| Oshima et al | 1971 | 12 | |
| Shohat et al | 1983 | 10 | Birth weight ≤1,250 g, no oxygen and 5 with <40% oxygen for few minutes at birth only |
| Yamamoto and Tabuchi | 1976 | 36 | Birth weight <2,500 g, born 1972–1975 |
| Zacharias | 1960 | 6 | |

**From Lucey JF, Dangerman B, A reexamination of the role of oxygen in retrolental fibroplasia.* Pediatrics *1984; 7B:1. (Used by permission.)*

with premature retinal development, leading to a process comparable to that in premature infants.[19, 21–24]

According to Lucey and Dangerman[19] the literature also challenges the contention that oxygen is the sole cause of RLF. They located 95 infants, most of low birth weight, who had RLF but who never received oxygen (see Table 3–10).

Although other workers were not able to prove the efficacy of the 40% oxygen directive clinically, because of its timing, method of publication, and ostensible clinical validity, it was to achieve clinical acceptance that set the standard for neonatal care.

Curiously, while this standard was in effect RLF decreased significantly.[13] However, the "less than 40% only" policy of oxygen treatment was reinforced by the knowledge that malpractice suits for RLF were increasing.[13] At the same time, however, total elimination of RLF could not be achieved. The possibility was accepted that 21% oxygen in ordinary room air can produce RLF.[13]

Avery and Oppenheimer,[25] Cross,[26] and Bolton and Cross[27] pointed out the increased frequency of hyaline membrane disease and neonatal death following restrictive oxygen therapy (Table 3–11). These authors concluded that "the increase in the number of deaths from hyaline membrane disease during the period of restricted oxygen use suggests that some infants with respiratory distress may need more oxygen than they have been receiving."[25]

**TABLE 3–11.**
Mortality and Occurrence of Hyaline Membrane Disease in Two 5-Year Periods (Johns Hopkins Hospital Premature Nursery)*

| | | | | Hyaline Membrane Disease§ | | |
|---|---|---|---|---|---|---|
| | | Deaths‡ | | | | |
| Years | Number of Births† | No. | % | No. | As % of Births | As % of Autopsies |
| 1944–1948¶ | 1152 | 95 | 8 | 17 | 2 | 24 |
| 1954–1958‖ | 1492 | 186 | 13 | 56 | 4 | 39 |

*From Avery ME, Oppenheimer EH: Recent increase in mortality from hyaline membrane disease. J Pediatrics 1957: 553–559. (Used by permission.)
†Birthweight 1.0–2.5 kg (2 lb 4 oz-5 lb 8 oz).
‡From 30 min to 6 days of age.
§Hyaline membrane disease was determined by the microscopic appearance of lungs. All slides were reviewed, retrospectively, by the same pathologist.
¶Oxygen concentration was not measured during this period but almost all premature infants received oxygen at a rate sufficient to produce a concentration of 60–80%. There was a high frequency of RLF during this period.
‖Because the role of oxygen in RLF was "defined," pediatricians were reluctant to raise the oxygen concentration in incubators to more than 40 percent.

Cross[26] and Bolton[27] associated the decrease in blindness with the rise of day of birth deaths during the two decades after the RLF epidemic was brought under control. If blindness had fallen from 50 cases per year (in England), and if there had been more than 700 deaths per year, then it seemed that each sighted baby gained may have cost some 16 deaths.[26, 27]

In 1962 McDonald[28] found that prolonged oxygen therapy may prevent diplegia in very immature infants who had cyanotic attacks. It was suggested that this treatment was of value and that RLF could be avoided.

In 1982 Kalina and Karr[29] reported two decades of experience at the University of Washington (Seattle) with RLF in infants weighing less than 2 kg. The incidence of retinopathy of prematurity (ROP) or RLF in surviving neonates from 1960 through 1967 was 14%. From 1968 through 1980, 20% of 140 infants developed cicatricial disease (Tables 3–12 and 13–13). Most of these neonates retained useful vision; however, in most of these eyes cicatricial RLF was mild and regression occurred spontaneously. Careful oxygen monitoring was thought to be a major factor in the favorable visual outcomes. Oxygen levels and durations were not specified.

## ANIMAL INVESTIGATIONS

Animal investigations showed slightly different results from those observed in neonates. In kittens, Ashton et al.[30] showed increased severity of oxygen vaso-obliterative effects with concentrations of 60% to 70% used for more than 4 days. Of interest, though, Ashton et al.[30, 31] were unable to produce the scarring and retinal detachments characteristic of the later stages of the disease in humans. They suggested that severe oxygen deficit might at times produce RLF in its early stages.

Gyllensten and Hellstrom[32] in 1956 and Patz and Eastham[33] in 1957, independently working with mice, showed that the severity and frequency of vascular changes increase with additional oxygen exposure during periods of slow tapering of supplemental oxygen.

Michaelson, in cats in 1948[34] and in humans in 1954[35]; Cogan in 1963,[36] and Ashton in 1970,[37] using India ink injection into retinal vessels and retinal digest, noted that the retinal vessels developed from primitive mesenchymal cells. The latter produced a capillary network with arteries and veins. These investigators showed that the retinal vessels were not derived from the primitive hyaloid system (as Terry[38] had theorized) but from early mesenchymal cells. The approach of these three scientists was in accord with that outlined by the noted ocular anatomist Ida Mann[39] in 1928.

Flower,[40] using the beagle puppy model, recently found similarities between the development of the canine and human retinal vasculatures. Primordial arterial vessels from spindle-shaped angioblasts were noted to develop in cystic spaces in the peripheral beagle puppy retina. The angioblasts may organize even distant to established endothelial cell cords. Müller cell processes provide the scaffolding throughout the avascular retina on which angioblasts differentiate and organize into a vascular network. Arteries develop from beds of primordial capillaries; vein formation later ensues. The entire artery-capillary-vein system subsequently matures. The primordial vessels from differentiating angioblast precursors also exist in peripheral retinal spaces at birth. These vessels form in a different manner from the process of neovascularization.[40]

Flower[40] was able to produce cicatricial ROP in the beagle puppy eye.

**TABLE 3–12.**
Severity of Cicatricial Retrolental Fibroplasia in Premature Infants by Birth Weight Category 1960–1980*

| Birth weight (gm) | Number of Infants | Mean grade CRLF† |
|---|---|---|
| ≥750 | 2 | 2.0 |
| 751–1000 | 14 | 3.2 |
| 1001–1250 | 12 | 1.4 |
| 1251–1500 | 5 | 1.2 |
| 1501–1750 | 1 | 1.0 |
| 1751–2000 | 1 | 1.0 |
| Total | 35 | 1.7 |

*From Kalina RE, Karr DJ: Retrolental fibroplasia: experience over two decades in an institution. Ophthalmol 1982; 89:291–295. (Used by permission.)
†CRLF = cicatricial retrolental fibroplasia.

**TABLE 3–13.**
Retrolental Fibroplasia in Premature Infants 1968–1980*

| Birth Weight (gm) | 1968–1974 | | | | | 1975–1980 | | | | | Total 1968–1980 | | | | |
|---|---|---|---|---|---|---|---|---|---|---|---|---|---|---|---|
| | PRLF* | | CRLF† | | %CRLF/PRLF | PRLF | | CRLF | | %CRLF/PRLF | PRLF | | CRLF | | %CRLF/PRLF |
| | No. | % | No. | % | | No. | % | No. | % | | No. | % | No. | % | |
| ⩾750 | 3 | 100 | 0 | 0 | 0 | 4 | 40 | 1 | 10 | 25.0 | 7 | 53.8 | 1 | 7.7 | 14.3 |
| 751–1000 | 12 | 30.0 | 2 | 5 | 16.7 | 32 | 42.1 | 9 | 11.8 | 28.1 | 44 | 37.9 | 11 | 9.5 | 25.0 |
| 1001–1250 | 21 | 18.9 | 5 | 4.5 | 23.8 | 25 | 13.5 | 6 | 3.2 | 24.0 | 46 | 15.5 | 11 | 3.7 | 23.9 |
| 1251–1500 | 15 | 8.6 | 1 | 0.6 | 6.7 | 10 | 3.5 | 2 | 0.7 | 20.0 | 25 | 5.5 | 3 | 0.7 | 12.0 |
| 1501–1750 | 7 | 3.7 | 1 | 0.5 | 14.3 | 7 | 2.5 | 0 | 0 | 0 | 14 | 3.0 | 1 | 0.2 | 7.1 |
| 1751–2000 | 1 | 0.6 | 1 | 0.6 | 100 | 2 | 0.6 | 0 | 0 | 0 | 3 | 0.6 | 1 | 0.2 | 33.3 |
| Total | 59 | 8.6 | 10 | 1.5 | 16.9 | 80 | 6.9 | 18 | 1.5 | 22.5 | 140‡ | 7.6 | 28 | 1.5 | 20.0 |

*From Kalina RE, Karr DJ: Retrolental fibroplasia: Experience over two decades in an institution. Ophthalmol 1982; 89:291–295. (Used by permission.)
†PRLF = proliferative retrolental fibroplasia.
‡CRLF = cicatricial retrolental fibroplasia.
§ = includes one hydropic infant > 2000 gm.

He hypothesized that during oxygen exposure the beagle and human retinae are more sensitive. Because they differentiate more slowly, they are less capable of sustaining oxygen-induced vascular damage. The more rapid differentiation of the kitten retina may make it less vulnerable to oxygen-induced vascular damage.

Flower could not determine whether the vascular damage was due to ischemia or to direct oxygen toxicity. However, oxygen-treated beagle puppies who had received aspirin did not develop vasoconstriction, yet they developed more severe retinopathy than the non-aspirin-treated group. Presumably, with less vasoconstriction there is greater blood flow. The increased blood flow raises capillary pressure. Elevated pressure within new capillaries produces ischemia, hemorrhages, and ultimately neovascularization and cicatricial ROP.[40]

## REFERENCES

1. Campbell K: Intensive oxygen therapy as a possible cause of retrolental fibroplasia: A clinical approach. *Med J Aust* 1951; 2:48–50.
2. Reese AB, Blodi FC: Retrolental fibroplasia. *Am J Ophthalmol* 1951; 34:1–24.
3. Gyllensten LJ, Hellstrom BE: Retrolental fibroplasia animal experiments. *Acta Pediatr* 1952; 41:577–582.
4. Jefferson E: Retrolental fibroplasia. *Arch Dis Child* 1952; 27:329.
5. Huggert A: Supply of oxygen to premature and appearance of retrolental fibroplasia. *Acta Pediatr* 1953; 42:147.
6. Szewczyk TS: Retrolental fibroplasia and related ocular diseases. *Am J Ophthalmol* 1953; 36:1336.
7. Crosse VM, Evans PJ: Prevention of retrolental fibroplasia. *Arch Ophthalmol* 1952; 48:83–87.
8. Patz A, Hoeck, LE, DeLaCruz E: Studies on the effect of high oxygen administration in retrolental fibroplasia. *Am J Ophthalmol* 1952; 35:1248–1252.
9. Patz A: Oxygen studies in retrolental fibroplasia. *Am J Ophthalmol* 1953; 36:1511–1522.
10. Patz A: Clinical experimental studies on role of oxygen in retrolental fibroplasia. *Trans Am Acad Ophthalmol Otalaryngol* 1954; 58:45–50.
11. Patz A: Experimental studies in symposium on retrolental fibroplasia. *Trans Am Acad Ophthalmol* 1955; 59:25–34.
12. Patz A: The role of oxygen in retrolental fibroplasia. *Pediatrics* 1957; 19:504–524.
13. Silverman WA: *Retrolental Fibroplasia: A Modern Parable.* New York: Grune & Stratton, 1980, pp 4–66.
14 Heath P: Pathology of retinopathy of prematurity. RLF. *Am J Ophthalmol* 1951; 34:1249–1259.
15. Kinsey VE, Hemphill FM: Etiology of retrolental fibroplasia and preliminary report of the Cooperative Study of retrolental fibroplasia. *Trans Am Acad Ophthalmol* 1955; 59:15–24.

16. Kinsey VE: Cooperative Study of retrolental fibroplasia and the use of oxygen. *Arch Ophthalmol* 1956; 56:481–543.
17. Bedrossian RH: Retinopathy of prematurity and oxygen. *Am J Ophthalmol* 1954; 37:78–86.
18. Lanman JT, et al: Retrolental fibroplasia and oxygen therapy. *JAMA* 1954; 155:223–225.
19. Lucey JF, Dangerman B: A reexamination of the role of oxygen in retrolental fibroplasia. *Pediatrics* 1984; 7B:1.
20. Gordon HH, Lucchenko L, Hix I: Observations on the etiology of retrolental fibroplasia. *Bull Johns Hopkins Hosp* 1954; 94:34–41.
21. Dixon JM, Paul EV: Separation of pars ciliaris retinae in retrolental fibroplasia. *Am J Ophthalmol* 1951; 34:182–190.
22. Patz A: The role of oxygen in retrolental fibroplasia. *Trans Am Ophthalmol Soc* 1968; 66:940–984.
23. Stefani FH, Ehalt H: Non-oxygen induced retinitis proliferans and retinal detachment in full term infants. *Br J Ophthalmol* 1974; 58:490–513.
24. Schulman J, Jampol LM, Schwartz H: Peripheral proliferative retinopathy without oxygen therapy in a full term infant. *Am J Ophthalmol* 1980; 90:509–514.
25. Avery ME, Oppenheimer EH: Recent increase in mortality from hyaline membrane disease. *J Pediatr* 1957:553–559.
26. Cross KW: Cost of preventing retrolental fibroplasia. *Lancet* 1973; 954–956.
27. Bolton DPG, Cross KW: Further observations on cost of preventing retrolental fibroplasia. *Lancet* 1974; 1:445.
28. McDonald AD: Neurological and ophthalmic disorders in children of very low birth weight. *Br Med J* 1962; 1:895–900.
29. Kalina RE, Karr DJ: Retrolental fibroplasia: Experience over two decades in an institution. *Ophthalmology* 1982; 89:291–295.
30. Ashton N, Ward B, Serpell G: Role of oxygen in the genesis of retrolental fibroplasia. *Br J Ophthalmol* 1953; 37:513–520.
31. Ashton N, Ward B, Serpell G: Effect of oxygen on developing retinal vessels with particular reference to the problem of retrolental fibroplasia. *Br J Ophthalmol* 1954; 38:397–432.
32. Gyllensten LJ, Hellstrom BE: The effects of gradual and rapid transfer from concentrated oxygen to normal air or oxygen induced changes in the eyes of young mice. *Am J Ophthalmol* 1956; 41:619–627.
33. Patz A, Eastham AB: Oxygen studies in retrolental fibroplasia. The effect of rapid versus gradual withdrawal from oxygen on mouse eye. *Arch Ophthalmol* 1957; 57:724–729.
34. Michaelson IC: Vascular morphogenesis in the retina of the cat. *J Anat* 1948; 82:167–174.
35. Michaelson IC: *Retinal Circulation in Man and Animals*. Springfield, IL: Charles C Thomas, 1954.
36. Cogan DG: Development and senescence of human retinal vasculature; *Trans Ophthalmol Soc UK* 1963; 83:465–489.

37. Ashton N: Retinal angiogenesis in the human embryo. *Br Med Bull* 1970; 26:103–106.
38. Terry TL: Fibroplastic overgrowth of persistent tunica vasculosa lentis in infants born prematurely. Studies in development and regression of hyaloid artery and tunica vasculosa lentis. *Am J Ophthalmol* 1942; 25:1409–1423.
39. Mann I: *Development of the Human Eye.* Cambridge: Oxford University Press, 1928.
40. Flower RW: Physiology of the developing ocular vasculature, in Flynn JT, Phelps DL (eds): *ROP: Problem and Challenge. Proceedings of Symposium Held at National Institutes of Health.* New York, Alan R. Liss, Inc. 1985, pp 129–146.

Chapter 4

# Historical Elements in Retinopathy of Prematurity, ACTH, and Light

Joseph W. Eichenbaum, M.D.

In the early 1950s, in controlled trials in New York City, one third of ACTH-treated neonates with retinopathy of prematurity (ROP) became blind in one or both eyes, but only one fifth of the controls became blind. Also, there were fewer deaths in the neonates not treated with ACTH. Thus, the ACTH-untreated group had a lower morbidity and mortality than the ACTH-treated group.[1]

In 1952, Locke and Reese[2] reported that light, mydriatics, and ophthalmoscopy were not contributory factors in RLF. These investigators were unable to prevent RLF in premature infants by patching one eye for amounts of time that varied from 1 to 75 days after birth.

Glass et al.[3] prospectively investigated the effect of infants' exposure to light in two intensive care nurseries. They compared the incidence of ROP among 74 infants in the standard bright nursery environment (median light level 60 ft-c) with the incidence among 154 infants of similar birth weight for whom the light levels were reduced (median 25 ft-c). The brighter-nursery-light infants with birth weights below 1,000 g had an 86% incidence of ROP, compared with a 54% rate of ROP in the comparable birth weight group under more dim illumination. However, healthy preterm and term infants showed no gross retinal damage when exposed to bright light in the nursery, as determined by electroretinographic, light threshold, and acuity screening.[4, 5] The Glass et al. ROP risk data emerged from neonates weighing 1,000 g or less who were exposed to bright light. They therefore concluded that safety standards regarding current nursery lighting practices should be reassessed.[3]

Hepner et al.[6] in 1948 and Locke and Reese[2] in 1952 had concluded that light was not an etiological factor in retrolental fibroplasia (RLF) in low birth weight neonates. From the data of Locke and Reese, short-term and prolonged monocular as well as binocular occlusion showed no significant decrease in the incidence of the disease. In 1985 Sisson,[7] in a *New England Journal of Medicine* editorial, cited the increased incidence of ROP in the high-illumination v. lower illumination setting from the Glass[3] report. He stated that cycled light in the nursery environment may have a protective effect, possibly relating to the preservation of circadian rhythms of the newborn.[8] However, one is left to wonder about utilization of natural circadian light in nurseries, or anywhere, and its relation to cyclic metabolic processes.

## INCIDENCE, ASSOCIATIONS WITH OXYGEN, AND CLASSIFICATIONS OF RETINOPATHY OF PREMATURITY

Despite the meticulous attention to oxygen levels in neonate nurseries in the 1970s, DeLeon[9] and Mushin[10] in 1974, and Phelps[11, 12] in 1981, reported a moderate rise in the incidence of RLF. Phelps indicated that the survival rate of infants weighing less than 1 kg increased from 8% in 1950 to 35% in 1980. In 1981, Phelps[11] found the estimated annual accrual of new ROP-blinded infants (397 in 1971 to 883 in 1981) comparable to the estimated number of cases that had occurred during the "epidemic years" 1943–1953. Silverman[1] estimated that in the United States, 7,000 cases occurred in the "epidemic years." Mushin[10] and Phelps[11, 12] suggested (as had Terry[13] in 1943) that prematurity itself produced neovascularization and RLF. It had been clear that oxygen toxicity was not a factor in Phelps' series.

All of the original studies associating RLF with oxygen administration were conducted prior to the availability of routine blood-gas monitoring. Also, their correlation between RLF and oxygen was not necessarily direct.[14, 15] Aranda and Sweet[17] and Gunn and associates[18] failed to document any correlation between hyperoxemia and RLF. Infants of lower than 1,750 g birth weight with elevated $PO_2$ values over a period of 24 hours or more were selected in their studies.[17, 18] Episodes of hyperoxemia to >100, >200, or >300 torr failed to correlate with later development of RLF.[14, 17]

Other authors[14, 16, 19–24] observed RLF in full-term infants not exposed to supplemental oxygen.

It has been suggested that these infants have an exaggerated response to oxygen arterial saturation at the time of birth.[20] It has also been suggested that, "numerous other complicating factors may place the very low birth weight infant at special risk even in the absence of hyperoxic stimulus."[14]

In 1949, Unsworth[25] and subsequent investigators[26–30] noted an inverse

**TABLE 4–1.**
Retrolental Fibroplasia (RLF) Among 177 Surviving Premature Infants*

| Birth Weight | | | |
|---|---|---|---|
| Grams | Pounds | No. | No. with RLF |
| ≥2,275 | ≥5 | 65 | 0 |
| 1,820–2,275 | 4–5 | 77 | 2 (2.6%) |
| 1,365–1,820 | 3–4 | 28 | 4 (14.3%) |
| 910–1,365 | 2–3 | 5 | 2 (40.0%) |
| 455–910 | 1–2 | 2 | 2 (100.0%) |

*From Unsworth AC: Retrolental fibroplasia or ophthalmic dysplasia of premature infants. Trans Am Ophthalmol Soc 1949; 47:738–771. (Used by permission.)

relationship between low birth weight and the incidence of RLF (Table 4–1): with progressively lower weight and gestational age both the incidence and the severity of retinal disease increase.[30–32] According to Lucey et al.[15] very low birth weight (VLBW) is the single most important variable determining the risk of ROP.

Sniderman et al.[29, 77] found that ROP now occurs in 7% of infants with a birth weight between 1,000 and 1,500 g, but increases to 42% among survivors who weigh between 500 and 700 g. "Others[27, 32, 33] have suggested that the risk may be as high as 75% among those weighing <1000 g."[14]

Aranda et al.[34] and Bard et al.[35] implicated blood transfusion or exchange transfusion during oxygen therapy for respiratory distress syndrome (RDS) in the development of ROP. Adamkin et al.[36] reported on a 36-week-old infant who had never received supplemental oxygen but who had received an exchange transfusion for hyperbilirubinemia. Stage 4 RLF was noted in this infant at five months.[14, 36]

Returning to the issue of safe arterial oxygen tension to decrease the risk of RLF, in 1977, Kinsey[37] reported on a five-hospital collaborative study. In 719 infants, most of whom had respiratory distress syndrome, no significant difference was found in the average oxygen tension in infants who developed cicatricial RLF.[37] Aranda et al.[38] found "there is no single $PO_2$ value at which premature infants will uniformly show these changes (of RLF) and by inference no uniform level at which RLF will develop."[38]

In 1971, Baum,[39] however, found residual retinal artery tortuosity in 35 of 52, or 67.3% of eyes of 18-year-olds who had been born prematurely, before the oxygen-restricted phase. Some degree of cicatricial scarring was shown in 14 of 52, or 27%.

A second cooperative oxygen study conducted from 1969 to 1972[40] showed a relationship between higher fraction of inspired oxygen ($FIO_2$) levels and the development of RLF only in those infants of less than 1,200 g birth weight. Despite study limitations, because of the intermittent nature and variable frequency of $PO_2$ sampling, and the postductal umbilical artery sampling site, the strongest correlations with RLF were again found for low birth weight and longer duration of oxygen.[14, 40]

Based on the fundus photographs and fluorescein angiograms of early RLF done by Baum,[41] Mushin,[10] Kingham,[42] Flynn,[43–45] and Kushner and Flynn[46] in 1977, the latter authors postulated that mesenchymal capillary precursors are involved in the "silver line" retinal structure in early RLF. Presumably, hyperoxia obliterates newly formed capillaries, forming arteriovenous shunts just behind the advancing mesenchyme. The mesenchyme is halted and set up as a demarcation line. Regression of vascular anomalous development occurs as new vessels bud from adjacent areas of the front. Persistence and progression of abnormal vessels lead to cicatricial RLF in 15% of the cases. However, the preshunt details and natural history of the disease remain obscure.

Although Reese[47] in 1953 had classified RLF into retinal vascular stages and later retino-vitreal cicatricial changes, others[42, 48–54] attempted further classifications. Each classification, according to Patz,[56] "refined our understanding of the acute disease, but failed in one respect or another to furnish the clinician with a complete picture of retrolental fibroplasia as observed today."[57]

The often-cited McCormick classification,[48] for example, defined the activity of RLF as follows: grade 1, retinal neovascularization; grade 2, neovascularization into the vitreous; grade 3, grade 2 plus dilatation and tortuosity of the posterior pole vessels; grade 4, retinal detachment.[48] However, this classification failed to elucidate the types of cicatricial disease and their relationship to vitreous and retinal involvement.

Therefore, in 1984, the International Committee for Retinopathy of Prematurity (ICROP) reclassified ROP. According to the Committee, the term retinopathy of prematurity described all phases of retinal change in premature infants, from early retinal changes through advanced vitreoretinal disease. The traditional term retrolental fibroplasia was reserved solely for those later cicatricial changes involving the eyes of the most severely affected infants. The ICROP system allowed the examiner to specify the location, extent, and grading of the vascular abnormality. Concise fundus photos with line drawings accompanied the article. This was the first international collaborative effort to categorize ROP.

Three zones of retinal involvement were recognized. They were all concentric with the disc and included (1) the 60-degree posterior pole arch, (2) the near midtemporal and complete nasal periphery, and (3) the entire remaining peripheral retina. The extent of the disease was specified in clock hours (as the observer viewed each eye). The staging of the disease addressed the level of abnormal vascular response. Each stage was defined, including (1) a demarcation line (separating the avascular retina anteriorly from the vascularized retina posteriorly); (2) ridge enlargment of (1) with isolated neovascular tufts; (3) ridge with extraretinal fibrovascular proliferation; and (4) retinal detachment. In addition, when vascular changes were sufficient to produce, for example, posterior retinal arteriole and vein enlargment, a "plus" disease category was added. (A later staging system is described in Chapter 10 of this text, by Dr. Rainer Mittl, and includes a discussion of advanced cicatricial disease.)

Flynn[58] reviewed the Miami experience using the ICROP system to classify ROP in 121 neonates over 17 months. The location, extent, and stage of the disease provided by the study were reliable and reproducible. A unifying principle underlying the classification was obtained: the more posterior the disease and the greater the number of retinal vessels involved, the worse the prognosis.[58]

## RECENT INCIDENCE OF ROP; OXYGEN RE-EXAMINED

In 1984, Tasman[59] indicated that retrolental fibroplasia still accounted for severe visual loss in 250 to 500 babies each year in the United States. About 16% or 37 of 221 premature infants had received physiologic vitamin E therapy. Eight patients (21.5%) went blind, and three other infants lost sight in one eye, accounting for a total of 19 sightless eyes (25.7%). The remaining 74% of eyes retained vision. All eight babies who became blind weighed under 1,000 g at birth. Babies who showed little change in ROP usually weighed more than 1,300 g. Predisposing factors likely to lead to dragged retina in the posterior pole or loss of sight included:

1. Birth weight (infants of less than 1,000 g had 100% visual loss).
2. Presence of peripheral retinal detachment, with detachment more common when a vascular zone extended posterior to the equator; of these cases, 50% developed traction of the retina, 5.6% had severe retrolental membrane formation, and 43.8% resolved with only minimal peripheral fundus changes, with revascularization of the avascular zone occurring prior to reattachment.
3. Dilation and tortuosity of vessels in the posterior pole; 4 of 16 eyes with peripheral detachment and posterior vascular tortuosity developed "dragged retinas"; one became blind; one resolved.
4. Extraretinal neovascularization (4 of 9 eyes with neovascularization had peripheral retinal detachment; when detachment and extraretinal neovascularization were associated with dragging of the retina,

blindness developed in two eyes; when neovascularization without detachment or posterior pole vessel tortuosity occurred, five eyes cleared without posterior pole changes).
5. Extent of mesenchymal shunt (5 of 13 eyes had 360-degree involvement; two of the five went blind; three resolved).

Zak[60, 61] and Kingham[42] cited a comparable incidence of ROP. However, Zak[60, 61] found the incidence of blindness and cicatricial RLF cited by Tasman to be extremely high, or 8 of 37 infants (22%), compared with the 4 of 97 (4%) found by Zak,[60, 61] and the 1 in 140 (.7%) found by Kalina.[62] Zak[60, 61] agreed, however, with the above-noted risk factors cited by Tasman for blindness in RLF. Tasman[59] and Zak[60, 61] both emphasized the importance of low birth weight in the natural history of ROP. This was consistent with the findings of Palmer,[63] McCormick,[64] and Phelps.[65]

Biglan et al.[66] in a retrospective study, reported on more than 1,012 premature infants who had been exposed to increased ambient oxygen during the period 1979 through 1981. Only 19 neonates were found to have acute RLF grade 3 or worse in at least one eye (which is more in line with the findings of Zak[60, 61] and Kalina[62] than with Tasman's[59] data). Unlike the findings of Flower[67] and Bauer,[68] elevated $PO_2$ was not shown to increase the risk of RLF. Infants with chronic lung disease, or chronic lung disease and seizures, had a high risk for developing RLF grade 3 (39% and 57% respectively).[66]

In 1986, Merrit and Kraybill[69] reported on 565 premature infants born in a tertiary perinatal center over a 5-year period. Of these, 110 (about 20%) had ROP. Ten of these infants developed grade 5 cicatricial RLF (about 2% blindness), whereas two fellow eyes remained stable at grade 2 RLF.

Lensectomy and vitrectomy failed to improve vision or reattach the retina in any of the infants with grade 5 RLF. (In three operated eyes and two unoperated eyes, secondary glaucomas developed.) Five vitrectomized eyes developed phthisis. Lower than 1,000 g birth weight, multiple apneic episodes with ventilatory assistance of 100% oxygen, and inadvertent hyperoxemia during general anesthesia may have been significant factors.[69]

From a study in England in 1986, Harden[70] emphasized that all low-birth-weight babies (less than 1.5 kg) should be seen by an ophthalmologist prior to discharge, as well as at nine months and then at $3^1/_2$ years if grade 1 or 2 retinopathy is found. Grade 3 and 4 retinopathy required more frequent ophthalmic supervision. In his series, 18 of 242, about 13%, showed retinopathy of prematurity; 14 were grade 1, 2 were grade 2, and 2 were grade 3 (or about 9% with somewhat advanced disease).

Reexamining the issue of hyperoxic ROP as well as the diagnosis, severity, and natural history of ROP, Flynn et al.[71, 72] conducted a randomized, prospective trial of transcutaneous oxygen monitoring in 214 low birth weight infants. The overall incidence of ROP in the constantly monitored group (51%) was not significantly different from the standard care group (59%). The incidence of cicatricial ROP was also similar in both groups. Thus, the use of continuous transcutaneous oxygen monitoring did not reduce the incidence of ROP in a high-risk premature infant group; i.e., continuously monitoring the oxygen and adjusting the $FIO_2$ did not alter the outcome of the disease.

Of the 214 infants with birth weight less than 1,300 g, ROP developed in 119 (55.6%); cicatricial ROP developed in 9 (7.6%). On the average, ROP was diagnosed at 8 to 9 weeks in infants weighing 900 to 1,300 g. In cases where the disease regressed, ROP lasted about 15 weeks. Low birth weight strongly correlated with the severity of the disease. Total duration of oxygen therapy was only weakly related to the extent of the disease.[71, 72]

The higher incidence of ROP in the 1987 studies by Flynn et al.,[71, 72] compared with the findings of Kalina et al.[62] (14% ROP 20% cicatricial disease) and Campbell et al.[73] and others[74–77] (Tables 4–2 and 4–3) for infants of similar gestational age, was attributed to frequent eye examinations during the hospital stay. Mild forms of ROP that might otherwise have been missed with less frequent examinations were detected with these series.[71, 72]

Isenberg,[74] in discussing the recent Flynn studies, noted that mortality was greater and sepsis occurred more frequently in the continuously monitored group: "Thus longer transcutaneous monitoring may somehow weaken newborns or increase the sepsis rate via the cutaneous route. These implications appear nowhere else in the medical literature and deserve further study."[74] By definition, however, the continuously monitored group was also more at risk and the infants were more ill to start with. Thus, higher morbidity and mortality might be expected.

## RETINOPATHY OF PREMATURITY: HISTOPATHOLOGIC, ANGIOGRAPHIC, AND CLINICAL STUDIES

In 1950, Heath studied autopsy eyes of premature infants with RLF.[78, 79] He noted three distinct stages: (1) primary retinal disease; (2) vitreous involvement and retinal detachment; and (3) late repair and atrophy. Heath stated that RLF was "primarily an edematous, hemorrhagic and proliferative process associated with hamartomatous neovascular tissue in the retina."[78] In 1951, Heath[78] first called RLF "retinopathy of prematurity."

In 1952, Patz[80] found retinal microvascular changes secondary to oxygen therapy. Similarly, Ashton[81–85] noted that in cats, increased oxygen concentration of 6 hours or more resulted in vasoconstriction, vaso-obliteration,

**TABLE 4–2.**
Cicatricial ROP (RLF)*

| Patient no. | 1 | 2 | 3 | 4 | 5 | 6 | 7 | 8 | 9 |
|---|---|---|---|---|---|---|---|---|---|
| Treatment status | CM | SC | CM | SC | CM | SC | CM | SC | SC |
| Birthweight (g) | 620 | 700 | 730 | 740 | 750 | 760 | 800 | 950 | 1240 |
| Gestational age (wk) | 28 | 26 | 26 | 27 | 27 | 27 | 26 | 26 | 29 |
| Sex | F | M | F | M | F | M | M | M | M |
| Total hrs of $O_2$ | 497.3 | 1169.3 | 879.3 | 977.8 | 831.4 | 333.7 | 609.1 | 985.0 | 1400.0 |
| Hrs >70% | 42.0 | 14.9 | 2.4 | 4.1 | 4.5 | 0.0 | 0.5 | 6.6 | 129.2 |
| Hrs 40–69% | 356.4 | 866.0 | 775.2 | 938.4 | 772.3 | 315.8 | 573.4 | 904.7 | 949.5 |
| Hrs 21–39% | 99.3 | 289.0 | 101.7 | 35.4 | 104.8 | 17.8 | 35.2 | 73.6 | 321.4 |
| First + examination | | | | | | | | | |
| Wks of age | 12 | 13 | 12 | 10 | 12 | 11 | 6 | 3 | 14 |
| Conceptual age | 40 | 39 | 38 | 37 | 38 | 38 | 32 | 29 | 43 |
| First cicatricial examination | | | | | | | | | |
| Wks of age | 50 | 13 | 23 | 17 | 86 | 44 | 33 | 21 | 33 |
| Conceptual age | 78 | 39 | 49 | 44 | 113 | 71 | 59 | 47 | 62 |
| Final cicatricial status (grade)† | | | | | | | | | |
| RE | I | V | V | I | V | V | V | III | I |
| LE | I | V | II | I | III | V | III | V | I |

*From Flynn JT, Bancalari E, et al: Retinopathy of prematurity: Diagnosis, severity, and natural history. Ophthalmol 1987; 94:620–629. (Used by permission.)

†Reese classification. ROP = retinopathy of prematurity; RLF = retrolental fibroplasia; RE = right eye; LE = left eye.

**TABLE 4–3.**
Incidence of ROP by Birthweight, Apgar Score, and Treatment Group (n = 214)*

| Birthweight (g) | Treatment Group | 5-min Apgar ≤7 No. of Infants | ROP | % ROP | Odds Ratios[22] (95% CI) | 5-min Apgar ≤8 No. of Infants | ROP | % ROP | Odds Ratios (95% CI) |
|---|---|---|---|---|---|---|---|---|---|
| 500–699 | SC | 3 | 3 | 100 | — | 0 | 0 | — | — |
| | CM | 0 | 0 | — | | 1 | 1 | 100 | — |
| 700–799 | SC | 8 | 8 | 100 | 1[†] | 4 | 3 | 75 | 2.0 |
| | CM | 4 | 4 | 100 | | 5 | 3 | 60 | (0.057–103.000) |
| 800–899 | SC | 3 | 3 | 100 | 1[‡] | 6 | 5 | 83 | 1.7 |
| | CM | 8 | 8 | 100 | | 4 | 3 | 75 | (0.03–102.00) |
| 900–999 | SC | 10 | 9 | 90 | 1 | 8 | 2 | 25 | 0.6 |
| | CM | 10 | 9 | 90 | (0.022–44.500) | 8 | 3 | 38 | (0.038–7.100) |
| 1000–1099 | SC | 11 | 8 | 73 | 0.8 | 9 | 4 | 44 | 2.4 |
| | CM | 13 | 10 | 77 | (0.089–7.100) | 8 | 2 | 25 | (0.21–31.80) |
| 1100–1199 | SC | 12 | 7 | 58 | 1.2 | 11 | 5 | 45 | 9.1[†] |
| | CM | 13 | 7 | 54 | (0.19–7.90) | 5 | 0 | 0 | |
| 1200–1300 | SC | 11 | 4 | 36 | 3.4 | 17 | 6 | 35 | 7.6 |
| | CM | 7 | 1 | 14 | (0.22–106.00) | 15 | 1 | 7 | (0.67–195.00) |

*From Flynn JT, Bancalari E, et al: Retinopathy of prematurity: Diagnosis, severity, and natural history. Ophthalmol 1987; 94:6,620–629. (Used by permission.)
†Estimated value ROP = retinopathy of prematurity; CI = confidence interval; SC = standard care; CM = constantly monitored.

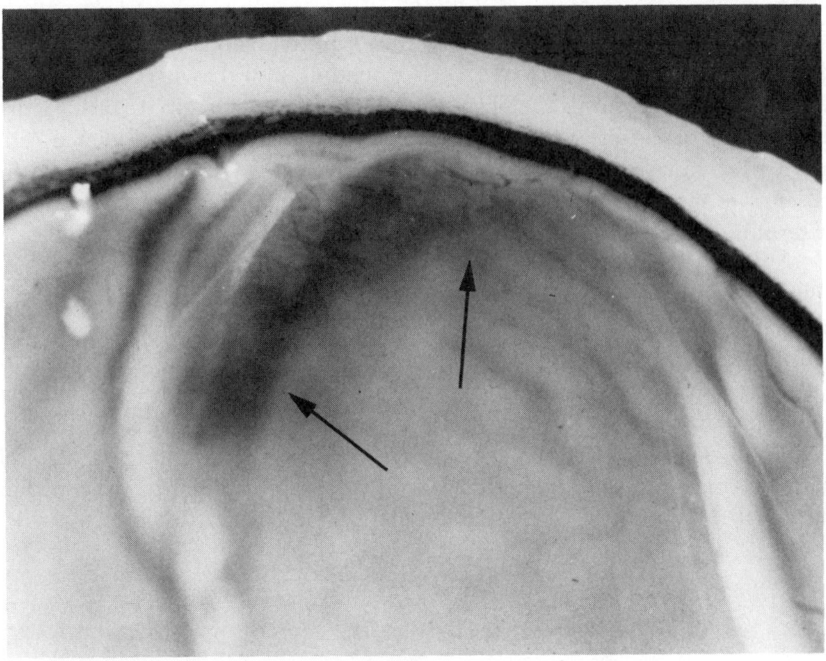

**FIG 4–1.**
Gross appearance of retina illustrating neovascularization with extension of vessels into vitreous *(arrows)*. Some vitreous hemorrhage is also present. *(From Karlsberg RC, Green WR, Patz A: Congenital retrolental fibroplasia.* Arch Ophthalmol *1973; 89:122–123. Used by permission.)*

and secondary arteriolovenous shunting. However, in a later study, using glass beads to occlude the retinal vessels of newborn kittens. Ashton[85] was able to demonstrate retinal vessel proliferation into the vitreous as a result of capillary obliteration, without the specific effect of hyperoxia.

Friedenwald et al.[86] first observed abnormal capillary budding in the nerve fiber layer in RLF patients. Serpell[87] indicated that these actively proliferating cells were mesenchymal, containing polysaccharide (glycogen) granules. They were spindle-shaped precursors of the retinal vascular system. Reese et al.[88, 89] showed that neovascularization began in the retina as canalized, proliferating endothelial cells which broke through the internal limiting membrane. This resulted in retinal edema and hemorrhage and then vitreous hemorrhage and eventually contracture and retinal detachment. Ashton's[90] histopathologic analysis was quite similar.

Karlsberg et al.[91] presented histopathologic findings in a full-term infant with hydrocephalus, other congenital defects, and retrolental fibroplasia. Figure 4–1[91] is the gross appearance of the retina illustrating neovascularization with extension of vessels into the vitreous. Some vitreous hemorrhage is also present. Figure 4–2[91] is a section of retina showing nodules of endothelial cells and thin-walled vessels extending into the vitreous. Extravasated blood is present in the nerve fiber, ganglion cells, and vitreous. Figure 4–3[91] is the anterior extent of the nodular proliferation of endothelial cells and vessels in vitreous. "The observation of typical ROP proliferation in the absence of oxygen therapy points to the need for further basic research to determine factors that control retinal vascularization."[91]

Utilizing trypsin digestions, Chui and Green[92] reported a second case of ophthalmoscopically documented retrolental fibroplasia. Kalina and Forrest[93] had reported in 1973 on the first trypsin digest of a documented case of retrolental fibroplasia. Figure 4–4[92] shows mesenchymal cell proliferation in the retinal nerve fiber layer. Figure 4–5[92] shows an area of neovascularization extending through the internal limiting membrane into the vitreous. Figure 4–6[92] shows a neovascular network demonstrating glomerular like tufts of mesenchymal and endothelial cells with abundant red blood cells within thin-walled capillaries. Chui and Green[92] postulated that hyperoxia results

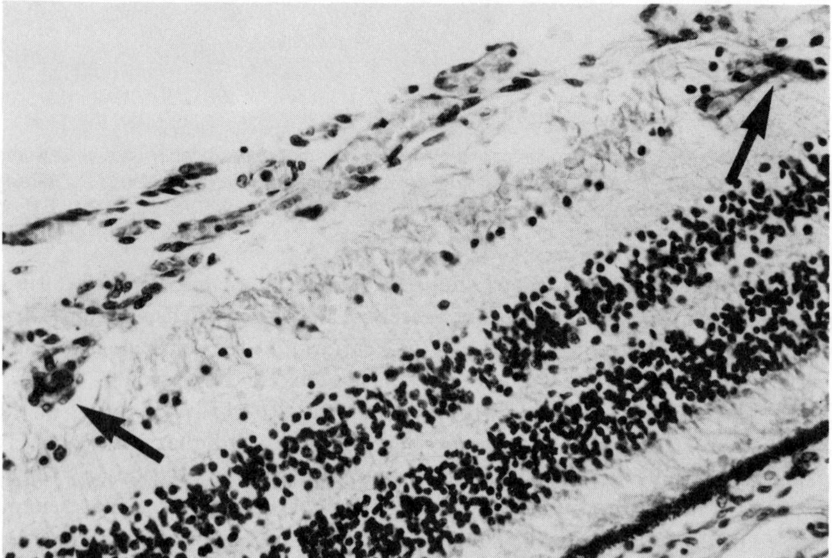

**FIG 4–2.**
Section of retina showing nodules of endothelial cells *(arrows)* and thinned walled vessels extending into vitreous. Extravasated blood is present in nerve fiber and ganglion cell layers and in vitreous (hematoxylin-eosin, original magnification ×275). *(From Karlsberg RC, Green WR, Patz A: Congenital retrolental fibroplasia.* Arch Ophthalmol *1973; 89:122–123. Used by permission.)*

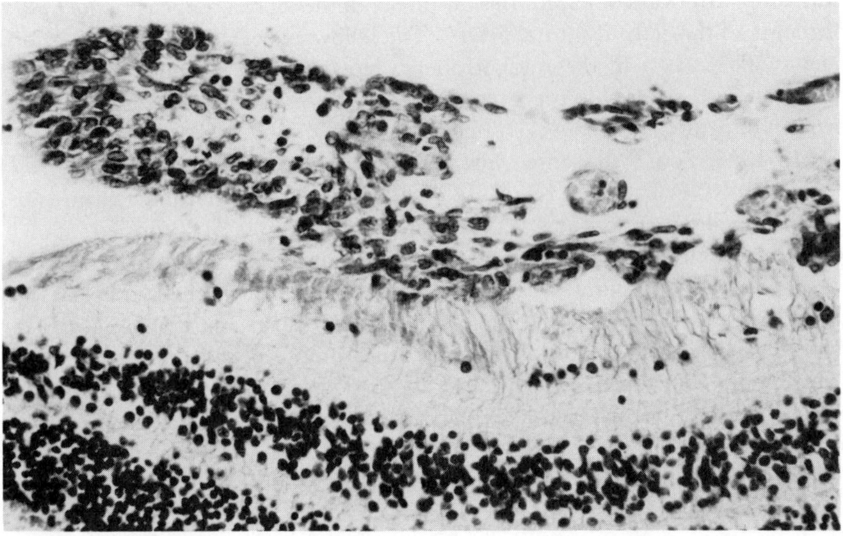

**FIG 4–3.**
Anterior extent of nodular proliferation of endothelial cells and vessels in vitreous (hematoxylin-eosin, original magnification ×275). *(From Karlsberg RC, Green WR, Patz A: Congenital retrolental fibroplasia.* Arch Ophthalmol *1973; 89:122–123. Used by permission.)*

in capillary obliteration. The reduction or loss of capillaries results in hypoxia. The hypoxia stimulates mesenchymal elements to proliferate in a compensatory fashion but with an excess amount. The trypsin digest and routine sections showed large masses of mesenchymal cells. Posterior to the front line of mesenchymal proliferation, neovascularization occurred.

In 1979, Naiman et al.[94] presented a case of RLF documented histopathologically in an infant born at 29 weeks. The baby was given supplemental oxygen, but because it had congenital heart defects, the arterial alveolar partial pressure of oxygen never increased above 91 mm Hg. Only on three isolated measurements was it greater than 80 mm Hg. Thus, RLF developed in this hypoxic infant. Figure 4–7[94] illustrates peripheral hypervascular and hypercellular venous areas with progressively increasing vascular anastomosis and arcades merging with a dense zone of endothelial cell proliferation. Nonvascularized strands of mesenchymal cells extend anteriorly from the endothelial zone and some of these join to form an arcade.

Figure 4–8[94] shows nodular anterior extensions of the proliferative endothelial zone with strands of mesenchymal cells streaming from its anterior extent.

Scanning electron microscopy[95] of the vascular development of a premature infant with respiratory distress syndrome showed the absence of branching arterioles or capillaries despite endothelial cell replicas in the main branches of the central retinal artery. The fellow eye of this baby had retinal neovascularization in the midperiphery. However, the authors themselves questioned whether this represented "true neovascularization or a normal process of growth at 27 weeks of gestation."[95]

In 1985, Foos[96] presented histopathologic changes of 40 autopsy cases of chronic ROP. Previous reports[97, 98] had documented anatomic features of normal development of the retinal vasculature in paranatal autopsied infants as well as pathologic features of the acute phase. A "vanguard zone" of mesenchymal cells and a "rear guard" zone of endothelial cells precede the development of primitive retinal vessels in man. In the acute phase of ROP, hyperplasia occurs sequentially, first in the vanguard and then in the rear guard zone. Extraretinal vasoproliferation, with retinal folding at that site and subsequent retinal scroll-like rolling anteriorly toward the lens, with foreshortening and detachment, constitute the chronic ROP phases. The scenario is complex: it is not clear if the mesenchymal cells of the vanguard

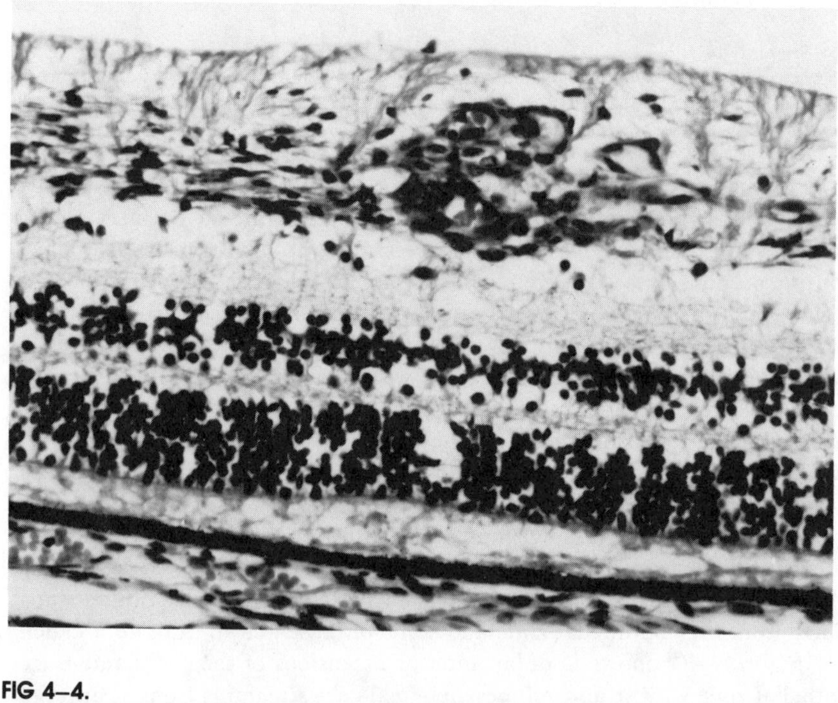

**FIG 4–4.**
Mesenchymal cell proliferation in the retinal nerve-fiber layer (hematoxylin-eosin, original magnification ×330). *(From Chui HC, Green WR: Acute retrolental fibroplasia: A clinicopathologic case report.* Maryland Med J *1977. Used by permission.)*

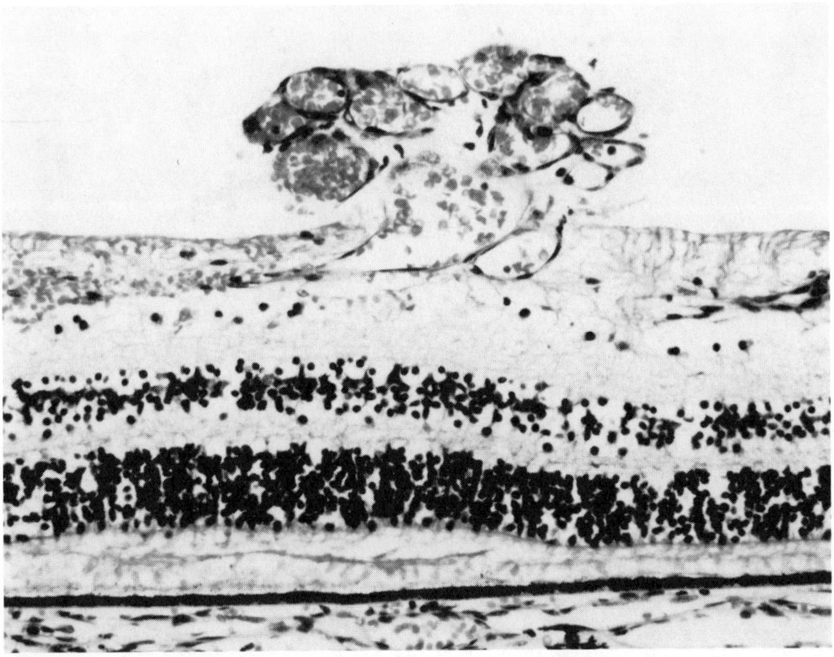

**FIG 4–5.**
Area of neovascularization extending through the internal limiting membrane into the vitreous. (hematoxylin-eosin, original magnification ×320). *(From Chui HC, Green WR: Acute retrolental fibroplasia: A clinicopathologic case report.* Maryland Med J *1977. Used by permission.)*

contain contractile proteins and if the detachment occurs after extraretinal vasoproliferative traction. Ridge elevation from contraction of the rear guard astrologliosis and contraction of the vanguard mesenchyme, contraction of vasoproliferative tissue itself, vitreolytic changes during the vasoproliferative phase with secondary retinal traction, as well as nonvascular components, e.g., from retinal pigment epithelial changes, are all possible additional factors in the retinal detachment scheme. Foos stated that although it is likely to be multifactorial in etiology, inflammation is not present during this process.

In the Foos[96] report on chronic ROP, 80 eyes from 40 autopsies were included; 35 patients had died in infancy, birth weight varied from 780 to 1,530 g and most had had some oxygen therapy. In all eight infants with patent ductus arteriosus, surgery had been performed; seven cases of anencephaly were included. Advanced cicatricial cases were excluded.

As had been indicated by Flynn et al.,[43] Kushner et al.,[46] Cantolino et al.,[52] Kingham,[42] and Foos,[96] the majority of the intraretinal lesions regressed. White, linear, retinal scars were left behind. In two cases, the extraretinal

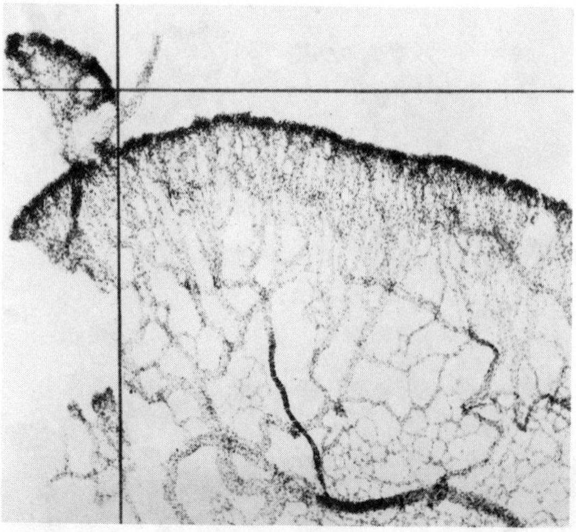

**FIG 4–6.**
Neovascular network demonstrating glomerular-like tufts of mesenchymal and endothelial cells with abundant red blood cells within thin-walled capillaries (trypsin digest, PAS-hematoxylin, original magnification ×130). *(From Chui HC, Green WR: Acute retrolental fibroplasia: A clinicopathologic case report.* Maryland Med J *1977. Used by permission.)*

vessels had the configuration of sea-fans, as seen in sickle-cell retinopathy. Lesions similar to those of ROP were seen in seven cases of anencephaly. Extramedullary erythropoiesis outside of extra retinal vasoproliferative sites were observed in four cases.[96]

Retrolental membranes were obtained from six premature infants, with birth weight ranging from 580 to 1,750 g. All presented with leukokoria and a history of treatment with 100% oxygen. The retrolental membranes showed, via fluorescent probe, filamentous actin.[99] Actin filaments in myofibroblasts also result from penetrating posterior ocular injuries.[100] These specialized cells have characteristics of fibroblast and smooth-muscle cells, and these qualities are felt to underlie the production of contractile forces in vitreoretinal traction and cicatricial ROP.[98, 101] Glial cells,[102, 103] retinal vascular pericytes,[104, 105] hyalocytes,[105] and ciliary epithelial cells[106] have all been implicated in the process of contractile force generation in vitreoretinal membranes. Thus, it is difficult to definitively identify the exact cellular source of actin and contractile forces in pathologic tissue.[99] However, Soong et al.[99] have suggested that the visualization of actin filament bundles prompts the potential use of pharmacologic inhibitors of cellular contraction strands as a nonsurgical alternative in vitreoretinal traction disease.[99]

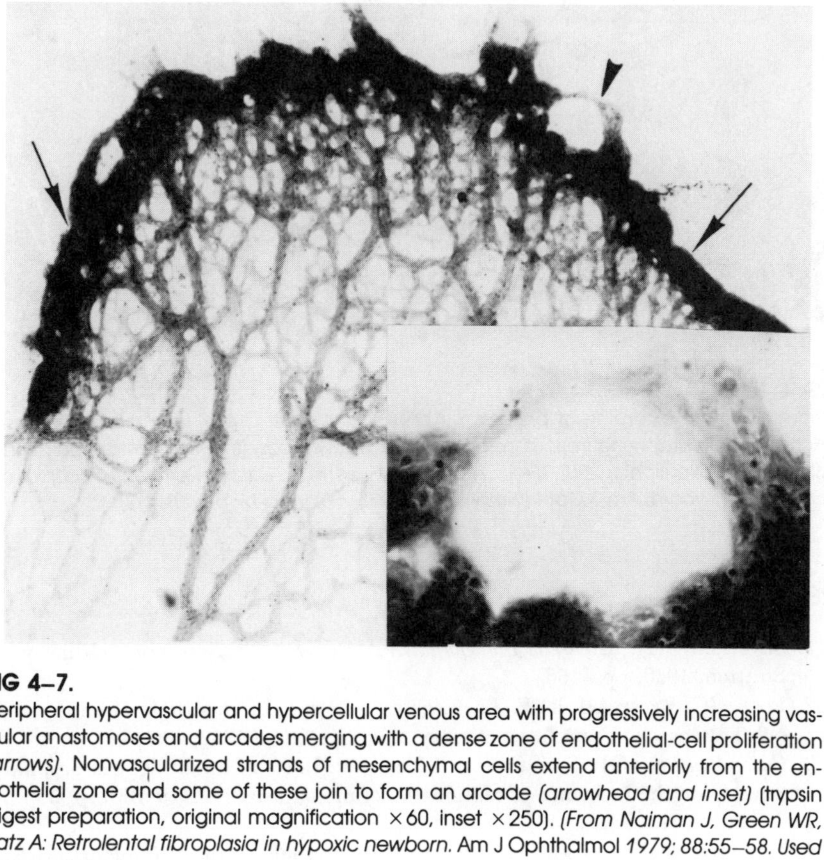

**FIG 4–7.**
Peripheral hypervascular and hypercellular venous area with progressively increasing vascular anastomoses and arcades merging with a dense zone of endothelial-cell proliferation *(arrows)*. Nonvascularized strands of mesenchymal cells extend anteriorly from the endothelial zone and some of these join to form an arcade *(arrowhead and inset)* (trypsin digest preparation, original magnification ×60, inset ×250). *(From Naiman J, Green WR, Patz A: Retrolental fibroplasia in hypoxic newborn.* Am J Ophthalmol *1979; 88:55–58. Used by permission.)*

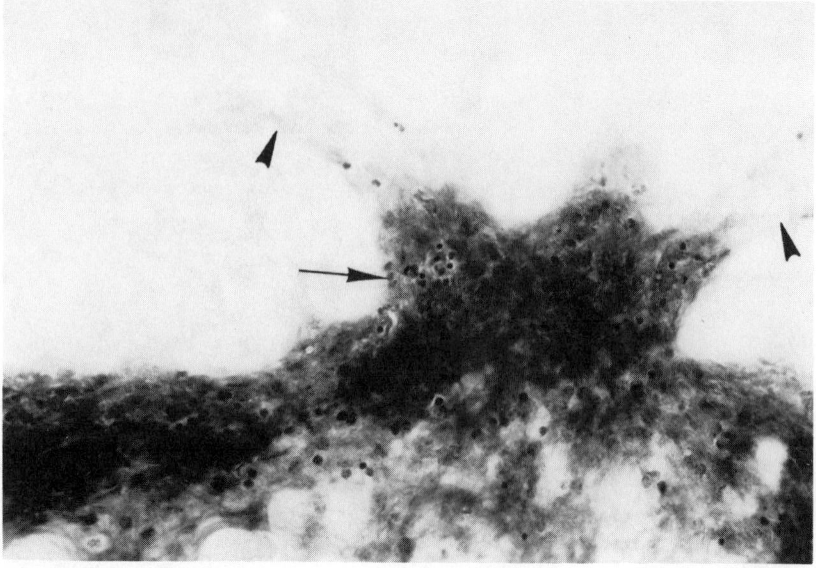

**FIG 4–8.**
Nodular anterior extension of proliferative endothelial zone *(arrow)* with strands of mesenchymal cells streaming from its anterior extent *(arrowheads)* (trypsin digest preparation, original magnification ×250). *(From Naiman J, Green WR, Patz A: Retrolental fiboplasia in hypoxic newborn.* Am J Ophthalmol *1979; 88:55–58. Used by permission.)*

## REFERENCES

1. Silverman WA: *Retrolental Fibroplasia: A Modern Parable.* New York: Grune & Stratton, 1980, pp 4–66.
2. Locke JC, Reese AB: RLF: The negative role of light, mydriatics, and the ophthalmoscope exam in its etiology. *Arch Ophthalmol* 1952; 48:44–47.
3. Glass P, Avery GB, Subramanan KNS, et al: Effect of bright light in hospital nursery on the incidence of retinopathy of prematurity. *N Engl J Med* 1985; 313:401–404.
4. Hamer R, Dobson V, Mayer M: Absolute thresholds in human infants exposed to continuous illumination. *Invest Ophthalmol Vis Sci* 1974; 25:381–388.
5. Dobson V, Riggs LA, Sigueland ER: Electroretinographic determination of dark adaptation functions of children exposed to phototherapy as infants. *J Pediatr* 1974; 85:25–29.
6. Hepner WR, Kraus AC, Davis ME: Retrolental fibroplasia and light. *Pediatrics* 1949; 3:824–828.
7. Sisson TRC: Hazards to vision in the nursery (editorial). *Engl J Med* 1985; 313:444–445.

8. Sisson TRC, Root AW, Kechavary-Oliali L, et al: Biologic rhythm of plasma human growth hormone in newborns of low birth weight, in Scheving L, Halberg F, Pauly J (eds): *Chronobiology*. Tokyo:Igaju-Shoin, 1974, pp 348–352.
9. DeLeon AS, Elliot JW, Jones DB: The resurgence of retrolental fibroplasia. *Pediatr Clin North Am* 1970; 17:309–322.
10. Mushin AS: Retinopathy of prematurity: A disease of increasing incidence. *Trans Opthalmol Soc UK* 1974; 94:251–257.
11. Phelps DL: Retinopathy of prematurity: An estimate of vision loss in the United States—1979. *Pediatrics* 1981; 67:924–926.
12. Phelps DL: Vision loss due to retinopathy of prematurity. *Lancet* 1981; 1:606.
13. Terry TL: Fibroplastic overgrowth of persistent tunica vasculosa lentis in premature infants. Report of cases: Clinical aspects. *Arch Ophthalmol* 1943; 29:36–53.
14. Lucey JF, Dangerman B: A reexamination of the role of oxygen in retrolental fibroplasia. *Pediatrics* 1984; 7B:1.
15. Kinsey VE: Cooperative Study of retrolental fibroplasia and the use of oxygen. *Arch Ophthalmol* 1956; 56:481–543.
16. Stefani FH, Ehalt H: Non-oxygen induced retinitis proliferans and retinal detachment in full term infants. *Br J Ophthalmol* 1974; 58:490–513.
17. Aranda JV, Sweet AY: Sustained hyperoxeonia without cicatricial retrolental fibroplasia. *Pediatrics* 1974; 54:434–437.
18. Gunn TR, Easdown J, Outerbridge EW, et al: Risk factor in retrolental fibroplasia. *Pediatrics* 1980; 65:1096–1100.
19. Foos RY: Acute retrolental fibroplasia. *Graefes Arch Clin Exp Ophthalmol* 1975; 18:87–100.
20. Brockhurst RJ: Christi MI: Cicatricial RLF: Its occurrence without oxygen administration and in full term infants. *Graefes Arch Clin Exp Ophthalmol* 1975; 195:113.
21. Kraushar MF, Harper F, Sia CG: Retrolental fibroplasia in full term infants. *Am J Ophthalmol* 1975; 80:106.
22. Kushner BJ, Gloeckner E: Retrolental fibroplasia in full term infants without exposure to supplemental oxygen. *Am J Ophthalmol* 1984; 97:148–158.
23. Alfano JE: Retrolental fibroplasia: A continuing program. *Trans Am Acad Ophthalmol Otolaryngol* 1970; 74:18.
24. Bruckner HL: RLF associated with intrauterine anoxia. *Arch Ophthalmol* 1968; 20:504.
25. Unsworth AC: Retrolental fibroplasia or ophthalmic dysplasia of premature infants. *Trans Am Ophthalmol Soc* 1949; 47:738–771.
26. Kinsey VE, Arnold HJ, Kalina RE, et al: $PaO_2$ levels and RLF: A report of the cooperative study. *Pediatrics* 1977; 60:655–667.
27. McCormick AQ: RLF: The future. *Can J Ophthalmol* 1976; 11 (suppl):13–15.
28. Pomerance JJ, Breger B, Brown S: Incidence of RLF. *Clin Res* 1982; 30:122A.
29. Sniderman SH, Riedel PA, Bert MD, et al: Influence of transcutaneous oxygen ($TcPO_2$). *Clin Res* 1982; 30:148A.
30. Katzman G, Satish M, Krishnan V, et al: Comparative analysis of lower and higher stage RLF (abstracted). *Pediatric Res* 1982; 16:294A.

31. Yamamoto M, Tabuchi A: Management of the retinopathy of prematurity. *Jpn J Ophthalmol* 1976; 20:372–383.
32. Phelps DL: Vitamin E and RLF in 1982. *Pediatrics* 1982; 70:420–425.
33. Shohat M, Reisner SH, Krikler R, et al: ROP: Incidence and risk factors. *Pediatrics* 1983; 72:159–163.
34. Aranda JV, Clark TE, Manniello R, et al: Blood transfusion: Possible potentiating risk factor in retrolental fibroplasia. *Pediatr Res* 1975; 9:633.
35. Bard H, Cornet A, Orquin J, et al: Retrolental fibroplasia exchange transfusions. *Pediatr Res* 1975; 9:634.
36. Adamkin DH, Shott RJ, Cook LN, et al: Non-hyperoxic retrolental fibroplasia. *Pediatrics* 1977; 60:828–829.
37. Kinsey VE, et al: $PaO_2$ levels and retrolental fibroplasia: Part of the cooperative study. *Pediatrics* 1973; 60:655–668.
38. Aranda JV, Saheb N, Stern L, et al: Arterial oxygen tension and retinal vasoconstriction in new born infants. *Am J Dis Child* 1971; 122:189–194.
39. Baum JD: Retinal artery tortuosity in ex-premature infants: 18 year follow-up on eyes of premature infants. *Arch Dis Child* 1971; 46:247–252.
40. Kinsey VE, Arnold HJ, Kalina RE, et al: $PaO_2$ levels and retolental fibroplasia: A report of the cooperative study. *Pediatrics* 1977; 60:655–668.
41. Baum JD: Retinal photography in premature infants forms fruste retrolental fibroplasia. *R Soc Med (Lond)* 1971; 64:777–779.
42. Kingham JD: Acute retrolental fibroplasia. *Arch Ophthalmol* 1977; 95:39–47.
43. Flynn JT: Acute proliferative retrolental fibroplasia: Evolution of the lesion. *Graefes Arch Clin Exp Ophthalmol* 1975; 195:101–111.
44. Flynn JT, O'Grady GE, Herrera J, et al: RLF I: Clinical observations. *Arch Ophthalmol* 1977; 95:217–223.
45. Flynn JT, Cassidy J, Essner D, et al: Fluorescein angiography in retrolental fibroplasia: Experience from 1969–1977. *Ophthalmology* 1970; 86:1700–1723.
46. Kushner BJ, Essner D, Cohen I, and Flynn JT: Retrolental fibroplasia II: Pathologic correlation. *Arch Ophthalmol* 1977; 95:29–38.
47. Reese AB, King MJ, Owens WC: A classification of retrolental fibroplasia. *Am J Ophthalmol* 1953; 36:1333–1335.
48. McCormick AQ: Retinopathy of prematurity: Current problems. *Pediatrics* 1971; 7:1–28.
49. Patz A: Retrolental fibroplasia. *Surv Ophthalmol* 1969; 14:1–29.
50. Schaffer DB, Johnson L, Quinn GE, et al: A classification of retrolental fibroplasia to evaluate vitamin E therapy. *Ophthalmol* 1979; 86:1749–1760.
51. Quinn GE, Schaffer DB, Johnson LA: A revised classification of retinopathy of prematurity. *Am J Ophthalmol* 1982; 94:744–749.
52. Cantolino SJ, Curran J, VanCaden TC, et al: Acute retrolental fibroplasia: Classification and objective evaluation of incidence, natural history and resolution by fundus photography and intravenous fluorescein angiography. *Perspect Ophthalmol* 1978; 2:175–187.
53. Uemura Y: Current status of retrolental fibroplasia: Report of the Joint Committee for the Study of RLF. *Jpn J Ophthalmol* 1977; 21:366–378.

54. Keith GL: Retrolental fibroplasia: A new classification of the developing and cicatricial changes. *Aust J Ophthalmol* 1979; 7:189–194.
55. Reference deleted in proof.
56. Patz A: The new international classification of retinopathy of prematurity. *Arch Ophthalmol* 1984; 102:1129.
57. Committee of the Classification of Retinopathy of Prematurity: An International Classification of ROP. *Arch Ophthalmol* 1984; 102:1130–1134.
58. Flynn JT: An international classification of ROP. *Ophthalmology* 1985; 92:987–994.
59. Tasman W: The natural history of active retinopathy of prematurity. *Ophthalmology* 1984; 91; 12:1499–1502.
60. Zak TA: Discussion of ROP & W. Tasman's paper #60. *Ophthalmology* 1984; 91:12:1502–1503.
61. Zak TA: Retinopathy of prematurity: An update on retrolental fibroplasia. *NY State of J Med* 1982; 82:1795–1796.
62. Kalina RE, Karr DJ: Retrolental fibroplasia: Experience over two decades in an institution. *Ophthalmology* 1982; 89:291–295.
63. Palmer EA: Optimal timing of examination for acute retrolental fibroplasia. *Ophthalmology* 1981; 88:662–668.
64. McCormick AQ: Retinopathy of prematurity. *Curr Probl Pediatr* 1977; 7:3–28.
65. Phelps DL: ROP: An estimate of vision loss in U.S. 1979. *Pediatrics* 1981; 67:924–926.
66. Biglan AW, Brown DR, Reynolds JD, et al: Risk factors associated with retrolental fibroplasia. *Ophthalmology* 1984; 91:1054–1511.
67. Flower RW: A new perspective on the pathogenesis of retrolental fibroplasia: The influence of elevated arterial $PCO_2$. *Retinopathy of Prematurity Conference*, Wash DC, Dec 1981, pp 20–45.
68. Bauer CR, Widmayer SM: A relationship between $paCo_2$ and retrolental fibroplasia. *Pediatr Res* 1981; 15:649.
69. Merrit JC, Kraybill EN: Retrolental fibroplasia: A five year experience in a tertiary perinatal center. *Ann Ophthalmol* 1986; 18:65–67.
70. Harden AF: Retinopathy of prematurity — A long term follow-up. *Trans Ophthalmol Soc UK* 1986; 105: 717–719.
71. Flynn JT, Bancalari E, et al: Retinopathy of prematurity: Diagnosis, severity, and natural history. *Ophthalmology* 1987; 94:620–629.
72. Flynn JT, Bancalari E, et al: Retinopathy of prematurity: A randomized, prospective trial of transcutaneous oxygen monitoring. *Ophthalmology* 1987; 94:630–637.
73. Campbell PB, Bull MJ, Ellis FD, et al: Incidence of ROP in a tertiary newborn intensive care unit. *Arch Ophthalmol* 1983; 101:686–688.
74. Isenberg SJ: Discussion of Flynn et al. *Ophthalmology* 1987; 94:637–638.
75. Pomerance JJ: Incidence of retrolental fibroplasia. Presented at Retinopathy of Prematurity Conference, Washington, DC Dec 1981.
76. Petersen RA: Six years experience with retrolental fibroplasia in the Joint Program for Neonatology at Harvard Medical School. Presented at Retinopathy of Prematurity Conference, Washington, DC, Dec 1981.

77. Sniderman SH, Riedel PA, Bert MD, et al: Factors influencing the incidence of retrolental fibroplasia. Presented at Retinopathy of Prematurity Conference, Wash., DC, Dec 1981.
78. Heath P: Pathology of retinopathy of prematurity, RLF. *Am J Ophthalmol* 1951; 43:1249–1259.
79. Heath P: Retrolental fibroplasia as a syndrome: Pathogenesis and classifications. *Arch Ophthalmol* 1950; 44:245–274.
80. Patz A, Hoeck LE, DeLaCruz E: Studies on the effect of high oxygen administration in retrolental fibroplasia. *Am J Ophthalmol* 1953; 36:1511–1522.
81. Ashton N, Ward B, Serpell G: Role of oxygen in the genesis of retrolental fibroplasia. *Br J Ophthalmol* 1953; 37:513–520.
82. Ashton N, Ward B, Serpell G: Effect of oxygen on developing retinal vessels with particular reference to the problem of retrolental fibroplasia. *Br J Ophthalmol* 1954; 38:397–432.
83. Ashton N: Personal communication cited in Tizard JPM: Indications for oxygen therapy in the newborn. *Pediatrics* 1964; 34:771–786.
84. Ashton N: Oxygen and growth and development of retinal vessels. *Am J Ophthalmol* 1966; 62:412–435.
85. Ashton N, Henkind P: Experimental occlusion of retinal arterioles: Using graded glass balloting. *Br J Ophthalmol* 1965, 49:225–235.
86. Friedenwald J, Owens WC, Owens EU: RLF in premature infants. III. The pathology of the disease. *Trans Am Ophthalmol Soc* 1951; 49:207–234.
87. Serpell G: Polysaccharide granules in association with developing retinal vessels and with retrolental fibroplasia. *Br J Ophthalmol* 1950; 44:245–274.
88. Reese AB, Blodi F, RLF: Fifth Francis I. Proctor Lecture. *Am J Ophthalmol* 1951; 34:1–24.
89. Reese AB, Blodi FC, Locke JC: The pathology of early retrolental fibroplasia with an analysis of the histologic findings in the eyes of newborn and stillborn infants. *Am J Ophthalmol* 1952; 35:1407–1426.
90. Ashton N: Pathological basis of RLF. *Br J Ophthalmol* 1954; 38:385–396.
91. Karlsberg RC, Green WR, Patz A: Congenital retrolental fibroplasia. *Arch Ophthalmol* 1973; 89:122–123.
92. Chui HC, and Green WR: Acute retrolental fibroplasia: A clinicopathologic case report. *Maryland Med J* 1977; 26:71–74.
93. Kalina RE, Forrest GL: Proliferative RLF in infant retinal vessels. *Am J Ophthalmol* 1973; 76:811–815.
94. Naiman J, Green WR, Patz A: Retrolental fibroplasia in hypoxic new born. *Am J Ophthalmol* 1979; 88:No. 1.
95. Frycykowski AW, Peiffer RL, Merrit JC, et al: Scanning electron microscopy of the ocular vasculature in retinopathy of prematurity. *Arch Ophthalmol* 1985; 103:224–228.
96. Foos RY: Chronic retinopathy of prematurity. *Ophthalmology* 1985; 92:563–574.
97. Foos RY, Kopelow SM: Development of retinal vasculature in para-natal infants. *Surv Ophthalmol* 1973; 18:87–100.

98. Foos RY: Acute retrolental fibroplasia. *Graefes Arch Clin Exp Ophthalmol* 1975; 18:87–100.
99. Soong HK, Ellen AW, Hirose T, et al: In situ actin distribution in excised retrolental membranes in retinopathy of prematurity. *Arch Ophthalmol* 1985; 103:1553–1556.
100. Ussman JH, Lazarides E, Ryan SJ: Traction retinal detachment: A cell mediated event. *Arch Ophthalmol* 1981; 99:869–872.
101. Gabbiani G, Hirsched BJ, Ryan GB, et al: Granulation tissue as a contractile organ: A study of structure and function. *J Exp Med* 1972; 135:791–734.
102. Laqua H, Machemer R: Glial cell proliferation in retinal detachment (massive periretinal proliferation). *Am J Ophthalmol* 1975; 80:602–618.
103. Rentsch F: Preretinal proliferation of glial cells after mechanical injury of the rabbit, retina. *Graefes Arch Clin Exp Ophthalmol* 1973; 188:79–90.
104. Wallon IH, Greaser ML, Steven TS: Actin filaments in diabetic fibrovascular preretinal membrane. *Arch Ophthalmol* 1981; 102:1370–1375.
105. Wallon IH, Stevens TS, Greaser ML, et al. Actin filaments in contracting preretinal membranes. *Arch Ophthalmol* 1984; 102:1370–1375.
106. Cleary PE, Minkler DS, Ryan, SJ: Ultrastructure of traction retinal detachment in rhesus monkey eyes after a posterior penetrating ocular injury. *Am J Ophthalmol* 1980; 90:829–845.

Chapter 5

# The Vitamin E Controversy

Joseph W. Eichenbaum, M.D.

Silverman cited the work of Kinsey and Zacharias[1] in 1949 as the first attempt to explain the increased frequency of retrolental fibroplasia (RLF) by correlating it to increased oxygen, iron, and water soluble vitamin therapy. Apparently, the occurrence of RLF related most closely with ferrous sulfate therapy in a retrospective study from the premature nursery at the Boston Lying-In Hospital, 1938–1947.[1]

In the early 1940s, artificial, mild mixtures made with a relatively low concentration of fat were administered, with the rationale that premature infants absorbed milk fat inefficiently. This mixture overcame the absorption difficulty.

Owens and Owens,[2] however, suggested that low-fat milk feedings would be deficient in necessary fat-soluble vitamins. After birth, with increased body demand, signs of deficiency would be expected to appear. They postulated that this might correlate with the earliest signs of RLF which occurred one month after birth. Of all the fat soluble vitamins, vitamin E was not administered routinely to premature infants at that time. Owens and Owens[2] suggested that vitamin E prophylaxis might play an antioxidant role in retinal neovascularization.

Owens and Owens[2] administered oral vitamin E (alphatocopherol acetate, 150 mg per day) at the time of the earliest changes of RLF; the condition appeared to be arrested in some infants. For 10 months, alternate infants admitted to the premature nursery of Johns Hopkins Hospital were given either 150 mg of vitamin E or no treatment.

During the study, eleven infants received vitamin E. None developed RLF. Of the 15 neonates in the untreated group, 5 developed RLF.

Woods and Friedenwald at Johns Hopkins Hospital persuaded Owens and Owens to abandon the controlled trial. Instead, all infants in the Baltimore nursery were given supplementary vitamin E. As word of this experience spread throughout the world, vitamin E prophylaxis was started in many hospitals. Unfortunately, the informal experience of nine other groups failed to confirm the Johns Hopkins experience. Owens and Owens were unable to demonstrate an impressive protective effect of vitamin E in the years following that curtailed formal trial.[3] In 1953, Owens[4] observed spontaneous regression in retrolental fibroplasia in noenates without antioxidant therapy.

About 20 years later, vitamin E was shown to have "antioxidant" and "free radical scavenger" function, as well as function as an organizer and stabilizer in cell membranes.[5] According to Puklin et al.,[6] for all these reasons interest in vitamin E therapy in RLF resurfaced. Johnson et al.,[7] in a preliminary study on infants, and work in kittens by Phelps et al.,[8, 9] suggested a therapeutic effect of vitamin E on the advance of RLF. On this basis, Puklin et al.[6] undertook a randomized, double-masked study of the effect of intramuscular vitamin E during the acute phase of therapy for respiratory distress syndrome (RDS) on the development of retinopathy of prematurity (ROP).

One hundred neonates with RDS received either vitamin E or placebo intramuscularly (IM) within the first 24 hours of birth and at 24, 48, and 168 hours respectively. Doses of 20 mg per kg (0.4 ml per kg) were administered intramuscularly. As long as the infant remained in the oxygen-enriched environment, additional doses were given twice weekly. Ventilatory assistance was adjusted to maintain an arterial $PO_2$ between 50 and 75 mm Hg and an arterial $PO_2$ between 30 and 45 mm Hg. All of the infants were exposed to nutritional sources of vitamin E. During the acute phase of RDS therapy they received an intravenous protein alimentation solution containing 2.5 IU vitamin E per liter. Each infant's hematocrit during supplemental oxygen therapy was maintained at more than 40% with packed red cell transfusion.[6]

Infants treated with parenteral vitamin E had significantly increased serum vitamin E levels as compared to placebo-treated infants (Table 5–1). Normal serum vitamin E levels were attained in most placebo-treated neonates during the second week of life because of nutritional sources of vitamin E. Infants treated with a placebo and vitamin E had respiratory distress syndrome of similar severity and all survived longer than ten days.

Puklin et al.[6] showed that the administration of vitamin E did not alter the incidence of active stages of early ROP. (Table 5–2). They noted that (1) none of the infants in whom retinal abnormalities were observed developed severe ROP changes, (2) spontaneous regression occurred in most infants with early ROP, and (3) the effect of vitamin E on the severity or healing of ROP was unclear.

**TABLE 5–1.**
Serum Vitamin E Levels*

| | Serum Vitamin E (mg/100 ml) | | | |
|---|---|---|---|---|
| Treatment | Pretreatment | + 24 hours† | + 72 hours | + 168 hours |
| Vitamin E | 0.45 ± 0.04‡ (37) | 2.18 ± 0.16 (31) | 5.48 ± 0.60 (14) | 3.89 ± 0.24 (30) |
| Placebo | 0.43 ± 0.03 (46) | 0.60 ± 0.05 (33) | 0.60 ± 0.06 (18) | 0.78 ± 0.08 (21) |

**From Puklin J, Simon RM, Ehrenkranz RA: Influence on RLF of intramuscular vitamin E administration during respiratory distress syndrome. Ophthalmol 1982; 89:96–102. (Used by permission.)*
*†Hours after the first dose.*
*‡Mean ± SEM of the number of determinations shown in parentheses.*

**TABLE 5–2.**
Influence of Vitamin E*

A. Retinal Findings in Vitamin E–treated and Placebo–treated Patients

| | Number of Patients | | | |
|---|---|---|---|---|
| Treatment | Normal | Stage I | Stage II | Total |
| Vitamin E | 28 | 8 | 1 | 37 |
| Placebo | 29 | 5 | 3 | 37 |

B. Retinal Findings† in Vitamin E–treated and Placebo–treated Infants with Retinopathy of Prematurity

| | Number of Eyes | | |
|---|---|---|---|
| Treatment | Normal | Stage I | Stage II |
| Vitamin E | 1 | 16 | 1 |
| Placebo | 1 | 10 | 5 |

**From Puklin J, Simon RM, Ehrenkranz RA: Influence on RLF of intramuscular vitamin E administration during respiratory distress syndrome. Ophthalmol 1982; 89:96–102. (Used by permission.)*
*†Classified according to Table 2.*

Puklin et al.[6] suggested that vitamin E may exert its protective effect against the development of extraretinal proliferative ROP when given after oxygen therapy is terminated.

Phelps and Rosenbaum[8, 9] found that vitamin E administration to kittens after the hypoxic insult significantly blocked vitreal neovascularization. They noted though, as did Ashton[10] and Patz,[11] that the kitten as a model of late cicatricial changes was not acceptable. Phelps et al.[8, 9] and Ashton[10] and Patz[11] all failed to obtain progression to retinal detachment in the cat after severe oxygen stress. However, vitamin E did retard the other earlier aspects of oxygen-induced retinopathy in kittens.[8, 9] They proposed that this was related to the ability of vitamin E to inhibit wound healing[12] and reduce inflammation.[13]

**TABLE 5–3.**
Incidence of RLF at Jackson Memorial Hospital, 1969–1980*

| | | |
|---|---|---|
| Infants examined | 1,087 | |
| Proliferative RLF | 233 | (21.4%) |
| Grade III cicatricial RLF + | 32 | (3.0%) |

**From Flynn JT: Discussion of two preceding papers. Ophthalmol 1982; 89:103. (Used by permission.)*

Thus, they suggested that vitamin E perhaps protects only against the cicatricial stigmata of ROP and not the early changes.[8, 9]

As previously described in the cooperative RLF study,[14, 15] Puklin et al.[6] found that birth weight and total time in oxygen were the most important risk factors for the development of ROP. Infants with birth weights of less than 1,200 g carried the greatest risk of developing cicatricial changes.

Gunn et al.,[16] however, reported that gestational age and duration of ventilatory assistance (rather than birth weight and duration of oxygen exposure) were highly correlated with active ROP and cicatricial ROP.

Procianoy et al.[17] noted an association of intraventricular hemorrhage in cicatricial ROP in very low birth-weight infants. However, gestational age, duration of oxygen exposure, and occurrence of patent ductus arteriosus did not correlate with cicatricial ROP.

In discussing Puklin's study in vitamin E for ROP, Flynn concluded, "The search to prevent RLF must continue. Vitamin E is not the answer . . . There is no current indication to change the standard neonatal nursery practice today as far as the administration of vitamin E to premature infants is concerned."[18] Also, in the discussion, Flynn[18] found a 3% incidence of grade 3 cicatricial RLF and 21.4% incidence of proliferative RLF (Table 5–3). This is in accord with Zak[19, 20] and Kingham's[21] data.

The conclusion of Flynn appeared despite his citation of the work of Monaco, Kretzer, and Hittner.[22] In the work of Monaco et al.,[22] five times the dosage of vitamin E (which Puklin employed in his study) had suppressed the development of grade 3 ROP.[22]

Finer et al.[23] (with 174 infants weighing less than 1,500 g who survived beyond 4 weeks of age), using stepwise multiple linear regression analysis, found that the lack of early vitamin E as well as the number of days of exposure to supplemental oxygen significantly correlated with the development of cicatricial RLF. In phase 1 of their study,[23] which was prospective, randomized, and controlled, all infants in the treated group were given vitamin E D/L-α-tocopherol acetate 25 mg IM, repeated in 12 hours and followed by 20 mg IM daily for 14 days, and then 20 mg IM every three days for another five doses. In phase 1, 48 infants received IM vitamin E. There was evidence of cicatricial RLF in 6.3% after about $3^1/_2$ years, compared with 51 controls, of whom 10% had cicatricial RLF.

Serum tocopherol rose to between 4 and 5 mg/dl in these infants after six days, while controls remained below 1 mg/dl. Insignificant differences were noted in occurrence rates of both acute and cicatricial RLF in the vitamin E and control groups. Finer et al. state that in subsequent follow-up visits, infants treated with vitamin E who had cicatricial RLF retained good visual function, whereas three infants in the control group were functionally blind.[23] The frequency of RLF in the Finer et al.[23] series was 17.7% for acute disease and 8.6% for cicatricial disease, with a follow-up period of approximately four years. The Finer et al.[23] phase I results for lower incidence of cicatricial RLF and blindness for infants receiving IM vitamin E were not significant by single variate analysis[23] (Table 5–4).

In phase 2, 44 infants received oral vitamin E within 12 hours of birth; 8 infants received vitamin E at 39 hours of age; 23 infants received no vitamin E at any time. No infants received the initial dose of vitamin E between 12 and 39 hours of age. The incidence of RLF, either acute or cicatricial, was not significantly related to the time of vitamin E administration. The incidence was, however, significantly greater in infants who did not receive vitamin E. None of the early vitamin E–treated infants had evidence of

**TABLE 5–4.**
Comparison of Early Parenteral Vitamin E with Controls Phase I*

| | Early (n = 48) | Control (n = 51) | *P* Value |
|---|---|---|---|
| Birth weight (g) | 1197.0 | 1207.5 | NS |
| Gestational age (wk) | 29.3 | 29.4 | NS |
| Survival greater than 8 weeks | 47 | 50 | NS |
| Duration of mechanical ventilation (days) | 29.0 | 29.0 | NS |
| Duration of $FIO_2$ >21 (days) | 24.1 | 27.8 | NS |
| Duration of $FIO_2$ >60 (hr) | 22.6 | 89.3 | NS |
| Number of $PAO_2$ >100 mm Hg | 4.5 | 2.7 | NS |
| Number of $PaO_2$ 75–99 mm Hg | 25.7 | 20.3 | NS |
| Number of capillary $PO_2$ >50 mm Hg | 42.8 | 21.4 | NS |
| Highest $PaCO_2$ (mm Hg) | 57.51 | 57.6 | NS |
| Number of $PaCO_2$ >50 mm Hg | 24.9 | 16.9 | NS |
| Volume of packed cells transfused (ml/kg birth weight) in first 12 weeks | 165.3 | 160.5 | NS |
| Number of continuous $PO_2$ >100 mm Hg | 4.52 | 2.74 | NS |
| NEC | 7 | 6 | NS |
| RLF—acute | 9 | 12 | NS |
| RLF—cicatricial | 3 | 5 | NS |

*From Finer, Schindler RF, Peters KL et al: Vitamin E and retrolental fibroplasia improved visual outcome with early vitamin E. Ophthalmol 1983; 90:5. (Used by permission.)
NS = not significant; NEC = necrotizing enterocolitis; RLF = retrolental fibroplasia.

**TABLE 5–5.**
Specific Eye Diagnosis at Follow-up All Infants With Cicatricial RLF*

| Case | Stage of Acute RLF | Surgery | Grade of Cicatricial RLF | Refractive Error (Diopters) in Spherical Equivalents | Age at Most Recent Examination (mo) |
|---|---|---|---|---|---|
| Early vitamin E (oral or parenteral) | | | | | |
| 1. | OD III | No | II | −13.50 | 31 |
| | OS III | Cryo | I | −13.50 | |
| 2. | OD III | No | II | −8.00 | 38 |
| | OS III | No | II | −6.50 | |
| 3. | OD I | No | I | — | 14 |
| | OS O | No | O | — | |
| No vitamin E (controls) | | | | | |
| 4. | OD II | No | II | +3.50 | 24 |
| | OS III+ | Cryo | O | Plano | |
| 5. | OD II | No | II | −8.50 | 11 |
| | OS II | No | II | −8.50 | |
| 6. | OD — | No | II | +1.25 | 21 |
| | OS — | No | IV | — | |
| 7. | OD — | No | I | — | 6 |
| | OS — | No | I | — | |
| 8. | OD II | | O | — | 6 |
| | OS II | No | I | | |
| 9. | OD V | No | V | — | 27 |
| | OS V | Vit | V | — | |
| 10. | OD V | No | V | — | 13 |
| | OS V | No | V | — | |
| 11. | OD V | Cryo | V | — | 15 |
| | OS V | Cryo | V | — | |
| 12. | OD V | No | V | — | 26 |
| | OS V | No | V | — | |
| Late oral vitamin E | | | | | |
| 13. | OD II | No | II | −2.00 | 14 |
| | OS IV | Cryo | III | −5.00 | |
| 14. | OD III | Cryo | II | — | 6 |
| | OS IV | Cryo X2, then RD | IV | — | Deceased |
| 15. | OD II | No | 0 | +0.50 | 11 |
| | OS II | No | I | +0.50 | |

**From Finer, Schindler RF, Peters KL, et al: Vitamin E and retrolental fibroplasia improved visual outcome with early vitamin E.* Ophthalmol *1983; 90:5. (Used by permission.)*
*RLF = retrolental fibroplasia; CRYO = cryopexy; RD = Retinal detachment repair; VIT = Vitrectomy; OD = right eye; OS = left eye.*

cicatricial RLF on follow-up examination.[23] The phase II experience was neither randomized nor controlled. (Tables 5–5 and 5–6).It is only "from the combined results of Phase I and II . . . a statistically significant reduction in the incidence of cicatricial RLF" was shown.

Hittner et al,[24] in a controlled double-blind study, administered oral vitamin E 100 mg/kg within 24 hours of birth and found a decreased incidence of stage 3 or more advanced retinopathy.

Hittner et al.,[24] as well as Finer et al.[25] suggested that an effective level of vitamin E could be obtained by oral administration of 100 mg/kg/day.

Finer et al.[25] previously reported that in a controlled trial a lower incidence of cicatricial RLF and blindness occurred in infants receiving intramuscular vitamin E.[25] By single variate analysis, these differences were insignificant. By multiple linear regression analysis, however, vitamin E was found to reduce the severity of RLF significantly.[25]

Contrary to the concern expressed by Sobel et al.,[26] Finer et al.[23] did not find any increased incidence of necrotizing enterocolitis associated with vitamin E therapy according to the diagnostic criteria of Bell et al.[27]

In addition, Finer et al.[23] noted no increased occurrence of intraventricular hemorrhage in infants receiving vitamin E, as suggested by Phelps.[28] However, all four infants with grade 5 cicatricial RLF, and six of seven infants with grade 3 or greater cicatricial RLF, had documented intraventricular hemorrhage. Finer et al.[23] pointed out that this rate of intraventricular hemorrhage is in line with the findings of Hittner et al.[24] and that intraventricular hemorrhage is a definite risk factor associated with RLF.[23]

Phelps[29] produced hepatosplenomegaly in kittens with serum concentration of 10.5 mg/dl of vitamin E and death at serum levels of 24.0 mg/dl.

In a discussion of the work of Finer et al.,[23] Tasman[30] pointed out that no median birth weight was given, making it difficult to assess whether lower birth weight and consequently increased RLF was more common in those

**TABLE 5–6.**
Risk Factors for Cicatricial RLF (Eye Diagnosis at Follow-up Eye Examination) Phase I and Phase II Univariate Analysis*

| | RLF | No RLF | *P* Value |
|---|---|---|---|
| Duration of $FIO_2$ >21 (days) | 67.6 | 21.6 | 0.002 |
| Duration of mechanical ventilation (days) | 61.3 | 21.1 | 0.005 |
| Discharge age (days) | 127.4 | 74.8 | 0.005 |
| Number of $PaO_2$s 75–99 mm Hg | 36.9 | 14.8 | 0.010 |
| Gestational age (weeks) | 28.5 | 29.7 | 0.011 |
| Number of $PaO_2$s >100 mm Hg | 5.8 | 2.5 | 0.019 |
| Birth weight (g) | 1124.8 | 1230.9 | 0.021 |
| Volume of packed cells (ml/kg birth weight) transfused in first 12 weeks | 183.8 | 115.3 | 0.024 |
| Number of capillary $PO_2$s >50 mm Hg | 113.7 | 34.9 | 0.029 |
| Highest $PaCO_2$s (mm Hg) | 62.5 | 53.2 | 0.031 |

**From Finer, Schindler RF, Peters KL, et al: Vitamin E and retrolental fibroplasia improved visual outcome with early vitamin E. Ophthalmol 1983; 90:5.*

infants who did not receive vitamin E. Also, Tasman[30] indicated that the risk factors (e.g., duration of mechanical ventilation, supplemental oxygen administration, number of recorded arterial oxygen concentrations greater than 100 mm Hg, units of packed red blood cells received in the first 12 weeks of life, and duration of hospitalization; see Table 5–6) were greater in the RLF group. Therefore, it may have been that as a whole, the RLF group of infants were more ill to begin with. Thus, the absence of vitamin E therapy may not have been the sole source of the increased RLF and blindness in four infants in the study by Finer et al.[25]

Tasman[30] stated that his own observations had included infants with RLF who were on early pharmacologic doses of vitamin E, but who later became blind.

The incidence of necrotizing enterocolitis was 15.3% for each of the groups in the study of Finer et al.[23] Blood levels of vitamin E above 3.5 mg/dl[30, 31] produced increased risk of sepsis and necrotizing enterocolitis. Finer et al.[23] showed blood levels in infants who received early intramuscular vitamin E to be above 3.5 mg/dl. Tasman[30] suggested that a larger series may have shown vitamin E patients with higher blood levels to have a greater prevalence of sepsis. Tasman advised that vitamin E levels be kept at "a physiologically sufficient level: between 1.5 mg and 2.0 mg/dl; blood levels of vitamin E should be checked twice a week."[30]

Tasman[30] concluded, in the final analysis, that Ehrenkranz and Puklin[6, 32] had raised one of the most important questions of all. If vitamin E is an effective agent in suppressing cicatricial retrolental fibroplasia, why should there not be a demonstrable effect in the earliest stages of the disease?

Hittner et al.[33] reported that continuous intramuscular vitamin E supplementation to adult physiologic levels 1.1 to 3.1 mg/dl from the first hours of life suppressed the development of severe ROP but did not alter the incidence of ROP. In the severe stages, vitamin E supplementation did not increase the incidence of necrotizing enterocolitis, sepsis, intraventricular hemorrhage, or mortality. Hittner et al.,[33, 36] using ultrastructural data, postulated that increased oxygen tension triggered extensive gap junctions between adjacent mesenchymal spindle cells. Within the first 4 days of life, the increased gap junction formation between spindle cells halted normal vascularization and triggered neovascularization. The latter became evident some 8 to 12 weeks later.

The oxygen-triggered spindle cell gap-junction formation mechanism contrasts with that proposed by Ashton[34] and Patz.[35] The latter investigators theorized that vasoconstriction, vaso-obliteration, and endothelial necrosis are the underlying events in RLF. None of the 71 pairs of whole-eye donations studied ultrastructurally had endothelial cell necrosis, according to Hittner et al.[36]

Reviewing spindle-cell kinetics in severe ROP and in control and vitamin E treated groups, Hittner et al.[33] found a 2-week lag in spindle cell maturation in adult physiologic range vitamin E–treated groups compared with controls. Thus, they advised that the treatment of cryopexy to the avascular region be delayed until after 2 weeks but before 10 weeks of life. In other cases where adult physiologic range vitamin E was maintained, gap junction formation was further suppressed and the clinical development of severe ROP was reduced. By linking the severity of ROP to spindle cell–gap junction formation, they suggested that the first retinal exam for ROP occur at 8 weeks of life.[33]

Hittner et al.[33, 36] argued that only multivariate analysis (Table 5–7), which considers all risk factors simultaneously, was appropriate for determining the efficacy of vitamin E in attenuating severe ROP. They stated that although numerous studies in the literature had attempted to identify risk factors in ROP, these reports stressed ROP in term infants, i.e., ROP not associated with oxygen administration and congenital ROP. They felt that many of these case reports were consequences of intrauterine insults or genetically altered cellular migration. The actual incidence of these atypical cases is low. The ROP they refer to is a disease of infants of less than 1,500 g birth weight, younger than 31 weeks gestational age, who require oxygen administration, and who have other neonatal complications and develop the disease at a predictable time.[33]

They proposed that the pathologic insult to spindle cells in severe ROP is triggered by oxygen tensions greater than the hypoxic in utero environment. They pointed out that patent ductus arteriosus, bronchopulmonary dysplasia, hyaline membrane disease, pneumothorax, and apnea (all of which are related to supplemental oxygen), are all factors that activate spindle cells by inducing gap junction formation. Similarly, spindle cell activation occurs in transfusion of packed cells, intraventricular hemorrhage, sepsis, low pH, and low temperature, all of which affect oxygen levels and gap junction formation. Thus, they rejected univariate analysis in favor of the multivariate analysis format.

Hittner et al.[33] believed that oral vitamin E administration, provided it was initiated within the first hour of life and given without interruption in adult physiologic dosages, protected the developing retina from free radical damage.

Hittner's 1983 study[37] failed to demonstrate an advantage of intramuscular administration over the oral route in suppressing the development of ROP. With interruption of infant feeding, intramuscular injections in the first week of life were suggested. In infants of less than 1,000 grams birth weight, the mortality was felt to be reduced in those who received the early intramuscular injections.[33, 36]

**TABLE 5–7.**
Risk Factors for Retrolental Fibroplasia, Identified by Multivariate Statistical Analysis of Control and Treatment Groups*

| Group-Risk Factor† | Significance of Factor Relative to Disease‡ | Statistical Value: Regression Coefficient (Beta) | Statistical Value: Cumulative Variance Explained (R) |
|---|---|---|---|
| Control infants | | | |
| Gestational age | <0.001 | $-0.21$ | 39% |
| Weighted oxygen score | 0.005 | $+1.2 \times 10^{-1}$ | 50% |
| Intraventricular hemorrhage | 0.019 | $+0.56$ | 57% |
| Sepsis | 0.047 | $+0.60$ | 61% |
| Birth weight | 0.100 | $-7.3 \times 10^{-4}$ | 62% |
| Control and treated infants | | | |
| Gestational age | <0.001 | $-0.17$ | 33% |
| Weighted oxygen score | <0.001 | $+6.8 \times 10^{-3}$ | 39% |
| Intraventricular hemorrhage | 0.002 | $+0.45$ | 45% |
| Vitamin E dose§ | 0.012 | $-0.30$ | 48% |
| Sepsis | 0.023 | $+0.41$ | 51% |
| Birth weight | 0.028 | $-8.8 \times 10^{-4}$ | 54% |

*From Hittner HM, Godio LB, Rudolph AJ, et al: Retrolental fibroplasia: Efficacy of vitamin E in a double-blind clinical study of preterm infants. N Engl J Med 1981; 305:1365–1370. (Used by permission.)
†Risk factors are given in order of their significance.
‡Partial F significance probabilities. The significance of all variables in both groups was $P<0.001$.
§The treatment dose (100 mg) significantly reduced the severity of retrolental fibroplasia.

Hittner et al.[33] suggested that in the preterm retina, the increase in gap junctions could be a cellular response to hyperoxia. Free radicals could produce membrane lipid peroxidations and change the membrane surface properties and result in increased gap junctions.

They indicated, however, that severe ROP may develop in infants despite continuous supplementation with vitamin E.[33] Apparently, if sufficient additional oxygen-related risk factors pertain, vitamin E only transiently suppresses gap junction formation. After a lag period of 2 weeks, gap junction levels are comparable to those seen in controls. This lag period perhaps explains the delayed clinical onset of severe ROP.[33]

In cases where severe ROP develops with or without vitamin E, Hittner et al.[33] believed that the effective ablation of avascular zones with cryopexy[38–42] is in line with their theory of destruction of activated gap junction–linked spindle cells.

Hittner et al.[33] provided the following recommendations: (1) Vitamin E prophylaxis is unnecessary in infants weighing more than 1,500 g birth weight and who are older than 31 weeks gestational age; these infants are not usually at high risk for the development of severe ROP; (2) Oral vitamin E (tocopherol or tocopherol acetate) supplementation to adult physiologic levels should be begun within the first hours of life in children less than 31 weeks of age; (3) Physiologic supplementation with continuus oral vitamin E should be maintained until retinal vascularization is complete; IM vitamin E (tocopherol) should be used if the infant has had nothing by mouth for three days or more and not to exceed a plasma vitamin E level of 3.5 mg/dl; and (4) A retinal screening exam should be performed at age 8 weeks and as necessary thereafter, depending on the severity of ROP observed. Early weekly screening is unnecessary and can be deceptive because an adverse clinical course may not be manifest despite the subclinical activation of spindle cells. Two additional recommendations regarding mortality, intraventricular hemorrhage (IVH) and cryopexy, are based upon the same clinical and ultrastructural studies: (1) three early IM injections of vitamin E should be given beginning on the first day of life to decrease infant mortality and intraventricular hemorrhage, and (2) if vitamin E supplementation does not prevent the development of severe ROP in infants 27 weeks gestational age or less, cryoretinopexy should be applied to the avascular retina while the spindle cells are activated.[33]

In their comments on Hittner et al.,[33] Rosenbaum and Phelps[43] pointed out that a randomized double-masked study is essential because of the complexities of ROP. Randomization spreads out poorly understood etiologic factors more evenly between treatment groups. Also, disease and observer variability (as well as observer subjectivity) are better counterbalanced with the double-blind technique. Because the number of patients who develop severe ROP is small, sample sizes can be statistically insignificant.[43]

Both the Hittner et al.[33] and Finer et al.[23] studies presented subsequent uncontrolled data which attempted to show that vitamin E was effective in ROP. They pooled their randomized, controlled data with noncontrolled, nonrandomized data. Rosenbaum and Phelps,[43] for reasons enumerated in the above paragraph, as well as because of the ever-changing methods of care in newborn intensive care units, questioned the validity of such conclusions about the efficacy of vitamin E.

In a table on ROP randomized controlled data, Rosenbaum and Phelps[43] pointed out that the number of cases in the Puklin et al.[6] and Finer et al.[23] series were not statistically significant, while the data of Hittner et al.[24] were (at $P < 0.03$) statistically significant with five cases in the control and none in the vitamin E group. However, "a trend does exist that suggests vitamin E may be effective in reducing the severity of acute ROP. The case numbers that point to such a conclusion are still painfully small, and a few cases one way or the other could alter that conclusion."[43] Vitamin E toxicity could also be an issue.[43]

It has been estimated that 22,000 premature infants under 1,500 g birth weight survive yearly.[43] Two thousand will develop cicatricial ROP, and the remaining 20,000 will not. However, the drug would be given to perhaps 90% of the infants who might not benefit. Although none of the above controlled studies (Hittner et al.,[24] Puklin et al.,[6] and Finer et al.[23]) mentioned any side effects of vitamin E, Johnson et al.,[44] in a randomized controlled clinical trial, reported a higher incidence of both necrotizing enterocolitis and bacterial sepsis in premature infants who received vitamin E therapy. The median serum level of vitamin E in their treated group was 4.5 mg/dl, while that in the placebo group was 0.9 mg/dl. It is assumed that these statistically highly significant differences in vitamin E and placebo group complications were probably related to high vitamin E serum levels.[44] It is unclear whether they would have occurred at lower levels in premature infants.[43]

Rosenbaum and Phelps[43] concluded, "Finally, whether vitamin E is or is not effective, it does not eliminate the possibility of blindness. Severe cases of retinal detachment and blindness from ROP have still occurred in cases treated with vitamin E."

Schaffer et al.,[45] in a randomized, prospective, masked study, found the incidence of RLF in infants treated with vitamin E to be 7.2% (with serum levels at 5 mg/dl) and 6.8% in placebo-treated infants. The incidences of hyperopia, myopia, anisometropia, strabismus, and amblyopia were also similar in placebo-and vitamin E–treated groups.[45] At variance with this, Kushner reported that cicatricial changes, high refractive errors, strabismus, and amblyopia increased in youngsters who have had ROP.[46] Also, more recently in cases of mild ROP, the absence of any sequelae to ROP and complete resolution have been reported.[47]

Similar to the nonsignificant outcome of vitamin E therapy in ROP reported by Schaffer,[47] Milner et al.[49] found a nonsignificant effect of vitamin E in RLF. The serum vitamin E levels in the placebo group were 0.8 to 0.9 mg/dl, while the target vitamin E group levels were 2 to 3 mg/dl. In the placebo group, 16.7% had mild RLF and 4.4% had severe RLF. Of the infants treated with vitamin E, 11.4% had mild disease, and 2.7% had severe RLF.

On the basis of their data, Schaffer et al.[45] stated, "We cannot support the treatment of infants from birth with prophylactic vitamin E to attain pharmacologic serum levels (>2 mg/dl). Currently, in our nurseries, we attempt to establish only vitamin E sufficiency early and monitor the serum E levels carefully." In an addendum, Schaffer et al. stated:

> Since this paper was read in November, 1984, the importance of the findings of Table 6 [Table 5–8] have been substantiated. The decreased severity of cicatricial disease among those infants who developed RLF is significantly associated with vitamin E ($P<.025$). Nine vitamin E treated infants had Grade 1

**TABLE 5–8.**
Grade of Cicatricial Retrolental Fibroplasia of Each Eye in Placebo-(P) and Vitamin E-(E) Treated Groups*

| Patient No. | E/P | Grade | | Patient No. | E/P | Grade | |
|---|---|---|---|---|---|---|---|
| | | OD | OS | | | OD | OS |
| 1179 | P | 1 | 1 | 1372 | E | 1 | 0 |
| 1177 | P | 0 | 1 | 2103 | E | 1 | 1 |
| 2404 | P | 1 | 5 | 3139 | E | 1 | 2 |
| 3511 | P | 3 | 1 | 2234 | E | 1 | 1 |
| 1061 | P† | 5 | 5 | 3502 | E | 1 | 1 |
| 1161 | P | 1 | 2 | 1273 | E† | 3 | 5 |
| 3135 | P | 2 | 2 | 1320 | E | 1 | 1 |
| 1066 | P | 2 | 3 | 3617 | E | 2 | 2 |
| 1095 | P | 2 | 1 | 2608 | E | 1 | 1 |
| 3620 | P | 1 | 1 | 3644 | E | 1 | 1 |
| 3742 | P | 5 | 1 | 3651 | E | 1 | 1 |
| | | | | 1331 | E | 1 | 1 |

**From Schaffer DB, Johnson L, Quinn GE, et al: Vitamin E and retinopathy of prematurity: Follow-up at one year. Ophthalmol 1985; 92: (Used by permission.)*
*† = bilaterally blind from retrolental fibroplasia. OD = right eye; OS = left eye.*

cicatricial, two had Grade 2 cicatricial, none had Grade 3 cicatricial disease, and only one was bilaterally blind. Among the placebo infants, there were three Grade 1 cicatricial and three Grade 2 cicatricial or worse.

On the basis of this and extensive analysis of confounding variables, we find only support for our current practice. In our nurseries, we try to establish E sufficiency early in life using the preparations of E acetate now available, i.e., parenteral multivitamin E infusate at standard doses and, after the initiation of oral feeding, oral E acetate (Aquasol E) in aliquots with feed. We believe it is essential to monitor E levels frequently to maintain as much as possible serum levels with in the physiologic range.

According to the Institute of Medicine report on vitamin E and retinopathy of prematurity, after detailed presentations by Drs. Hittner, Kretzer, Schaffer, Quinn, and Phelps the Committee found "no conclusive evidence either of benefit or harm from vitamin E administration."[48] Conclusions were not possible (as of June 1986) with regard to the effect of vitamin E and intraventricular hemorrhage, necrotizing enterocolitis, or late sepsis. The Committee also stated that "risks from vitamin E appear to be minimal for premature infants provided that doses are kept moderate to achieve a blood level no higher than 3 mg/dl."[48]

## ROP 1989

ROP continues to challenge medical thinking. Very low birth weight, chronic lung disease, duration of mechanical ventilation, oxygen administration, units of packed red blood cells received in the first 3 months of life, patent ductus arteriosus, duration of hospitalization, seizures, xanthine administration,[50] and as yet multivariate factors of prematurity seem to be strongly implicated as causes. Weaker satellite factors such as oxygen concentration and duration of vitamin E, oxygen exchange transfusions, ambient light levels, and arachidonic acid metabolites[51–53] all hover in the background. It is as if many pieces of the puzzle are missing, or at least do not fit together well.

Initially, the effort to implicate oxygen toxicity as the etiology of ROP was received with intense enthusiasm. However, the significance of the oxygen hypothesis has receded as reports have emerged on nonhyperoxic ROP, along with careful scrutiny of the national cooperative study, and the fact that the incidence of ROP has increased in spite of strict oxygen control. Indeed, ROP has been reported even in a hypoxic clinical setting. Curiously, cautious oxygen use to counteract potential ROP has resulted in an increase in cerebral palsy and brain damage. Excess oxygen restriction could be a contributing factor in exacerbating neonatal respiratory distress syndrome.

The role of vitamin E deficiency in ROP, if any, is unclear. Even high dosages of vitamin E have failed to totally eliminate advanced stages of ROP. Most authorities agree that mild cases usually resolve spontaneously. In fact, the potential complications of retinal and intraventricular hemorrhage, as well as necrotizing enterocolitis, may outweigh any benefit of vitamin E therapy.

Perhaps further studies with cryotherapy will elucidate hidden pathways in the pathogenesis of ROP. More important, however, is the advance of our understanding of the embryologic, cellular, and biochemical changes in normal and premature infants, which are helping us track the course of events in retinal detachment and retinovitreal scarring. Further details of normal and abnormal biochemical cytologic mechanisms will play a decisive role in unraveling the mystery of ROP.

## REFERENCES


1. Kinsey VE, Zacharias L: RLF: Incidence in different localities in recent years and a correlation of the incidence with treatment. *JAMA* 1949; 139:572–578.
2. Owens WC, Owens EU: Retrolental fibroplasia in premature infants: Studies on the prophylaxis of the disease. *Am J Ophthalmol* 1949; 32:1631–1637.
3. Silverman WA: *Retrolental Fibroplasia: A Modern Parable.* New York, Grune & Stratton, 1980, pp 4–66.
4. Owens WC: Spontaneous repression in retrolental fibroplasia. *Trans Am Ophthalmol Soc* 1953; 51:555–579.
5. Nair PP, Kayden HJ: International conference on vitamin E and its role in cellular metabolism. *Ann NY Acad Sci* 1972; 203.

6. Puklin J, Simon RM, Ehrenkranz RA: Influence on RLF of intramuscular vitamin E administration during respiratory distress syndrome. *Ophthalmology* 1982; 89:96–102.
7. Johnson L, Shaffer D, Boggs TR: The premature infant: Vitamin E deficiency and RLF. *Am J Clin Nutr* 1974; 27:1158–1173.
8. Phelps DL, Rosenbaum AL: The role of tocopherol in oxygen induced retinopathy. *Pediatrics* 1977; 59:998–1005.
9. Phelps DL, Rosenbaum AL: Vitamin E in kitten oxygen induced retinopathy. II. Blockage of vitreal neovascularization. *Arch Ophthalmol* 1979; 97:1522–1526.
10. Ashton N, Ward B, Serpell G: Effect of oxygen on developing retinal vessels with particular reference to the problem of retrolental fibroplasia. *Br J Ophthalmol* 1954; 38:397–432.
11. Patz A: Experimental studies. *Am J Ophthalmol* 1955; 40:174.
12. Ehrlich HP, Tarver H, Hunt TK: Inhibitory effects of vitamin E on collagen synthesis and wound repair. *Ann Surg* 1972; 175:235–240.
13. Levy L: The anti-inflammatory action of some compounds with antioxidant properties. *Inflammation* 1976; 1:333–345.
14. Kinsey VE: Cooperative Study of retrolental fibroplasia and the use of oxygen. *Arch Ophthalmol* 1956; 56:481–543.
15. Kinsey VE, Arnold HJ, Kalina RE, et al: PaO2 levels and RLF: A report of the cooperative study. *Pediatrics* 1977; 60:655–667.
16. Gunn TR, Easdoun J, Arterbridge EW, et al: Risk factors in retrolental fibroplasia. *Pediatrics* 1980; 65:1096–1100.
17. Procianoy RS, Garcia Prats JA, Hittner HM, et al: An association between retinopathy of prematurity and intraventricular hemorrhage in very low birth weight infants. *Acta Paediatr Scand* 1981; 70:473–477.
18. Flynn JT: Discussion of two preceding papers. *Ophthalmology* 1982; 89:103.
19. Zak TA: Discussion of ROP and Dr. Tasman's paper #60. *Ophthalmology* 1984; 91:1502–1503.
20. Zak TA: Retinopathy of prematurity: An update on retrolental fibroplasia. *NY State J Med* 1982; 82:1795–1796.
21. Kingham JD: Acute retrolental fibroplasia. *Arch Ophthalmol* 1977; 95:39–47.
22. Monaco W, Kretzer F, Hittner H: Evidence that vitamin E suppresses the development of grade III retinopathy of prematurity. *Invest Ophthalmol Vis Sci* 1981; 20(suppl):58.
23. Finer NN, Schindler RF, Peters KL, et al: Vitamin E and retrolental fibroplasia: Improved visual outcome with early vitamin E. *Ophthalmology* 1983; 90:428–435.
24. Hittner HM, Godio LB, Rudolph AJ, et al: Retrolental fibroplasia: Efficacy of vitamin E in double-blind clinical study of preterm infants. *N Engl J Med* 1981; 305:1365–1370.
25. Finer NN, Schindler RF, Grant G, et al. Effect of intramuscular vitamin E on frequency and severity of retrolental fibroplasia. A controlled trial. *Lancet* 1982; 1:1087–1091.
26. Sobel S, Guerigian J, Troendle G, et al: Vitamin E in retrolental fibroplasia (letter). *N Engl J Med* 1982; 306:867.

27. Bell MJ, Teinberg JL, Feigin RD, et al: Neonatal necrotizing enterocolitis: Therapeutic decisions based upon clinical staging. *Ann Surg* 1978; 187:1–7.
28. Phelps DL: Local and systemic reactions to parenteral administration of vitamin E. *Dev Pharmacol Ther* 1981; 2:156–171.
29. Phelps DL: Vitamin E and retrolental fibroplasia in 1982. *Pediatrics* 1982; 70:420–425.
30. Tasman W: Discussion of Finer et al, Vitamin E and RLF. *Ophthalmology* 1983; 90:434–435.
31. Weiter JJ: Retrolental fibroplasia: An unsolved problem. *N Engl J Med* 1981; 305:1404–1406.
32. Ehrenkranz RA, Puklin JE: (Reply to letter). *Ophthalmology* 1982; 89:988–989.
33. Hittner HM, Rudolf AJ, Kretzer FL: Suppression of severe retinopathy of prematurity with vitamin E supplementation. *Ophthalmology* 1984; 91:12.
34. Ashton N: Retinal angiogenesis in the human embryo. *Br Med Bull* 1970; 26:103–106.
35. Patz A: Current status of retrolental fibroplasia. *Metab Pediatr Syst Ophthalmol* 1982; 6:185–187.
36. Hittner HM, Godro LB, Speer ME, et al: Retrolental fibroplasia: Further clinical evidence and ultrastructural support for efficacy of vitamin E in preterm infants. *Pediatrics* 1983; 71:423–432.
37. Hittner HM, Speer ME, Rudolph AJ, et al: Retrolental fibroplasia and vitamin E in preterm infant: Comparison of oral versus intramuscular administration. *Pediatrics* 1984; 73:238–249.
38. Hindle NW and Leyton J: Prevention of cicatricial retrolental fibroplasia: Cryotherapy. *Can J Ophthalmol* 1978; 13:277–282.
39. Hindle NW: Cryotherapy for retinopathy of prematurity to prevent RLF. *Can J Ophthalmol* 1982; 17:207–211.
40. Ben-Sira, Nissenkorn I. Grenwald E, et al: Treatment of acute RLF by cryopexy. *Br J Ophthalmol* 1980; 64:758–762.
41. Gaynon M: Subclassification of cryotherapy of acute proliferative stage three retinopathy of prematurity. *Invest Ophthalmol Vis Sci* 1983; 24(suppl):113.
42. Mousel DK, Hoyt CS: Cryotherapy for retinopathy of prematurity. *Ophthalmology* 1980; 87:1121–1127.
43. Rosenbaum AL, Phelps DL: Discussion. *Ophthalmology* 1984; 91:1522–1523.
44. Johnson L, Bowen F, Herrmann N, et al: The relationship of prolonged elevation of serum vitamin E levels to neonatal bacterial sepsis (SEP) and necrotizing enterocolitis (NEC), (abstract). *Pediatr Res* 1983; 17:319A.
45. Schaffer DB, Johnson L, Quinn GE, et al: Vitamin E and retinopathy of prematurity: Follow-up at one year. Ophthalmology 1985; 92:1005:1011.
46. Kushner BJ: Strabismus and amblyopia associated with regressed retinopathy of prematurity. *Arch Ophthalmol* 1982; 100:256–261.
47. Schaffer DB, Quinn GE, Johnson L: Sequelae of arrested mild retinopathy of prematurity. *Arch Ophthalmol* 1984; 102:373–376.
48. Vitamin E and Retinopathy of Prematurity. Report of a Study from the Institute of Medicine, Division of Health Sciences Policy. National Academy Press, Washington, DC, June 1986.

49. Milner RA, Watts JL, Paes B, et al: RLF in 1500 gram neonates: Part of a randomized clinical trial of the effectiveness of vitamin E. Presented at Retinopathy of Prematurity Conference, Washington, DC, Dec, 1981, pp 2703–2716.
50. Hammer ME, Mullen PW, Ferguson JG, et al: Logistic analysis of risk factors in acute retinopathy of prematurity. *Am J Ophthalmol* 1986; 102:1–6.
51. Flower RW, Blake DA, Wajer SD, et al: Retrolental fibroplasia: Evidence for a role of the prostaglandin cascade in the pathogenesis of oxygen-induced retinopathy in newborn beagle. *Pediatr Res* 1981; 15:1293–1302.
52. Karper CW, Merola AJ, Trewyn RW, et al: Modulation of platelet thromboxane $A_2$ and arterial prostacyclin by dietary vitamin E. *Prostaglandins* 1981; 22:651–661.
53. Stuart MJ, Graeberg JE, Clark DA: Neonatal vascular prostaglandin $I_2$ and plasma prostaglandin $I_2$ regenerating activity. *Retinopathy of Prematurity Conference,* Washington, D.C., Dec 1981, pp 194–203.

Chapter 6

# Retinopathy of Prematurity

John T. Flynn, M.D.

## DEFINITION

Retinopathy of prematurity (ROP) is a vasoproliferative retinopathy that occurs principally, but not exclusively, in premature infants. It occurs in two somewhat overlapping phases: (1) an acute phase in which normal vasculogenesis is interrupted and a response to injury is observable in the retina and (2) a chronic[1] or late proliferation of membranes into the vitreous during which tractional detachments of the retina, ectopia, and scarring of the macula and significant visual loss occur. More than 90% of cases of acute ROP go on to spontaneous regression, healing with minimal scarring and little or no visual loss. Fewer than 10% of the involved eyes go on to significant cicatrization.[2]

## INTRODUCTION

The following is a brief background of ROP. Although not recognized as such, ROP occurred sporadically prior to 1940. During the decade following Terry's initial report,[3] ROP burst onto the consciousness of the pediatric and ophthalmological communities as an epidemic of blindness among premature infants. Silverman[4] estimated that in the decade 1943–1953, 7,000 children in the United States and 10,000 worldwide were blinded by ROP. A hectic, disorganized search for possible causes, ranging from light to lack of iron and vitamins, led nowhere.[5] A pediatrician in Melbourne, Australia,[6] provided the first substantial clinical clue by comparing the frequency of occurrence of ROP in three nurseries, each differing in the ease of access to supplemental oxygen. She noted that each produced different attack rates of ROP. This pointed to a possible etiologic role for oxygen. The study of Patz et al.[7] followed promptly, and supported this conclusion. A randomized prospective trial of oxygen therapy, the Kinsey study,[8] was quickly organized. It was the first application of the then new science of biostatistics in ophthalmology. Its results clearly established that the incidence of ROP was related inversely to birth weight. The study further established that the incidence of cicatricial retrolental fibroplasia (RLF) (as the end-stage disease was then called) was 23% in prematures kept for 28 days in an oxygen environment of more than 50%, and 7% in infants given oxygen only when clinically necessary and in concentrations below 50%. Finally, its results seemed to indicate no apparent differences in the mortality and the morbidity between the two groups. There seemed to be no relationship between the concentrations of inspired oxygen and ROP. No "safe" level of inspired oxygen was established in this benchmark study, but the conclusion was not based on a formal test: Infants were not assigned to specific concentrations of oxygen (e.g., 30%, 40%, 50%). Shortly before its publication, a single, hospital-based, randomized trial was published.[9] This study (which suffered from a number of design flaws identified in the years that followed) suggested that if oxygen was used in inspired concentrations of 40% or less, the incidence of cicatricial RLF was zero. Subsequent papers[10–12] promoted this optimistic view, although Kinsey argued to the contrary that no safe level had been established and that oxygen should be given in the lowest concentrations for the shortest duration possible. Having emerged from that decade and from the frightful epidemic, the state of medical knowledge at that time seemed secure: ROP was related causally to birth weight and exposure to oxygen. If oxygen exposure was kept under 40%, the disease disappeared. And so, it seemed, it did.[13]

Unfortunately, the book was closed too soon for the full significance of the one pioneering study — the randomized prospective trial[8] of the early 1950s — to be realized. The consequences of this premature abandonment of the scientific method soon had to be faced. Although severe end-stage ROP all but disappeared with the restriction of inspired oxygen to 40% or less, the disease was replaced by brain damage and death among premature infants. By the mid-1960s, the published studies of Avery and Oppenheimer[14] and MacDonald[15] suggested that the incidence of both rose inversely as ROP's fell. Cross[16] estimated that for every prevented case of blindness from ROP, 16 infants died in the United States. A more rational and liberal policy of oxygen use in premature nurseries began in the mid-1960s. ROP reappeared.[17]

Modern technology played a role in this reappearance, because one of its most striking and immediate benefits was the development of superb life-support systems, which resulted from many lines of research, including space technology, cardiovascular and pulmonary physiology, and surgery. With miniaturization, these life-support systems could be applied to the tiniest premature infants whose lives could now be saved. However, it is these same infants who are at greatest risk for ROP, and for this reason as well, ROP reappeared. Although the actual occurrence today of the disease is unknown, Phelps[18] has suggested both a relative and an absolute increase in its incidence. Data from recent studies[19, 20] indicate that this estimate may be too high.

## A MODEL OF NORMAL VASCULOGENESIS

Because ROP is a proliferative disease of newly formed blood vessels, it is important to review briefly modern theories of how blood vessels are formed in the retina. According to the theory of Ashton,[21] mesenchyme, the vascular precursor, pours out of the optic disc at 16 weeks of gestation and grows across the surface of the retina in a wavelike fashion, reaching the edge of the retina, the ora serrata, on the nasal side, at about 36 weeks of gestational age. Because of the greater distance, it does not reach the temporal ora until about 40 weeks, which probably accounts for the preponderance of the disease in the temporal retina. The vascular precursor, mesenchyme, grows in the nerve fiber layer of the retina (Fig 6–1). On its trailing edge is a delicate meshwork of capillaries that looks like chicken wire (Fig 6–2) which, by absorption and remodeling, results in mature arteries and veins surrounded by a capillary meshwork. This sequence, Mesenchyme → Capillary Meshwork → Mature Arteries and Veins, is the central thesis of Ashton's theory and is what differentiates it from those of Michaelson[22] and Cogan,[23, 24] who theorize that capillaries arise by budding from mature arteries and veins. The clinical and pathological findings of ROP appear to indicate that Ashton is correct, but it should be emphasized that the question remains open to investigation.[24]

## A MODEL OF ABNORMAL VASCULOGENESIS

To account for the ophthalmoscopic observations, Flynn and coworkers[25, 26] postulated the following sequence of events in vascular injury and response (Fig 6–3):

1. An *injury* from unidentified noxious agent(s) destroys vascular endo-

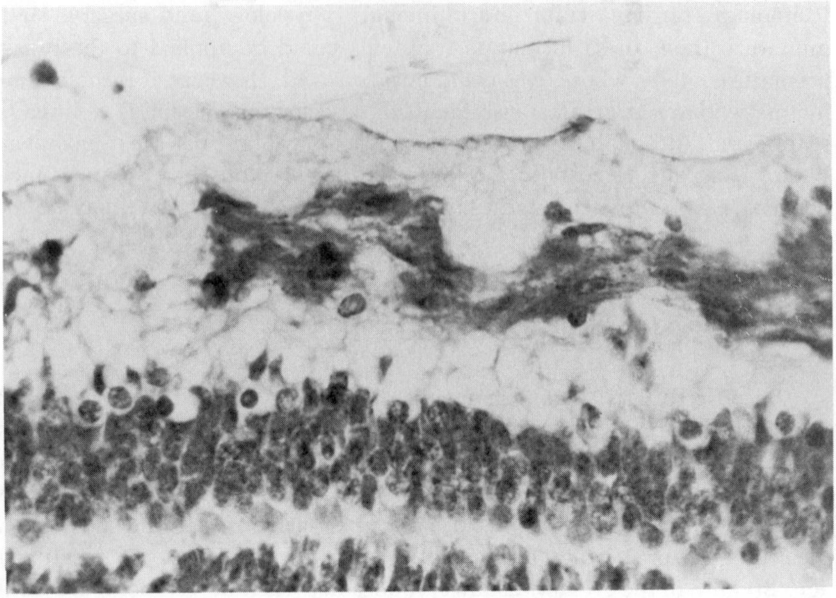

**FIG 6–1.**
Mesenchyme, the precursor of capillaries, growing in the nerve fiber layer. (PAS-hematoxylin; × 100.)

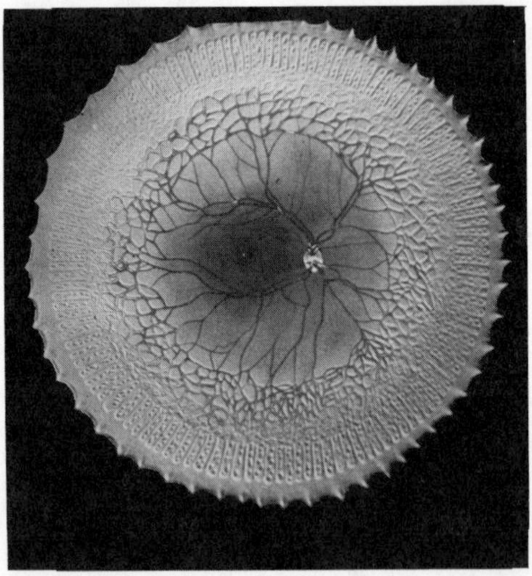

**FIG 6–2.**
Normal vasculogenesis. Mesenchymal vanguard growing toward the ora serrata followed by a capillary meshwork (enlarged for emphasis) which, by remodeling, forms mature arteries and veins. (Used by permission.)

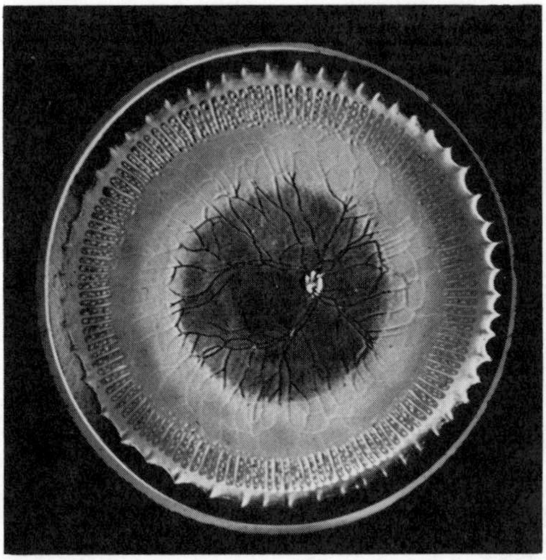

**FIG 6–3.**
Vascular injury results in obliteration of capillary meshwork with survival of mesenchyme and mature arteries and veins. (Used by permission.)

thelium where it is most vulnerable, namely, where it has just differentiated from mesenchyme to form the primitive capillary meshwork.

2. Two tissues, the mesenchyme, and mature arteries and veins, *survive* and *unite* via the few remaining vascular channels. The survival of these tissues constitutes the vascular response to injury. They form a structure that replaces the destroyed capillary bed — the mesenchymal arteriovenous shunt.

3. The *mesenchymal arteriovenous (AV) shunt* (Fig 6–4, A-C). This unique vascular structure, seen in no other retinopathy, forms a distinct demarcation line between vascular and avascular retina. It is composed of a nest of primitive mesenchymal and maturing endothelial cells, fed by mature arteries and veins. No capillaries are found in the region of the shunt. It is this structure that is the pathognomonic lesion of acute ROP. It has certain characteristics: First, it has a *location* and an *extent* in the retina; the more posterior the location and the more the circumference of the developing vasculature involved, the more severe the prognosis for the eye (Fig 6–5). Second, there is a sessile period after the injury when all vascular development of the eye ceases. This period may last from days to months, during which there are few changes in the ophthalmoscopic findings. Then the tissues that form the shunt begin to thicken, and the originally gray-white structure changes from pink to salmon to red in color. During this period, when vasculogenic activity resumes in the retina, in a very real sense the fate of the eye is decided. If the cells inside the shunt *divide* and *differentiate* into normal capillary endothelium, they then form primitive endothelial tubes, and on fluorescein angiography it is possible to see, instead of a thick, lu-

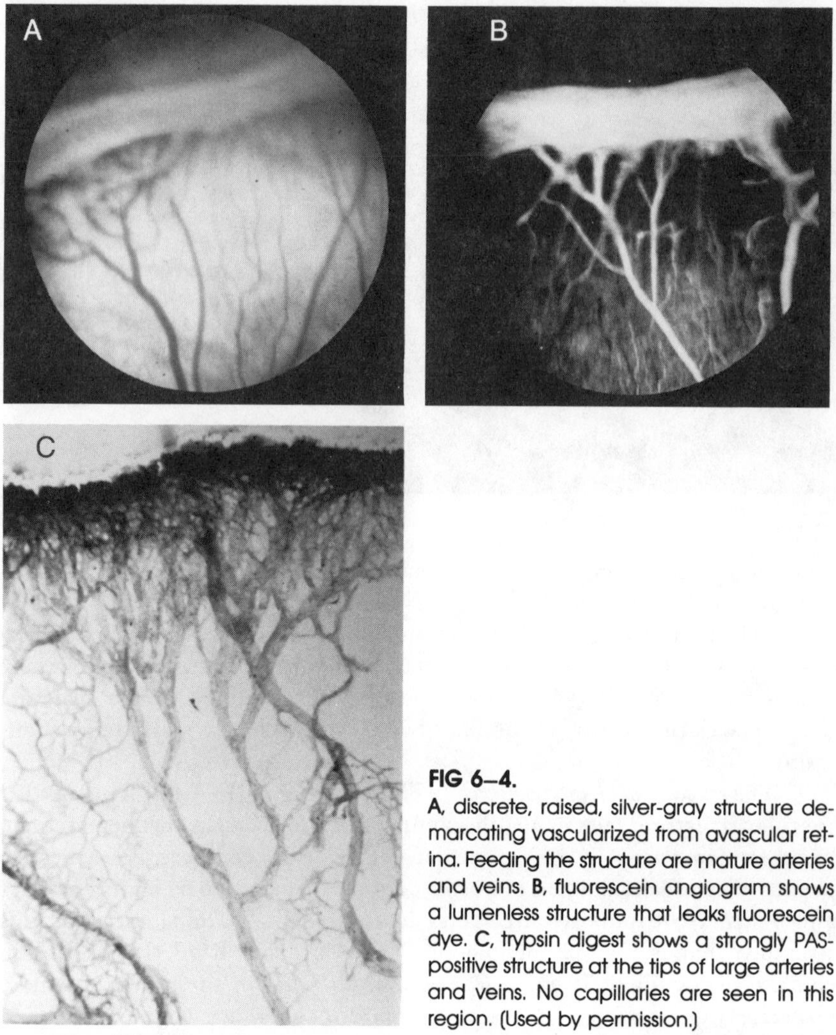


**FIG 6–4.**
**A**, discrete, raised, silver-gray structure demarcating vascularized from avascular retina. Feeding the structure are mature arteries and veins. **B**, fluorescein angiogram shows a lumenless structure that leaks fluorescein dye. **C**, trypsin digest shows a strongly PAS-positive structure at the tips of large arteries and veins. No capillaries are seen in this region. (Used by permission.)

menless structure that outlines the shunt, a regular "brush" border of capillaries, which over time grow into the avascular retina and provide a blood supply (Fig 6–6, A and B). This is the essence of the process of regression (vide infra) which, fortunately, occurs in more than 90% of cases of ROP.

If, however, the primitive cells inside the shunt multiply and break through the internal limiting membrane of the retina but do not differentiate into normal endothelium, they grow into the vitreous body, over the surface of the retina (Fig 6–7) and the ciliary body, to the equator of the lens. It is this *lack of differentiation* and *destructive proliferation* of cells and their invasion into spaces and tissues where they do not belong that are the chief events in the process of *membrane proliferation* that lead to *traction detachment*. This process can either be slow but inexorable, occurring over weeks to months (Fig 6–8 A, and B), or, as described by the Japanese,[27] as "rush" disease during which its progress can be compressed into a matter of days to weeks. In either event, the outcomes are identical: A partial or total traction retinal detachment occurs, with accompanying visual loss.

The factors that control the process are largely unknown. What is apparent clinically, as stated above, is that the more posterior the disease and the more of the developing vasculature involved, the worse the prognosis for the eye. Kretzer et al.[28] and Hittner et al.[29] have suggested that the gap-

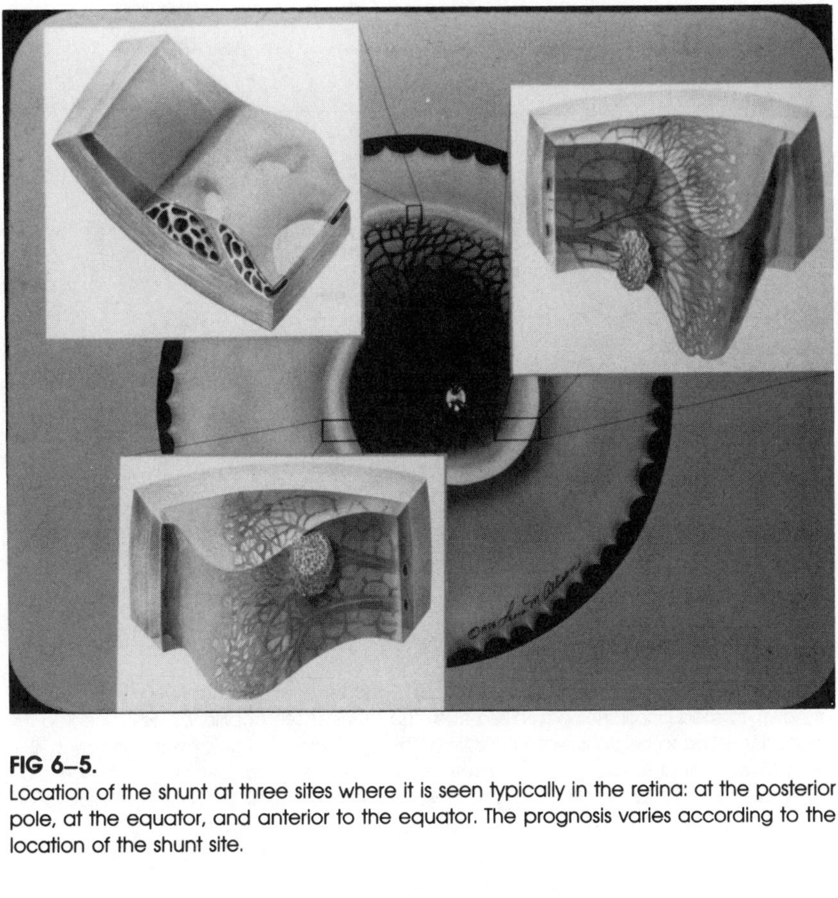

**FIG 6–5.**
Location of the shunt at three sites where it is seen typically in the retina: at the posterior pole, at the equator, and anterior to the equator. The prognosis varies according to the location of the shunt site.

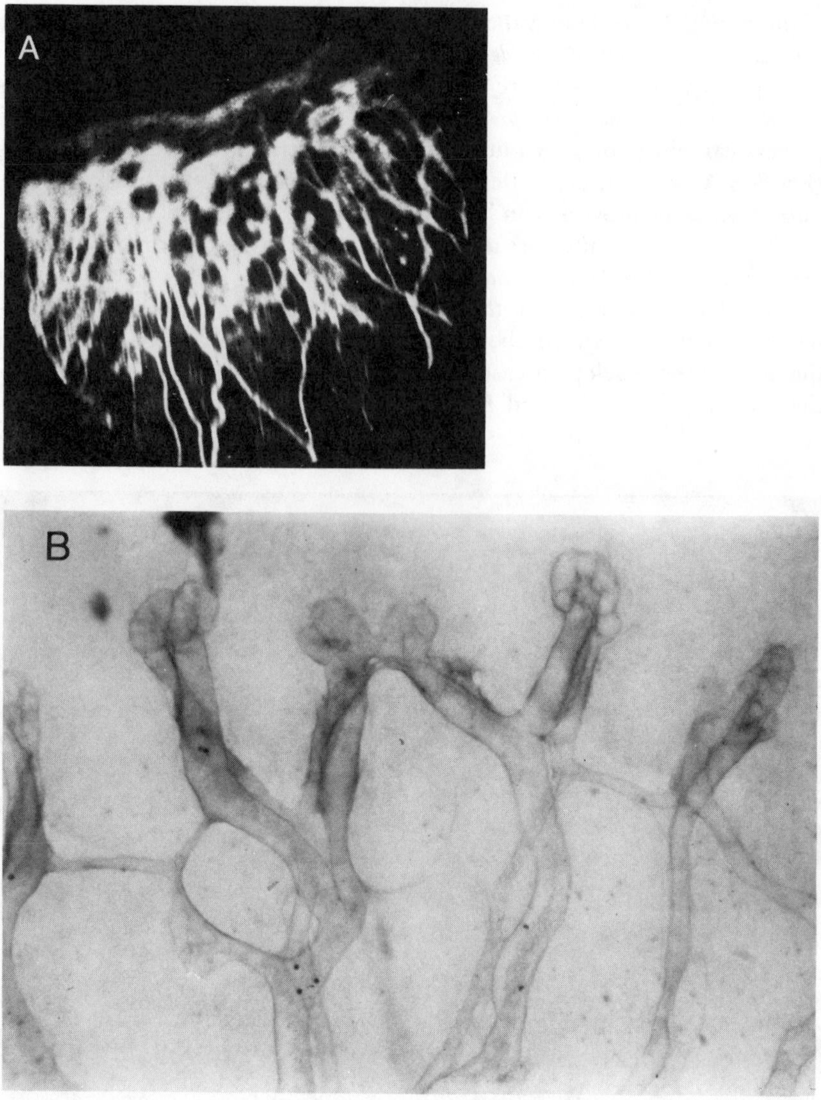


**FIG 6–6.**
**A,** fluorescein angiogram of regression of the RLF showing development of a "brush border" of newly formed capillaries organized from the shunt. These capillaries advance into the avascular retina to begin its vascularization. This is the essential process in regression. **B,** a PAS-stained retinal whole mount to show a slightly more advanced stage of regression. The vessels consist of an arteriole and a venule with a bridging tuft of proliferating endothelium at their tips.

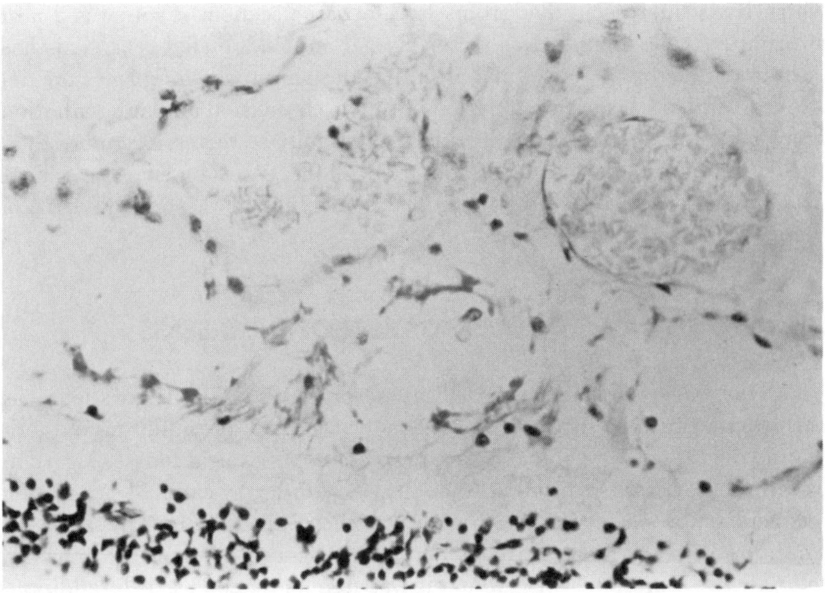

**FIG 6–7.**
Massive proliferation of tissue from the surface of the retina extending into vitreous gel and over the surface of the retina. (Hematoxylin and eosin; ×50.)

junction surface area between mesenchymal cells exposed to hyperoxic environment is increased. According to this theory, this increase in gap-junction area and presumably the activity it represents play a significant role in the genesis of neovascularization. The identification of the electron-dense surfaces as gap junctions is not accepted by all,[30] and furthermore, the hypothesis in its present form does not account for the traction and proliferative aspects of this disease, which seem to be its most devastating aspects.

To summarize, normal vasculogenesis presents on overall matrix in which many of the events of abnormal vasculogenesis can be placed. In the time domain, normal vasculogenesis begins at 16 weeks and is completed to the ora serrata by 40 weeks of gestation. The wavelike process spreads from the optic disc where mesenchyme originates from the primitive hyaloid system. An injury to this process results in directly observable consequences. First, vasculogenesis is arrested and there is cessation of the development of observable arteries, veins and, presumably, capillaries. Second, instead of a gradual, gentle blending of vascularized and avascular retina where it is not possible to distinguish the border between the two, an abrupt, observable structure is seen between the two zones. At first this is a line within the plane of the retina which gradually thickens into a ridge without a lumen and which leaks fluorescein dye profusely. On tissue section, it contains a nest of primitive cells identified as mesenchymal and endothelial cells. This has been designated a mesenchymal arteriovenous shunt which replaces the destroyed capillary bed. After a period of time, cell division and differentiation occur once more in this structure, either normally to regression (more than 90%) or abnormally to the proliferation of the tissue outside the retina, detachment of the retina, and loss of visual function (fewer than 10% of cases of ROP).

## THE NEED FOR A NEW CLASSIFICATION OF THE DISEASE

"Have we a satisfactory classification for ROP?" To this question, it is necessary to turn to history. In 1952, after a decade of confusion and ambiguity over the nature of the disease process and its clinical course, Algernon Reese and coworkers[31] brought some degree of order by carefully separating retrolental fibroplasia (as the disease was then called) from a hyperplastic condition of the primary vitreous and from falciform folds in the newborn retina,[32] two conditions with which it was frequently confused. In addition,

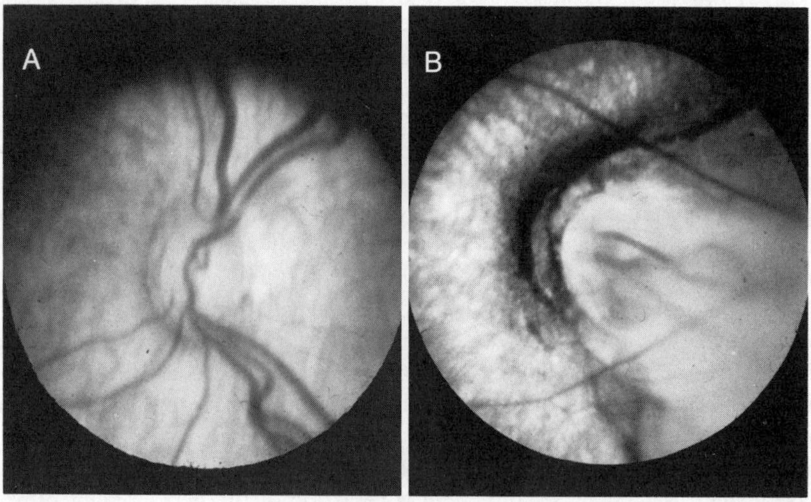


**FIG 6–8.**
The disc region in an infant shows the organization of a traction fold in the retina. The process begins at 8 weeks of age (*A*) and has reached stability at 23 weeks of age (*B*).

they classified the new disease[33] in a way that was accepted immediately by ophthalmologists and pediatricians, as their classification described succinctly the observations all were making with the mononuclear direct ophthalmoscope, the only instrument then available for observing the fundus of the eye. With the curtailment of the use of oxygen and the consequent subsiding of ROP as an epidemic, at least, further classification seemed both illogical and impractical because the Reese classification encompassed all that was necessary for a description of the disease. When ROP emerged again in the 1960s[34] and 1970s, clinicians possessed better tools to observe and describe what they saw. Chief among these were the binocular indirect ophthalmoscope, and fluorescein angiography,[35] a simple, practical technique of visualizing in vivo the vascular anatomy of the retina with surrounding retinal and choroidal tissues effectively subtracted from the image. In addition, Patz[36, 37] had made important observations on the role of oxygen in the kitten model, where excessive levels of oxygen caused severe vasoconstriction of retinal vessels. This added an earlier stage to a revised classification of ROP.[38] Patz then drew attention to the practical usefulness of this early vasoconstriction as a guide to hyperoxia.[39] Because sampling arterial $PO_2$ was not yet widespread, he suggested that ophthalmologists might use vasoconstriction as a clinical guide to hyperoxia. Although this latter suggestion proved clinically impractical,[40] it was a stimulus for a series of findings by several observers[41–46] that resulted in a clearer picture of ROP as it progressed in the retina, and that led to several classifications of acute ROP.[41–43, 46] These new classifications did not stray far from the ground broken earlier by Reese, and it seemed to at least one observer[47] that all classification systems failed to unify today's observations in as useful a manner as had Reese's earlier system. First, and most important, all classification systems current at the time failed to specify two critically important observable characteristics of the disease: the *location* in the retina, and the *extent* of the developing retinal vasculature involved.

A group of ophthalmologists representing eleven countries and sharing a common interest in ROP developed a new classification system.[48, 49] The advance that this classification system represents is the specification of location and extent of the disease, its accurate staging, and its evolution to retinal detachment or regression.

For specification of the *location* of the disease, the retina is divided into three zones (Fig 6–9):

1. Zone 1: The inner zone extends from the optic disc to twice the disc-macular distance, or 30 degrees in all directions from the optic disc.
2. Zone 2: The middle zone extends from the outer border of zone 1

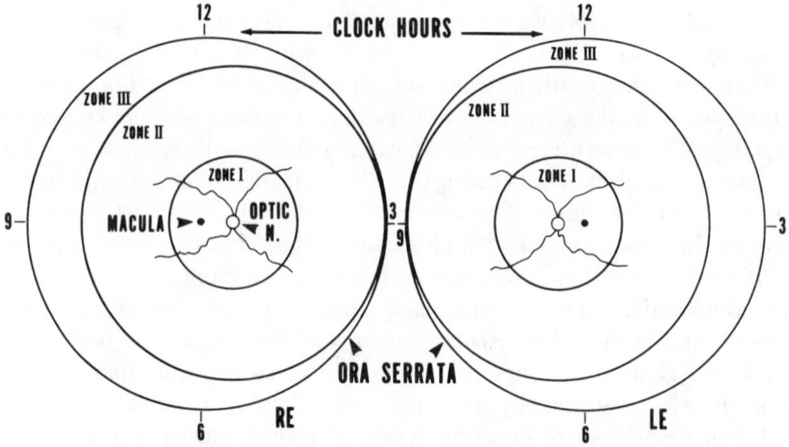


**FIG 6–9.**
Zones of retinal involvement. Illustration of the fundus with the zoning employed in conjunction with the new classification of ROP.

to the ora on the nasal side and to approximately the equator on the temporal side.

3. Zone 3: The outer zone extends from the outer edge of zone 2 in a crescentic fashion to the ora serrata.

The *extent* of the vascular involvement is simply coded by the number of clock hours involved. For example, disease extending from the 7 o'clock to 12 o'clock position in the right eye and from the 5 o'clock to 12 o'clock position in the left eye would mean 5 clock hours' involvement of the temporal retinal vasculature of both eyes in zone 2, as illustrated (Fig 6–10).

*Staging:* The retinopathy may be staged for each clock hour involved. It is more than likely that one or two stages of the disease may be present at any given time. The recognized stages are:

1. Stage 1. *Demarcation line*: A simple border or line seen at the edge of vessels dividing vascular from avascular retina.

2. Stage 2. *Ridge*. The line structure of the previous stage will have now acquired a volume and risen above the surface of the retina to become a ridge.

3. Stage 3. *Ridge with extraretinal fibrovascular proliferation:* From the surface of the ridge, this extraretinal tissue extends chiefly through the internal limiting membrane of the retina into the vitreous gel and back over the

surface of the vascularized retina; in later stages it may be seen proliferating forward over the surface of the avascular retina, the ciliary body, and the equator of the lens.

4. Stage 4. *Subtotal retinal detachment:* Traction forces developed from proliferating tissue in the vitreous gel or on retinal surfaces result in a traction-type of retinal detachment. This is further subdivided into: (1) subtotal retinal detachment not involving the fovea (Fig 6–11). This type of peripheral detachment generally carries a relatively good prognosis for vision, as the macula and fovea are uninvolved; and (2) subtotal retinal detachment involving the fovea (Fig 6–12). This detachment results in poor vision because it involves the macula and fovea. It is the typical traction fold through the macula that causes this (Fig 6–13).

5. Stage 5. *Total retinal detachment:* In contrast to the previous stage, in which some retina remains attached, this stage encompasses the total, funnel-shaped retinal detachment (Fig 6–14), and has very poor visual prognosis. Most commonly, the funnel assumes an open or closed form, although variants do occur.

In addition to classifying ROP, the committee also provided a computer-compatible examination record to facilitate data recording and communication between clinics, and to create a matrix for research into the disease.

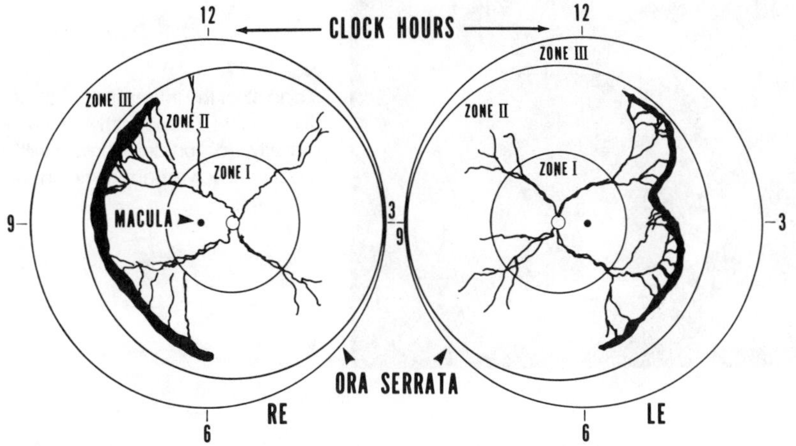


**FIG 6–10.**
Extent of involvement. Bilateral zone 2 retinopathy of prematurity of 5 clock hours in the temporal retina of both eyes.

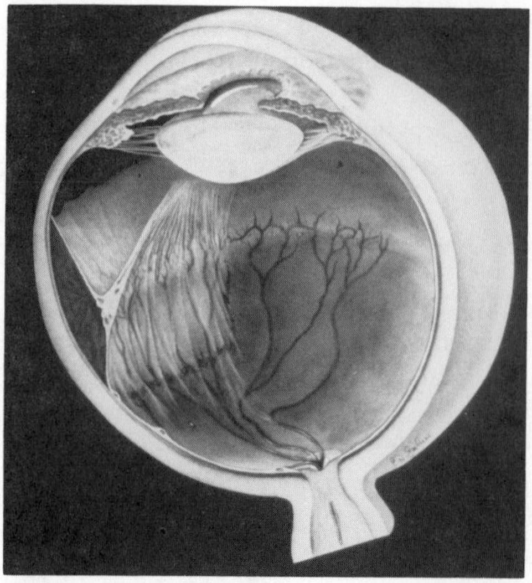

**FIG 6–11.**
Stage 4A of the International Classification of Retinopathy of Prematurity. Subtotal traction retinal detachment without macular involvement is shown.

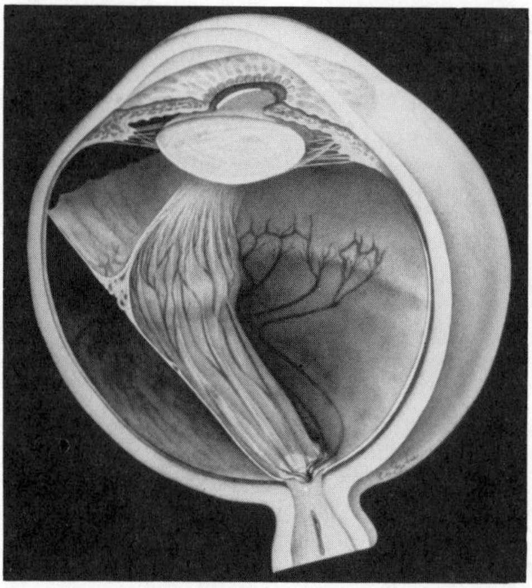

**FIG 6–12.**
Stage 4B of the International Classification of Retinopathy of Prematurity. Traction detachment with macular involvement is shown.

The above classification incorporates the best observational data on ROP available today. This classification has as its unifying idea a simple but powerful principle: The more posterior the zone, the more of the developing vasculature involved, and the more hours of the clock encompassed, the worse the prognosis for the eye.

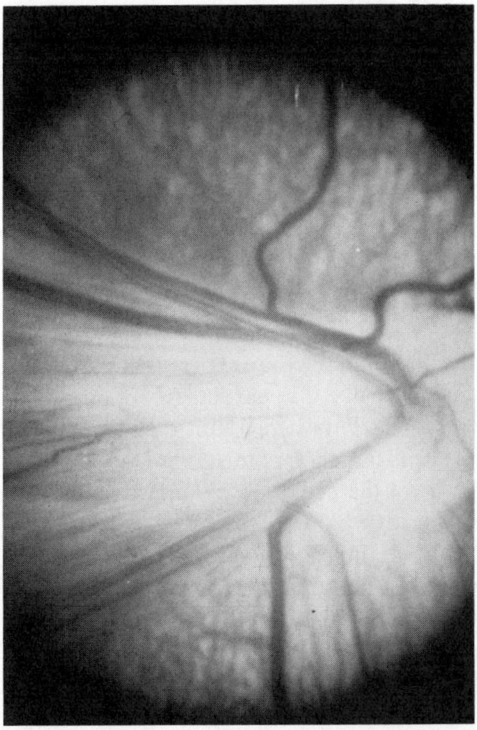

**FIG 6–13.**
Fundus photograph of stage 4B of the International Classification of Retinopathy of Prematurity.

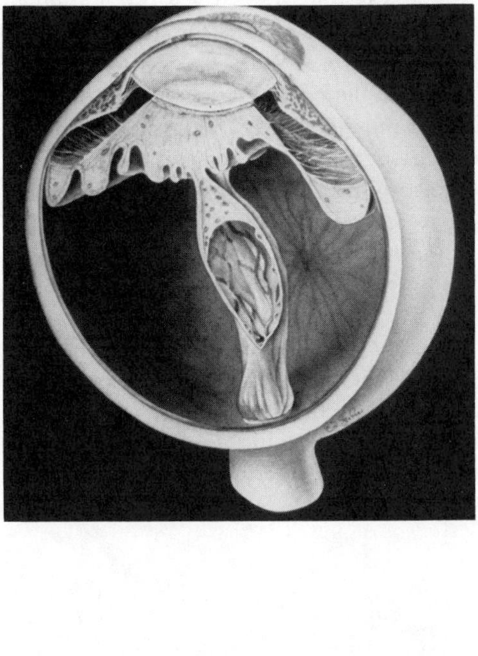

**FIG 6–14.**
Stage 5 of the International Classification, with total retinal detachment, closed-funnel type.

We began this section with the query: "Do we need a new classification?" If we are to present this fascinating disease in all of its various forms, the answer is that we do. To begin any rational, scientific examination of the merits of any of today's proffered therapies, we do. Finally, to communicate intelligently with each other about our experiences and observations with ROP, we do.

## CURRENT PROBLEMS

### Current Incidence and Course of the Disease

Implicit in this discussion is the notion that we are experiencing a relative and perhaps absolute rise in the incidence of ROP, particularly of the partial or total traction retinal detachments in ROP that inevitably damage vision.[50] What is the evidence on this point? It is largely circumstantial, and without specific efforts by interested members of the pediatric and ophthalmological communities, the evidence is destined to remain obscure. The first leg of the circumstantial case arises from the known improvement in neonatal mortality statistics over the past two decades.[51–55] Although these are most striking in developed countries, over time they may spread to developing countries as the technology of modern neonatal care diffuses through various societies of the world. The result is a pool of infants at risk, born under 1,500 gm birth weight. In an attempt to set limits on the dimensions of this problem, Phelps[18] reviewed current incidence figures for the western world. The data are meager and scattered, and consist for the most part in anecdotal incidence figures from various centers. Nevertheless, she was able to set at least some rational boundaries for what the figures may currently be in the United States. The annual accrual of new cases of stage 4B or worse ROP may vary from a low of 397 to a high of 883. These limits, it should be noted, are of the same order of magnitude as those arrived at retrospectively by Silverman[4] for the decade 1943–1953. Certainly, there are figures to challenge these. Kalina,[19] in presenting two decades of experience with severe disease at the University of Washington, reported an incidence of 1.2%, below the lowest figure of Phelps. McCormick's[56] figures on the number of blind children registered with the Canadian Society for Blindness have failed to demonstrate any significant rise over the decades of the 1960s and 1970s. More recently, Johnson et al.'s[20] figures on the reduction of incidence and severity of ROP in a large neonatal nursery offer grounds for guarded optimism. Further, the work in Switzerland of Treu et al.[57] supports this conclusion.

The fact remains that we do not know the number of children being visually handicapped and blinded by the disease today, and we are as lacking in basic epidemiological data of varying rates of incidence in geographic areas and socioeconomic strata as we were in the 1940s and 1950s. Nevertheless, a revolution in other areas of neonatal care has occurred in that time interval without any obvious benefit regarding ROP. It would seem incumbent on interested neonatologists and ophthalmologists who care for infants in tertiary care nurseries in the United States to organize their own ad hoc system using that very network as the basis for its organization and for gathering regional (rather than hospital-based) data on the frequency of occurrence. National organizations (Centers for Disease Control), state organizations (Bureau of Blind Services) and various service organizations (Lighthouse for the Blind, Research to Prevent Blindness) are not helpful in this regard. The model of tumor registries established in various medical schools and university hospitals might furnish useful insights into the mechanics of a nationwide reporting system through the tertiary care network. Without knowing the true dimensions of the problem of ROP today, it is difficult to convince financially hard-pressed governmental and private agencies to part with the scarce dollars necessary to support research into the problem.

## Specification of the Vulnerable Infant

In contrast to the decade between 1940 and 1950, when the healthiest infants subjected to an oxygen-rich environment seemed the most susceptible, in today's newborn intensive care units the sickest infants of lowest birth weight are the most susceptible to ROP. Birth weight literally swamps all other risk variables in accounting for the disease. The lower the birth weight the higher the risk of the disease. Indeed, in most studies of risk factors associated with ROP, it is necessary to stratify on this variable when looking at other potential risk variables. The relationship between birth weight and severe end-stage disease, while suggestive, is not firmly established.[2, 58] In neither case can anything be done about this demographic variable until methods of prolonging preterm pregnancies, especially very low birth weight pregnancies, are perfected. As pointed out by McCormick,[59] this is a social and economic as well as a medical problem.

## Specification of the Injurious Agent

### *Clinical Use of Oxygen*

Because of its early association with the occurrence of ROP in the 1940s and 1950s and because it is, of all therapeutic variables in the premature's environment, the most pervasive and among the most easily manipulated by the physician, oxygen heads the list of agents suspected of causing the initial insult that leads to ROP. Because of the recurrence of ROP in the late 1960s and 1970s, a case control study of prematures at five centers was begun in 1969 in an attempt to better define oxygen involvement. Intermittent sampling of arterial oxygen tension ($PO_2$) was employed; some 1,373 infants were admitted into the study through 1972. Data were analyzed and the results were published in 1977.[60] They were, however, disappointing to both the pediatric[61, 62] and ophthalmologic communities. As was already known, birth weight proved to be the single most powerful predictor of ROP. Duration of oxygen therapy rather than the concentration also seemed to be implicated. No clear relationship could be established between any intermittently sampled $PO_2$ and ROP. In one group of babies under 1,250 gm birth weight, there was a suggestive relationship between the number of $PaO_2$ values above 150 mm Hg and ROP. Failure to define a quantitative relationship between oxygen and ROP has led Silverman to sharply question the "oxygen dogma."[63] It has, in fact, been clear for some time that birth weight and oxygen are by no means the sole parameters determining the occurrence of ROP. The condition has been reported to occur without oxygen administration[64] in full-term infants,[65–68] in anencephalic infants who expire at birth,[45, 69] and in infants with cyanotic heart disease.[70] Conversely, sustained hyperoxygenation[71] in preterm infants may not result in ROP. The problem remains, however, to define for most premature infants the relationship between oxygen and ROP. Over the past decade, the transcutaneous oxygen monitor, which permits the almost continuous monitoring of warmed, arterialized capillary blood through the skin, has become available.[72, 73] Recently, Horbar and coworkers[74] have added microprocessor capabilities which enable the transcutaneous $PO_2$ ($tcPO_2$) values to be plotted in the form of hourly histograms. A randomized prospective trial[75] employing this technology on a population of high-risk premature infants (birth weight $\leq$1,300 gm) compared constant to $PO_2$ monitoring of oxygen vs. standard intermittent monitoring for their effects on the incidence of ROP. No protective effect of constant monitoring was found except in the heaviest strata of infants (birth weight 1,100 to 1,300 gm) where ROP is likely to be the mildest and least frequent. In an accompanying report, this same group[76] found significant correlations between hours of tc values in excess of 80 mm Hg for weeks 1 and weeks 2 to 4, and both incidence and severity of ROP while controlling for important predictive variables such as birth weight, 5-minute Apgar score,[77] and the duration of oxygen exposure. The relationship between the tc oxygen variable and ROP was not robust, and accounted for less than 11% of the variance in the outcome variable, ROP. Nevertheless, the study does represent a first step in defining this elusive relationship. It suggests a number of strategies for control of oxygen that might predict ways of lessening risk exposure for ROP for the most vulnerable infants, and that might be testable in the newborn intensive care unit (ICU). On a clinical level, then, the problem of oxygen and its relation to ROP remains only partially solved at best, and is still with us.

### *Basic Research Studies of Oxygen*

Although much has been learned about the enzymatic mechanisms by which oxygen in its various forms are handled, the exact specification of a mechanism of injury remains elusive. On a biochemical level, oxygen is seen as a two-edged sword: on the one hand vital for the existence of the organism, but capable of insidious cellular destruction on the other. At the heart of this apparent paradox are a series of chemical reactions whereby oxygen is converted to a number of transient free radicals, highly reactive substances that contain unpaired electrons. The substances, among them singlet oxygen, the superoxide anion radical ($O_2^-$), the hydroxyl radical ($OH^-$), and hydrogen peroxide ($H_2O_2$) are thought to be responsible for producing irreversible damage to biopeptides such as enzyme proteins and membrane lipoproteins.[78, 79] Cytochromes, catalases, peroxidases, and particularly superoxide dysmutase are the front line of enzyme systems active in handling these various states of oxygen. Any or all of these may be deficient, particularly in association with other glycolytic and respiratory enzymes in experimental animals subjected to hyperoxia.[80–82] The relationship between the enzyme-deficient retina in a premature's eye and the quantities of dissolved oxygen and hemoglobin-bound oxygen circulating in the newly mature vessels is, in principle, easy to visualize as the potential mechanism of oxygen damage. But much more work of a basic nature remains to be done in the experimental animal, in the biochemical laboratory, and in humans before it is possible to ascertain that it is, in fact, the mechanism of oxygen damage that occurs in the infant's eye.[83]

In summary, although oxygen has a long tradition of being implicated as a cause of ROP, it is clearly neither a necessary nor a sufficient cause of the disease.[84] The problem remains, however, of defining further the relationships among exposure, duration, and concentration of oxygen and ROP on the clinical level. The sequence of events that occurs at the biomolecular level will probably be elucidated at the same time as well.

### *Vitamin E**

This vitamin, first described in human nutrition by Evans and Bishop[85] in 1922 and chemically characterized by Evans & Emerson[86] in 1936, was reported in 1949 to have a promising protective effect against ROP in a group

---

**Vitamin E is taken up here separately from other forms of therapy because of its relation to oxygen and because it is the only form of therapy that purports to be preventative and noninvasive when given as a supplement to the premature.*

of premature infants, 1,360 gm birth weight and under, when given 50 mg three times a day by mouth as soon as oral feedings began.[87] However, Kinsey and Chisholm[88] failed to confirm this relationship, and interest in the vitamin, a known antioxidant, waned because there was no overwhelming evidence that limiting oxygen exposure was an effective means of preventing ROP. Interest in the vitamin reawakened with the human studies of Johnson et al.,[89] and in the kitten model of Phelps and Rosenbaum.[90] There followed in quick succession several trials[91–94] on generally similar infants ($\leq$1500 gm and requiring supplemental oxygen) of vitamin E given by several routes and dosage schedules. The outcome variable, ROP, was classified under different systems of classification. Although the samples were marginal in size, in three of four studies an ameliorating effect of vitamin E on the severity rather than the incidence of the disease was noted. As pointed out by Phelps,[95] in her excellent review of the topic of vitamin E therapy, the statistical manipulations necessary to make even this statement were formidable; the effect is clearly not very robust, and careful consideration must be given to recommendations about vitamin E therapy because it may have significant side effects in the dosage levels employed in some of these studies. The reports of Johnson[96] on the statistical association of high blood levels of circulating vitamin E and necrotizing enterocolitis and sepsis, and of Phelps et al.[97] on intraventricular hemorrhage anjd retinal hemorrhages[98] in infants weighing less than 1 kg even with normal blood levels of the vitamin, are cases in point. The alteration of the immune response[99, 100] and depression of leukocyte bacteriostatic activity,[101] both of which are known complications of excessive vitamin E therapy in adults, may well have serious consequences for prematures who receive massive doses of the vitamin. In addition, small prematures may be susceptible to complications[102] of therapy not yet described in adults. The recently issued report of the Institute of Medicine[103] on this subject seems definitive.

What then may be said of vitamin E therapy in ROP? Certainly, it has failed to live up to the claims originally made by its proponents. Any effect that it may have is small, and will require a large multicenter trial to demonstrate an effect of the magnitude suggested. None of its adherents who claim that vitamin E must be given early (right after birth) to be effective, have explained why, if this is so, it affects only the severity and not the incidence of the disease. It would seem today that prudence dictates the administration of no more vitamin E than is necessary to maintain serum levels between 1.2 and 3.0 μg/dl, which is E sufficiency.

### Carbon Dioxide

In interesting and challenging basic research papers, Flowers[104, 105] detailed the results of his group's study of the effects of aspirin and $CO_2$ retention on the production of ROP in beagle pups. In essence, both of these agents proved capable of enhancing the effect of oxygen damage in this animal model, producing pictures and fluorescein angiograms quite similar to those seen in acute ROP in infants. In one animal, cicatricial disease was produced, which was another first for that animal model. In the discussion of his work, Flowers also introduced the concept that vasoconstriction, rather than being an early form or stage of ROP, was instead a protective reflex designed to prevent damage to the infant's vasculature by oxygen. The latter statement is probably the most challenging aspect of his work. Flowers demonstrated the aspirin effect as causing inhibition of vascular prostacyclin (a vasodilator) and platelet thromboxane (a vasoconstrictor). The balance of these two was a net vasodilatation that exposed the animal's primitive endothelium to the toxic effects of oxygen. $CO_2$ retention worked in a similar fashion, resulting in vasodilitation.[106, 107] This vasodilitation presumably occurs because reflex vasoconstriction to oxygen is inactivated and the result is oxygen damage. Bauer and Widmayer[108] followed up on this clinically, and noted that in a retrospectively analyzed group of infants under 100 gm birth weight, $PaCO_2$ was the single most important variable in distinguishing infants who developed ROP from those who did not. However, recent studies of Biglan and coworkers[109] and Brown et al.[110] have failed to confirm this association.

#### *Indomethacin*

This nonsteroid anti-inflammatory agent, which is similar to aspirin, is currently used in the treatment of patent ductus arteriosus. It shares many aspirin-like effects on the prostacyclin-thromboxane system. Following up once again on Flowers' lead, Sun et al.[111] performed a retrospective chart review that seemed to substantiate the thesis that severe ROP was associated with indomethacin employed in the treatment of the ductus. The question of the influence of this medication and others like it on the etiology or ROP remains open until each of these medications is tested in turn by a masked, prospective, randomized trial against a placebo. Only then will the neonatal community possess sufficient information for weighing the potential risks of the drug against its benefits in the treatment of ROP. The recently published indomethacin collaborative study[112] is not adequate as far as ROP incidence is concerned. First, from the ophthamological standpoint, the follow-up on patients raises concerns that patients with milder or more moderate forms of the disease may have escaped detection. Second, the decreased incidence of ROP found in the indomethacin-treated group was not predicted before the trial began. The result found may simply illustrate the fallacy of the enumeration of favorable circumstances (if enough association of independent variables are sought, the laws of chance guarantee that some will be found).

### *Blood and Blood Products*

Fetal hemoglobin has a strong avidity for oxygen, and adult hemoglobin a weaker one. Hence, there is a shift to the left of the fetal hemoglobin dissociation curve. Transfusion of blood containing adult hemoglobin, both to treat the anemias associated with prematurity[113] and to replace blood volume drawn for laboratory determinations, may result in the replacement of a sick premature's blood volume several times during the course of the infant's hospital stay. This has led to the suggestion that the anemia[114] or transfusion[89, 115–118] of blood containing adult hemoglobin could conceivably play a role in potentiating the risk of ROP. The hypothesis is attractive: Oxygen bound loosely to the adult hemoglobin molecule might be more readily released in the vicinity of newly formed capillary endothelium, resulting in more damage than would oxygen bound more tightly to fetal hemoglobin. Unfortunately, studies done thus far have failed to demonstrate this, particularly in those controlled for other variables that might potentially confound the oxygen–adult hemoglobin variable. It would seem that a definitive study of the relationship should include serial hemoglobin electrophoresis determinations of the amounts of adult vs. fetal hemoglobin in the at-risk infant population. This would clarify whether any quantitative relationship exists between the putative risk variable, adult hemoglobin, and the outcome variable, acute ROP, apart from the former's relationship to oxygen and birth weight.

### *Miscellaneous Factors*

A review of the current literature on ROP reveals its resemblance to the literature reviewed exhaustively by Zacharias[5] in 1952, prior to the discovery of oxygen's role in ROP. Intraventricular hemorrhage,[119] multiple spells of apnea-bradycardia, respiratory distress syndrome,[92] chronic in utero hypoxia,[66] and acidosis[121] are among some of the factors implicated, either anecdotally or associated in a univariate statistical sense. The problem of teasing out the true role of any of these many potential risk variables, while controlling for the powerful confounding effects of low birth weight, gestational age, and duration of oxygen therapy, is formidable and as yet unsolved. It is likely that until oxygen's role is fully defined quantitatively, the association of any of these risk factors with the outcome variable, acute ROP, is suspect.

In the realm of treatment, actual or potential, nursery light levels[122] and D-penicillamine[123] have been reported to reduce the incidence of the disease. Both are interesting therapeutic approaches, and both await further study in clinical trials.

## Timing, Technique and Precautions for the Ophthalmological Examination

These critical issues have received far less attention than they deserve in either the ophthalmological or pediatric literature. Palmer,[124] in a retrospective analysis of 175 infants, concluded that the optimal age for the screening examination to detect ROP in the premature infant was between seven and 9 weeks of age. Flynn,[58] in his series of 639 infants, found that the vast majority of diagnoses of ROP were made between 32 and 44 weeks postconceptional age (gestational age at birth plus weeks of life postbirth). In a previous study of 861 infants, the Miami group[120] noted that infants were examined, on average, 13 days prior to discharge from the hospital. Non-ROP babies were 28 days old and ROP babies were 55 days old at that point ($P < 0.001$). Recently, Brown et al.[125] suggested as a guideline 1,600 gm birth weight and under for examination of premature infants for ROP, rather than the current 2,000 gm standard, on the basis of analysis of their own material of the past decade. The only exceptions to this guideline are infants receiving more than 50 days of supplementary oxygen therapy. Clearly, there still exists a lack of definition about which babies to examine, and when and how often. Both neonatology and ophthalmology should address themselves to the mundane but vital task of providing safe and sensitive guidelines for examining these infants.

After surviving the rigors of life-threatening illnesses, the premature is a resilient yet still fragile creature. The ophthalmic examination, carried out with the indirect ophthalmoscope, the infant lid speculum, and dilating drops, constitutes a stress for the infant. As part of a research protocol, serial examinations on some 296 premature infants (birth weight ≤1,300 gm) were performed from 1981 through 1984.[2] These examinations began at 32 weeks postconceptional age and were repeated every 2 weeks until discharge if the infant's condition permitted.Adequate dilatation of the pupils was obtained with 1 drop of 0.5% cyclopentolate and 1 drop of 2.5% phenylephrine administered 30 minutes prior to the examination. Care was taken by the neonatal nurse in instilling the drops not only to occlude the puncta but also to hold the lids apart for 30 seconds following instillation, to pool the drops in the conjunctival sac (Fig 6–15). The excess was then wiped off the infant's face after the lids were closed. It has been noted that the eyes of infants with chronic lung disease do not dilate as well with this regimen and require two or more instillations of cyclopentolate (0.50% to 1.0%). Each examined infant was attached to a portable pulse-audio monitor and kept on a warmer during the examination (Fig 6–16). A neonatal nurse was in attendance during the examination, which lasted about 5 minutes. A subset of these infants[126] were attached to a tc monitor during the examination and no

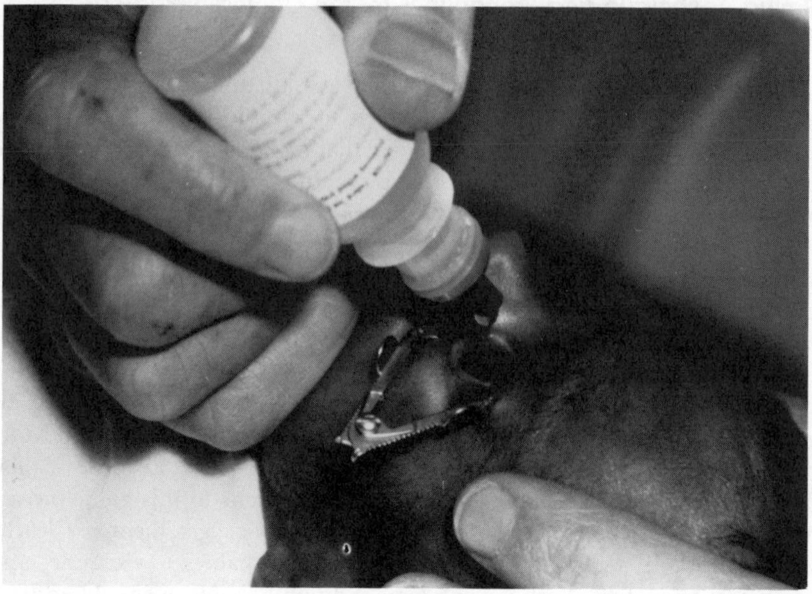

**FIG 6–15.**
Technique for instillation of drops. The lids are held apart with a speculum for 30 seconds to pool the medication in the conjunctival sac.

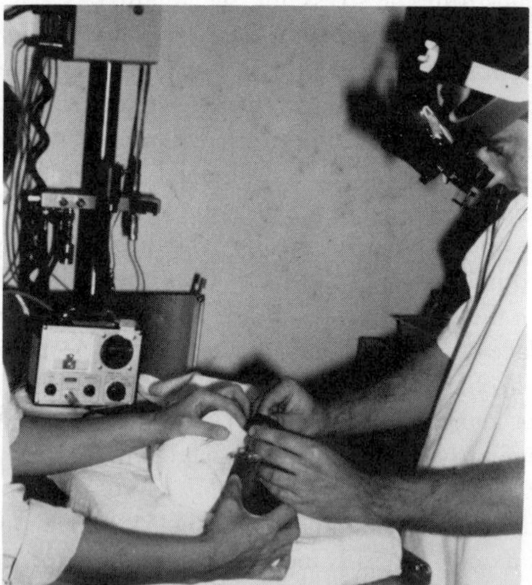

**FIG 6–16.**
Examination of a premature infant attached to a monitor; a neonatal nurse is in attendance.

hyperoxia or hypoxia was noted to occur during ophthalmoscopy, which was gently and quickly performed. When these simple precautions were observed more than 1,000 examinations were performed in this project without complications to the infants. Following the examination, abdominal girth and vital signs were observed hourly, bearing in mind the toxicity of cyclopentolate[126] and phenylephrine.[127]

For the ophthalmologist and neonatologist in clinical practice interested in thoroughly and safely screening infants in their neonatal units for the presence of ROP, the following would seem to be commonsense guidelines: The premature infant should be examined when its clinical condition is stable and the risk to the infant is acceptably small. For the vast majority of infants, this probably means that the examination should be conducted 1 to 2 weeks prior to discharge. For the rare, very sick infant with extremely low birth weight or a long history of perinatal disease and therapy, the examination can be judiciously done earlier, but only after the infant is no longer on life-support systems. For the ophthalmologist, the key question to be answered as a result of this examination is: What is the state of the developing vasculature? If, for example, vascularization has proceeded well past the equator of the eye temporally (zone 3 in ICROP notation), that is, if the ora can be visualized in the indirect lens field together with the ends of the vessels and no abnormality can be seen at the tips of the developing vessels, that infant carries essentially no risk for developing ROP and need not be seen again. If vascularization is at or just beyond the equator (border zone 2 to 3) but abnormalities are not visualized at the tips of the vessels, the infant probably is at low or no risk; however, an examination in 4 to 6 weeks would be prudent to be sure that the vascularization is complete. If vascularization has not progressed this far, then the infant should be examined biweekly. If, on the other hand, ROP is discovered, its location and extent should be carefully determined. If the disease in the infant's retina is anterior to the equator (in zone 3 by ICROP notation), plus disease is always absent and the outcome of regression is almost universal, in my experience. If, on the other hand, disease occupies part or all of the temporal aspect of zone 2, examinations every 2 to 3 weeks are indicated. Plus disease may develop in these infants, and some degree of traction on posterior pole structures may occur. Disease between the macula and equator (inner zone 2, outer zone 1) and more posterior disease is uniformly 12 clock hours in extent; it is in this group of patients that serial follow-up is mandatory at intervals of no more than 1 week. Consultation with a retina-vitreous specialist is probably indicated for disease posterior to the equator and occurring over more than one-half the circumference of the developing vasculature. If lesser disease is encountered, it will in all likelihood regress spontaneously. The infant must be kept under ophthalmological supervision for the complications of regressed ROP, as stressed by Kushner[128] and by others.[129–131]

## Regression

Data on this very important outcome are scarce, as noted above. Both its clinical description and a complete description of its spectrum[2, 25] are just beginning to emerge (Fig 6–17, A and B). Quantitative data on the duration of the disease from onset through complete regression would suggest in a small series that the disease, diagnosed on average at least 8 to 9 weeks after birth, lasts until about 25 to 26 weeks, when the process is ophthalmolscopically complete.[2] Collection of more data on this subject is one of the needs of a thorough clinical research protocol on ROP (see Chapter 9).

## Treatment

In the past two decades, an unprecedented development in technology has been quickly and successfully applied to the treatment of adult eye disease. The therapy of diabetic retinopathy[132] with light and laser coagulation, and treatment of vitreous disease with sophisticated instrumentation[133] to permit the removal of blood, membranes, and tissue from the vitreous gel have led to the natural and logical hope of extending these modalities to the premature infant. Articles reporting the use of photocoagulation,[44, 134] laser,[135] the application of cryotherapy,[129, 136–140] and scleral buckling procedures[141, 142] have appeared. Infants with stage 5, total retinal detachment, who are essentially blind if left untreated, have been approached surgically with the most modern techniques of retina-vitreous surgery.[143–149] In evaluating this literature, particularly that dealing with the application of modalities such as photocoagulation, laser, cryotherapy, and local scleral buckling, it is well to bear in mind that these therapies are all advocated for acute disease, which has a spontaneous regression rate of more than 90%. The burden of proof is then on the advocate of the particular therapy to prove that the proffered therapy is better, in fact, than the natural history of the disease. So far, none of the reported studies has met this test. The only scientifically sound way to meet it is by carrying out a carefully designed, randomized, prospective trial of therapy X, Y, or Z against no therapy. Such a trial, modeled on the diabetic retinopathy study, has been carried out at multiple centers in the United States.[150]

With regard to stage 5 disease[49] and its treatment by retina-vitreous surgery, no randomized trial would seem necessary, because these infants are blind from their disease. Among the proper questions any future studies of the modality must answer are: What is the proper time to undertake such surgical intervention? Presuming that surgery is successful and the retina is at least partially reattached anatomically, does it function and does the infant regain vision? These are difficult questions that can only be answered in the future by the most careful research designed to study the response of the

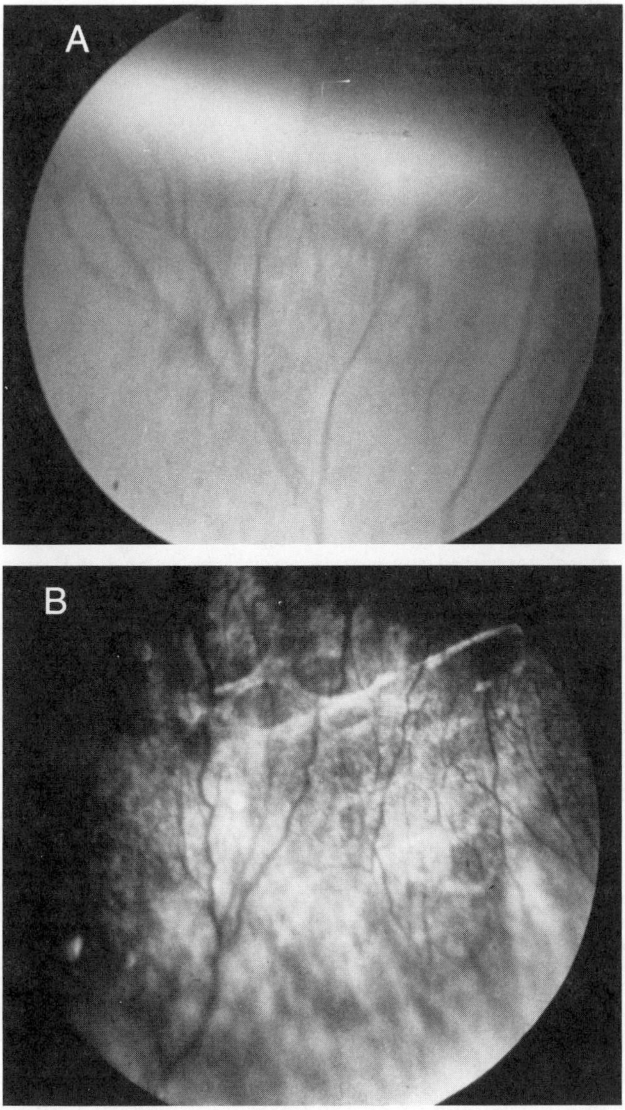


**FIG 6–17.**
**A**, fundus photograph of early regression of ROP with new vessel formation just breaking into the avascular retina. **B**, fundus photograph of late regression, showing the vitreoretinal interface changes at the site of the old shunt.

retina to this sophisticated form of surgery performed on the organ of sight.

In summary, then, therapy would have had no place in a review article on ROP even a decade ago. Today, it has a place. While the results of therapy are encouraging, it is necessary to maintain a healthy skepticism until the advantages of therapy for the premature infant are more clearly demonstrated.

## Medicolegal Aspects

Although the medicolegal aspects of ROP are perhaps not germane in a strictly scientific sense to a review of this type, I offer a few thoughts on this troubling and painful issue. Over the past 15 years it has been my unpleasant task to be involved in differing ways in over 30 malpractice actions against physicians, nurses, departments of pediatrics and divisions of neonatology, hospitals, and incubator manufacturers in the matter of ROP. Because of a simplistic equation firmly established in the literature dating back to the 1950s, that is, Prematurity + Oxygen = ROP, tort lawyers have taken the next step and rewritten the equation with the variation Prematurity + Oxygen = ROP = Malpractice. The questions debated in many of these legal proceedings, depositions, pre-trial hearings, and trials are often extraordinarily difficult scientific ones, for which the answers are not always available. Decisions of juries turn on evaluation not so much on the quality of the scientific information with which they are presented, but the *way* in which it is presented. In any event, no physician today, pediatrician or ophthalmologist, is immune from suit over ROP. Although it is not possible to be suit-proof, it is my belief that barring catastrophically incompetent legal representation, it is possible to be judgment-proof by maintaining, as a first step, careful records of the infant's in-hospital course, clearly noting the seriousness of the condition, and by justifying the necessity of the use of oxygen, both in durations and concentrations necessary to preserve both the infant's life and the quality of that life. Second, prompt diagnosis of any ROP should be carefully recorded, and when serious disease is present, there should be consultation with the best retina-vitreous surgeon available in the community. Third, there should be prompt and continuous communication with support of the parents by all the physicians involved with treating an infant with this tragic and difficult disease. For parents, perhaps no burden is heavier to bear than the lifetime responsibility for a child who is blind. It is my belief that with attention paid to these important details, many, if not all, lawsuits can be avoided, with primary attention focusing on the very real and challenging scientific aspects of this disease.

## SUMMARY

ROP has been a challenging disease in the 1980s and will continue to be challenging in the 1990s. Answers — even partial answers — to many of its questions may provide information that bears on those same questions in other blinding vascular retinopathies, such as diabetes and sickle cell disease. Answers that more clearly define the role of oxygen, ventilation, antioxidants, blood transfusions, and a host of diseases of the premature infant will lead to better care of these infants. This chapter has attempted to present the boundaries of the problem, a theory of its genesis and progression, and a review of the major issues that ROP continues to present to the pediatric, ophthalmological, and basic science communities. I have not hesitated to "editorialize" where I believe it is indicated. I have tried to make it clear to the reader when I was doing so. Because the field of ROP is growing rapidly I have used information liberally from studies under way and from those in the planning stages in order to make the reader aware of what is being done, even if this work has not yet reached fruition. Finally, I have tried to point out directions that I believe clinical and experimental work should take on certain critical issues. I have done this because I believe these issues are important, and therefore, make bold to add my say to what has been said and written about them. In so doing, I make no claim to infallibility, merely to a sense of curiosity and wonderment, as well as thought and concern about this disease that has fascinated me for almost 20 years.

## REFERENCES


1. Foos R: Chronic retinopathy of prematurity. *Ophthalmology* 1985; 92:563–574.
2. Flynn JT, Bancalari E, Bawol R., et al: Retinopathy of prematurity: Diagnosis, severity and natural history. *Ophthalmology* 1987; 94:620–629.
3. Terry TL: Extreme prematurity and fibroblastic overgrowth of persistent vascular sheath behind each crystalline lens. *Am J Ophthalmol* 1942; 25:203–204.
4. Silverman W: *Retrolental Fibroplasia: A Modern Parable.* New York, Grune & Stratton, 1980.
5. Zacharias L: Retrolental fibroplasia: A survey. *Am J Ophthalmol* 1952; 35:1426–1458.
6. Campbell K: Intensive oxygen therapy as a possible cause of retrolental fibroplasia: A clinical approach. *Med J Aust* 1951; 2:48–50.
7. Patz A, Hoech LE, DeLaCruz E: Studies on the effect of high oxygen administration in retrolental fibroplasia. I: Nursery observations. *Am J Ophthalmol* 1953; 35:1245–1253.
8. Kinsey VE: Retrolental fibroplasia. Cooperative study of retrolental fibroplasia and the use of oxygen. *Arch Ophthalmol* 56:481–543.

9. Lanman JT: Retrolental fibroplasia and oxygen therapy. *JAMA* 1954; 155:223–226.
10. Guy LP, Dancis J, Lanman JT: Retrolental fibroplasia. *NY State J Med* 1953; 53:2999–3002.
11. Guy LP, Lanman JT, Dancis J: The possibility of total elimination of retrolental fibroplasia by oxygen restriction. *Pediatrics* 1956; 17:247–251.
12. Slobody LB, Wasserman WE: *Survey of Clinical Pediatrics.* New York, McGraw-Hill, 1963, p 160.
13. Dunham EC, in Silverman WA (ed): *Premature Infants,* ed 3. New York, B Hoeber, 1961.
14. Avery ME, Oppenheimer EH: Recent increase in mortality from hyaline membrane disease. *J Pediatr* 1960; 57:553–559.
15. MacDonald AD: Neurological and ophthalmic disorders in children of very low birthweights. *Br Med J* 1962; 1:895–900.
16. Cross KW: Cost of preventing retrolental fibroplasia? *Lancet* 1973; 2:954–956.
17. American Academy of Pediatrics Committee on Fetus and Newborn: History of oxygen therapy and retrolental fibroplasia. *Pediatrics* 1976; 57(suppl 2):591–642.
18. Phelps DL: Retinopathy of prematurity: An estimate of vision loss in the United States in 1979. *Pediatrics* 1981; 67:924–926.
19. Kalina RE, Karr DJ: Retrolental fibroplasia: Experience over two decades in one instution. *Ophthalmology* 1982; 81:91–95.
20. Johnson L, Quinn G, Abassi S, et al: Decreasing incidence of retinopathy of prematurity (ROP) within birthweight groups. *ARVO Abstracts* 1987; p 119.
21. Ashton NW: Oxygen and the growth and development of retinal vessels. *Am J Ophthalmol* 1966; 62:412–435.
22. Michaelson IC: The mode of development of the vascular system of the retina with some observation on its significance for certain retinal diseases. *Trans Ophthalmol Soc UK* 1949; 68:137–180.
23. Cogan DG: Development and senescence of the human retinal vasculature. *Trans Ophthalmol Soc UK* 1963; 83:465–489.
24. Cogan DG, Kuwabara T: Accessory cells and vessels of the perinatal human retina. *Arch Ophthalmol* 1986; 104:747–752.
25. Flynn JT, O'Grady GE, Herrera J, et al: Retrolental fibroplasia. I: Clinical observations. *Arch Ophthalmol* 1977; 95:217–223.
26. Kushner B, Essner D, Cohen IJ, et al: Retrolental fibroplasia. II: Pathological correlation. *Arch Ophthalmol* 1977; 95:29–38.
27. Uemura Y: Current status of retrolental fibroplasia: Report of the Joint Committee for the Study of RLF: *Jpn J Ophthalmol* 1977; 21:366–378.
28. Kretzer FL, Hittner HM, Johnson AT, et al: Vitamin E and retrolental fibroplasia: Ultrastructural support of clinical efficacy. *Ann NY Acad Sci* 1982; 393:145–166.
29. Hittner HM, Godio LB, Speer ME, et al: Retrolental fibroplasia: Further clinical evidence and ultrastructural support for efficacy of vitamin E in the pre-term infant. *Pediatrics* 1983; 71:423–432.

30. Gole GA, Henderson D, Mukherjee T, et al: Vitamin E effect questioned. *Pediatrics* 1984; 73:734.
31. Reese AB: Persistence and hyperplasia of primary vitreous. Retrolental fibroplasia: Two entities. *Arch Ophthalmol* 1949; 41:527–552.
32. Reese AB: *Tumors of the Eye,* ed 2. New York, Harper & Row, 1963, pp 112–121.
33. Reese AB, King M, and Owens WC: Classification of retrolental fibroplasia. *Am J Ophthalmol* 1953; 38:1333–1335.
34. Kalina RE: Ophthalmic examination of children of low birthweight. *Am J Ophthalmol* 1962; 67:134–136.
35. Novotny HR, Alvis DL: A method of photographing fluorescence in circulating blood of the human eye. *Am J Ophthalmol* 1960; 50:176.
36. Patz A: The role of oxygen in retrolental fibroplasia. *Trans Am Ophthalmol Soc* 1968; 66:940–985.
37. Patz A: Retrolental fibroplasia. *Surv Ophthalmol* 1969; 14:1–29.
38. Patz A: Retrolental fibroplasia (retinopathy of prematurity). *Am J Ophthalmol* 1982; 94:552–554.
39. Patz A: A new role of the ophthalmologist in prevention of retrolental fibroplasia. *Arch Ophthalmol* 1967; 78:565–568.
40. Cantolino SJ, O'Grady GE, Herrera JA, et al: Ophthalmoscopic monitoring of oxygen therapy in premature infants. *Am J Ophthalmol* 1971; 72:322–331.
41. Cantolino SJ, Curran JS, Van Caden TC, et al: Acute retrolental fibroplasia: Classification and objective evaluation of incidence, natural history and resolution by fundus photography and intravenous fluorescein angiography. *Perspect Ophthalmol* 1978; 2:175–187.
42. Kingham JD: Acute retrolental fibroplasia. *Arch Ophthalmol* 1977; 95:39–47.
43. Uemura Y, Akiyama K: Classification of active retinopathy of prematurity. *Retinopathy Prematurity Conf* 1981; 1:253–263.
44. Nagata M, Tsuruoka Y: Treatment of acute retrolental fibroplasia with xenon arc photocoagulation. *Jpn J Ophthalmol* 1972; 16:131–143.
45. Foos RY: Acute retrolental fibroplasia. *Graefes Arch Clin Exp Ophthalmol* 1975; 195:87–100.
46. McCormick AQ: Retinopathy of prematurity: Current problems. *Pediatrics* 1977; 7:1–28.
47. Flynn JT: Notes on a classification of acute proliferative retrolental fibroplasia (retinopathy of prematurity). *Retinopathy Prematurity Conf* 1981; 1:247–252.
48. Committee on Classification of Retinopathy of Prematurity: An international classification of retinopathy of prematurity. *Arch Ophthalmol* 1984; 102:1130–1134.
49. An international classification of retinopathy of prematurity. II: The classification of retinal detachment. Committee for Classification of Late Stages of Retinopathy of Prematurity. *Arch Ophthalmol* 1987; 105:906–912.
50. Altman LK: Premature children show rise in a baffling eye disorder. *The New York Times,* Feb 28, 1984.
51. Gordon HH: Perspectives on neonatology, in Avery JB (ed): *Neonatology,*

*Pathophysiology and Management of the Newborn,* ed 2. Philadelphia, JB Lippincott, 1981, pp 3–12.
52. Jones RA, Cummins M, Davis PA: Intensive care and the very low birthweight infant. *Lancet* 1979; 2:523.
53. Hack H, Fanaroff AA, Merkatz IR: The low birthweight infant—Evolution of a changing outlook. *N Engl J Med* 1979; 301:1162–1165.
54. LaGamma EF, Auld PAM: Mortality patterns in the infant under 1000 grams. *Pediatr Res* 1980; 14:603.
55. Wegman ME: Annual summary of vital statistics — 1978. *Pediatrics* 1979; 64:835–842.
56. McCormick AQ: Personal communication, 1985.
57. Treu A, Bossi E, Koerner F: Epidemiological study of severe vision impairment in Swiss children with special reference to retrolental fibroplasia. *Schweiz Med Wochenschr* 1987; 117:359–364.
58. Flynn JT: Acute proliferative retrolental fibroplasia: Multivariate risk analysis. *Trans Am Ophthalmol Soc* 1983; 81:549–591.
59. McCormick M: Contribution of the low birthweight infant to mortality and morbidity, submitted for publication.
60. Kinsey VE, Arnold HJ, Kalina RE, et al: $PaO_2$ levels and retrolental fibroplasia: A report of the cooperative study. *Pediatrics* 1977; 60:655–668.
61. Commentaries: Caution about statistics of retrolental fibroplasia Study. *Pediatrics* 1977; 60:754–756.
62. Commentaries: Oxygen and retrolental fibroplasia: The questions persist. *Pediatrics* 1977; 60:753–754.
63. Silverman WA: Retinopathy of prematurity: Oxygen dogma challenged. *Arch Dis Child* 1982; 57:731–733.
64. Adamkin DH, Shott RJ, Cook LN, et al: Non-hyperoxic retrolental fibroplasia. *Pediatrics* 1977; 60:828–830.
65. Karlsberg RC, Green WR, Patz A: Congenital retrolental fibroplasia. *Arch Ophthalmol* 1973; 89:122–123.
66. Stafani FH, Ehalt H: Non-oxygen induced retinitis proliferans and retinal detachment in full-term infants. *Br J Ophthalmol* 1974; 58:490–513.
67. Kraushar MF, Harper RG, Siag C: Retrolental fibroplasia in a full-term infant. *Am J Ophthalmol* 1975; 80:106–108.
68. Brockhurst RJ, Chisti MI: Cicatricial retrolental fibroplasia: Its occurrence without oxygen administration and in full-term infants. *Graefes Arch Clin Exp Ophthalmol* 1975; 195:113–128.
69. Addison DJ, Font FL, Manshot WA: Proliferative retinopathy in anencephalic babies. *Am J Ophthalmol* 1972; 74:967–976.
70. Kalina RE, Hodson WA, Morgan BC: Retrolental fibroplasia in a cyanotic infant. *Pediatrics* 1972; 50:765–768.
71. Aranda JV, Sweet AY: Sustained hyperoxemia without cicatricial retrolental fibroplasia. *Pediatrics* 1974; 54:434–437.
72. Huch A, Huch R: New method for arterial blood sampling. *Arch Dis Child* 1973; 48:982–983.

73. Huch A, Lubbers DW, Huch R: Continuous $PO_2$ and heart rate recording in the human newborn. *Adv Exp Med Biol* 1976; 75:737–745.
74. Horbar JD, Clark JT, Lucey JF: The newborn oxygram: Automated processing of transcutaneous oxygen data. *Pediatrics* 1980; 56:848–851.
75. Bancalari E, Flynn JT, Goldberg R, et al: Influence of continuous transcutaneous oxygen monitoring on the incidence of retinopathy of prematurity. *Pediatrics* 1987; 79:663–669.
76. Flynn JT, Bancalari E, Gillings D, et al: Retinopathy of prematurity: A randomized prospective trial of transcutaneous oxygen monitoring. *Ophthalmology* 1987; 94:630–637.
77. Catlin, Carpenter MW, Brand BS, et al: The Apgar score revisited: Influence of gestational age. *J Pediatr* 1986; 109:865–868.
78. Feeney L, Berman ER: Oxygen toxicity: Membrane damage by free radicals. *Invest Ophthalmol* 1976; 15:789–792.
79. Fridovich I: The biology of oxygen radicals. *Science* 1978; 201:875–880.
80. Michaelson PE, Patz A, Howell RR: Oxygen studies in retrolental fibroplasia. *Ann Ophthalmol* 1970; 2:773–780.
81. Gerke E, Spitzhas M: Retinal enzyme activities under hypoxic conditions prior to neovascularization. *Graefes Arch Clin Exp Ophthalmol* 1977; 202:101–107.
82. Bougle D, Vert P, Reichart E, et al: Retinal superoxide dysmutase activity in newborn kittens exposed to normobaric hyperoxia: Effects of vitamin E. *Retinopathy Prematurity Conf* 1981; 1:227–242.
83. Katz M: Protection against autoxidante damage to the retina: Molecular and cellular mechanisms, submitted for publication.
84. Rothman JM: Causes. *Am J Epidemiol* 1976; 104:587–592.
85. Evans HW, Bishop KS: On the relationship between fertility and nutrition: The ovulatory rhythm of rats with inadequate nutrition. *J Metab Res* 1922; 1:319–356.
86. Evans HW, Emerson G: Isolation from wheat germ oil of an alpha tocopherol alcohol having properties of vitamin E. *J Biochem* 1936; 113:319–332.
87. Owens WC, Owens EU: Retrolental fibroplasia in premature infants. II. Studies on the prophylaxis of the disease. The use of alpha tocopherol acetate. *Am J Ophthalmol* 1949; 32:1631–1637.
88. Kinsey VE, Chisholm JF: Retrolental fibroplasia: Evaluation of several changes in dietary supplements of premature infants with respect to the incidence of the disease. *Am J Ophthalmol* 1951; 34:1259–1268.
89. Johnson LH, Schaffer DB, Goldstein DE: Influence of vitamin E treatment and adult blood transfusion on mean severity of retrolental fibroplasia in premature infants. *Pediatr Res* 1971; 11:534.
90. Phelps DL, Rosenbaum AL: Vitamin E protection in experimental retrolental fibroplasia in kittens. *Clin Res* 1976; 24:194(N).
91. Hittner HM, Godio LB, Rudolph AJ, et al: Retrolental fibroplasia: Efficacy of Vitamin E in a double blind clinical study of pre-term infants. *N Engl J Med* 1981; 305:1365–1371.

92. Puklin JE, Simon RM, Ehrenkrantz RA: Influence on retrolental fibroplasia of intramuscular vitamin E during respiratory distress syndrome. *Ophthalmology* 1982; 89:96–103.
93. Milner RA, Watts JL, Paes B, et al: Retrolental fibroplasia in 1500 gram neonates: Part of a randomized clinical trial of the effectiveness of Vitamin E. *Retinopathy Prematurity Conf* 2:703–716.
94. Finer NN, Schindler RE, Grant G, et al: Effect of intramuscular Vitamin E on the frequency and severity of retrolental fibroplasia: A controlled trial. *Lancet* 1982; 1:1087.
95. Phelps DL: Vitamin E and retrolental fibroplasia in 1982. *Pediatrics* 1982; 70:420–424.
96. Johnson L, Bowen FW, Abbasi S, et al: Relationship of prolonged pharmacologic serum levels of Vitamin E to incidence of sepsis and necrotizing enterocolitis in infants with birth weight 1,500 grams or less. *Pediatrics* 1985; 4:619–638.
97. Phelps DL, Rosenbaum A, Isenberg S, et al: Tocopherol efficacy and safety for preventing retinopathy of prematurity: A randomized, controlled, double-masked trial. *Pediatrics* 1987; 79:489–500.
98. Rosenbaum A, Phelps D, Isenberg S: Retinal hemorrhage in retinopathy of prematurity associated with tocopherol treatment. *Ophthalmology* 1985; 92:1012–1014.
99. Roberts HJ: Perspectives of vitamin E as therapy. *JAMA* 1981; 246:129–131.
100. Biesel WR, Edelman R, Nauss K, et al: Single nutrient effects on immunologic functions: Report of a workshop sponsored by the Department of Food and Nutrition Advisory Group of the American Medical Association. *JAMA* 1981; 245:53–58.
101. Prasad JS: Effect of vitamin E supplementation on leukocyte function. *Am J Clin Nutr* 1980; 33:606–608.
102. Smith TJ, Buchanan MF, Goss I: Vitamin E in retrolental fibroplasia. *N Engl J Med* 1983; 390:669–670.
103. Committee of the Institute of Medicine: *Vitamin E and Retinopathy of Prematurity.* Washington, DC: National Academy of Medicine Press, 1986, pp 1–24.
104. Flowers R: A new perspective on the pathogenesis of retrolental fibroplasia: The influence of elevated arterial $CO_2$. *Retinopathy Prematurity Conf* 1981; 1:20–45.
105. Flowers R, Blake DA, Waser SD: Retrolental fibroplasia: Evidence for a role of the prostaglandin cascade in the pathogenesis of oxygen-induced retinopathy in the newborn beagle. *Pediatr Res* 1982; 15:1293–1302.
106. Hickam JB, Fraser R: Studies on the retinal circulation in man: Observations on vessel diameter, arteriovenous oxygen difference and mean circulation time. *Circulation* 1966; 33:302–316.
107. Tsacoupoulas M, David NJ: The effect of arterial $PO_2$ on relative retinal blood flow in monkeys. *Invest Ophthalmol* 1973; 12:335–347.
108. Bauer CR, Widmayer SM: A relationship between $PaCO_2$ and retrolental fibroplasia (RLF). *Pediatr Res* 1981; 15:649.

109. Biglan AW, Brown DR, Reynolds JD, et al: The interrelationship of blood oxygen, carbon dioxide and ph level and the production of retrolental fibroplasia. *Ophthalmology* 1984; 91:1504–1511.
110. Brown DR, Milley JR, Repipi U, et al: Retinopathy of prematurity: Risk factors in a five year cohort of critically ill premature neonates. *Am J Dis Child* 1987; 141:154–160.
111. Sun XC, Aranda Z, Kamtorn V, et al: Indomethacin and retrolental fibroplasia. *Retinopathy Prematurity Conf* 1981; 2:522–525.
112. Gersony WM, Peckham GJ, Ellison RC: Effects of indomethacin in premature infants with patent ductus arteriosus: Results of a national collaborative study. *J Pediatr* 1983; 102:895–906.
113. Oski FA: Hematologic problems, in Avery GB (ed): *Neonatology: Pathophysiology and Management of the Newborn* ed 2. Philadelphia, JB Lippincott, 1981, pp 544–582.
114. Majima A: Problems on retinopathy of prematurity: Statistical analysis of factors related to occurrence and progression of retinopathy and fundus appearance and ocular functions in prematurely born subjects. *Jpn J Ophthalmol* 1977; 21:404–420.
115. Aranda JV, Clark TE, Maniello R, et al: Blood transfusions: Possible potentiating risk factor in retrolental fibroplasia. *Pediatr Res* 1975; 9:362.
116. Sacks LJ, Schaffer DB, Anday EK, et al: Retrolental fibroplasia and blood transfusion in very low birthweight infants. *Pediatrics* 1981; 68:770–774.
117. Clark C, Gibbs JH, Maniello R, et al: Blood transfusions: A possible risk factor in retrolental fibroplasia. *Acta Paediatr Scand* 1971; 70:535–543.
118. Mittelman D, Cronin C: Relationship of blood transfusion and retrolental fibroplasia. *Retinopathy Prematurity Conf* 1981; 2:526–535.
119. Procianoy RS, Garcia-Pratis JA, Hittner HM, et al: An association between retinopathy of prematurity and interventricular hemorrhage in very low birthweight infants. *Acta Paediatr Scand* 1981; 70:473–477.
120. Flynn JT, Cassady J, Essner D, et al: Fluorescein angiogram in retrolental fibroplasia: Experience from 1969–1971. *Ophthalmology* 1979; 86:1700–1723.
121. Bossi E, Koerner F, Zulaf M: Retinopathy of prematurity: Risk factors — a statistical analysis of matched pairs. *Retinopathy Prematurity Conf* 1981; 2:536–539.
122. Glass P, Avery GB, Siva Subramanian KN: Effect of bright light in the hospital nursery on the incidence of retinopathy of prematurity. *N Engl J Med* 1985; 333:401–404.
123. Lakatos L, Hatvani I, Oroszlan G, et al: Controlled trial of D-Penicillamine to prevent retinopathy of prematurity. *Acta Paediatr Hung* 1986; 27:47–56.
124. Palmer EA: Optimal timing of examination for acute retrolental fibroplasia. *Ophthalmology* 1981; 88:662–668.
125. Brown DR, Biglan A, Stretavsky M: Screening criteria for the detection of ROP in patients in a neonatal intensive care unit, submitted for publication.
126. Bauer CR, Trottier MCT, Stern L: Systemic cyclopentolate (Cyclogyl) toxicity in the newborn infant. *J Pediatr* 1973; 82:501–505.

127. Borromeo-McGrail V, Bordiuk JM, Keitel H: Systemic hypertension following ocular administration of 10% phenylephrine in the neonate. *Pediatrics* 1973; 51:1032–1036.
128. Kushner BJ: Strabismus and amblyopia associated with regressed retinopathy of prematurity. *Arch Ophthalmol* 1982; 100:256–261.
129. Ben-Sira I, Nissenkorn I, Weinberger D, et al: Long term results of cryotherapy for active stages of retinopathy of prematurity. *Ophthalmology* 1981; 93:1423–1428.
130. Stark DJ, Manning LM, Lenton L: Retrolental fibroplasia today. *Med J Aust* 1981; 1:278–280.
131. Schaffer DB, Quinn GE, Johnson L: Sequelae of arrested mild retinopathy of prematurity. *Arch Ophthalmol* 1984; 102:373–377.
132. Diabetic Retinal Research Study Group: Photocoagulation treatment of proliferative diabetic retinopathy. *Ophthalmology* 1981; 88:583–601.
133. Machemer R: *Vitrectomy: A Pars Plana Approach.* New York, Grune & Stratton, 1975.
134. Nagata M, Kobayashi Y, Fukuda H, et al: Photocoagulation for the treatment of retinopathy of prematurity. *Jpn J Clin Ophthalmol* 1968; 22:419–427.
135. Payne JM, Patz A: Treatment of acute proliferative retrolental fibroplasia. *Trans Am Acad Ophthalmol Otolaryngol* 1972; 76:1234–1241.
136. Kingham JD: Acute retrolental fibroplasia. II: Treatment by cryosurgery. *Arch Ophthalmol* 1978; 96:2044–2053.
137. Mousel KD, Hoyt CS: Cryotherapy for retinopathy of prematurity. *Ophthalmology* 1980; 87:1121–1127.
138. Harris GS, McCormick AQ: The prophylactic treatment of retrolental fibroplasia. *Mod Probl Ophthalmol* 1977; 18:364–367.
139. Hindle NW, Leyton J: Prevention of cicatricial retrolental fibroplasia by cryotherapy. *Can J Ophthalmol* 1978; 13:277–282.
140. Ben-Sira I, Nissenkorn I, Grunwald E, et al: Treatment of acute retrolental fibroplasia by cryopexy. *Br J Ophthalmol* 1980; 64:758–762.
141. McPherson A, Hittner HM: Scleral buckling for 2 1/2 to 11 month-old premature infants with retina detachments associated with acute retrolental fibroplasia. *Ophthalmology* 1979; 86:819–835.
142. McPherson A, Hittner HM, Lemos R: Retinal detachment in young prematures with acute retrolental fibroplasia: Thirty-two new cases. *Ophthalmology* 1982; 89:1160–1169.
143. Machemer R: Closed vitrectomy for severe retrolental fibroplasia in the infant. *Ophthalmology* 1983; 90:426–441.
144. Machemer R: Description and pathogenesis of late stages of retinopathy of prematurity. *Ophthalmology* 1985; 1000–1004.
145. Tasman W: Late complication of retrolental fibroplasia. *Ophthalmology* 1979; 86:1724–1740.
146. Charles S: Vitreous surgery for retinopathy of prematurity (ROP). *Retinopathy Prematurity Conf* 1981; 2:858–863.
147. Charles S: *Vitreous Microsurgery.* Baltimore, Williams & Wilkins, 1981, pp 159–160.

148. Paulman H: Pars plana vitrectomy in retrolental fibroplasia. *Retinopathy Prematurity Conf* 1981; 2:893–902.
149. Hirose T, Schedens DL, Lopahsri C: Subtotal open sky vitrectomy for severe retinal detachment occurring as late complication of ocular trauma. *Ophthalmology* 1981; 88:1–9.
150. Multicenter trial of cryotherapy for retinopathy of prematurity. Preliminary results. Cryotherapy for Retinopathy of Prematurity Cooperative Group. *Arch Ophthalmol* 1988; 106:471–479.
151. Editorial: Retrolental fibroplasia (RLF) unrelated to oxygen therapy. *Br J Ophthalmol* 1974; 58:487–489.
152. Flynn JT, Bancalari E, Bawol R, et al: Retinopathy of prematurity: A randomized, prospective trial of transcutaneous oxygen monitoring. *Ophthalmology* 1987; 94:630–637.
153. Johnson L, Schaffer D, Boggs TR: The premature infant, vitamin E deficiency and retrolental fibroplasia. *Am J Clin Nutr* 1974; 27:1158–1171.

Chapter 7

# Rationale for Successful Treatment of Retinopathy of Prematurity: Historical Analysis

Albert L. Ackerman, M.D.
Harvey W. Topilow, M.D.

The treatment of retinopathy of prematurity (ROP) can be divided historically into two periods: an early stage, from 1940 to 1960, when the condition was known as retrolental fibrolasia (RLF), and a recent stage, from the 1970s to the present, when the terminology was changed to ROP.[1] While sharing a common end-stage of cicatricial fibrosis, the etiologies of the conditions are different (Table 7–1).

In 1942, the classic paper of Terry,[2] described a condition in premature babies that resulted in blindness caused by retrolental fibrosis. The treatment that evolved during the 1950s was aimed at prevention by carefully monitoring and restricting oxygen. This was based on epidemiologic, experimental, and statistical evidence suggesting that oxygen toxicity was the prime factor in RLF. By controlling the duration and concentration of the oxygen, it was believed the condition could be prevented.

The investigative techniques available in that era included histologic examination of the retina, direct ophthalmoscopy, and experimental animal models. Certain facts were established. Blood vessels are not present in the human retina prior to four months gestation. The retina is not completely vascularized until term. Nasally, the retina is fully vascularized at eight months gestation, and temporally it is fully vascularized at 9 months. Immature retinal vessels are sensitive to oxygen and respond by vasoconstric-

**TABLE 7–1.**
Historical Phases and Treatment of Retinopathy of Prematurity

| | Phase I 1940–1960 | Phase II 1960–Present |
|---|---|---|
| Terminology | Retrolental fibroplasia (RLF) | Retinopathy of prematurity (ROP) |
| Cause | Oxygen toxicity | Prematurity |
| Birth weight (gm) | >1,500 | <1,500 |
| Treatment | Oxygen monitoring | Cryotherapy |

tion.[3] This primary vasoconstriction response is proportional to the concentration and duration of oxygen, as demonstrated in kittens.[4]

The rapid accumulation of clinical cases with retrolental fibroplasia was the result of a number of factors, including the development and increased availability of incubators, and the prevailing attitude that more oxygen was healthier. Consequently, in major hospital centers where oxygen was easily available, cases of RLF reached epidemic proportions, compared to smaller, regional institutions where cost was a factor and oxygen was restricted.

The Campbell report from Australia[5] contrasted the low incidence of RLF in hospitals not supplying oxygen because of additional expense with the very high incidence in those hospitals in which oxygen was used more extensively. Controlled series by Lanman[6] and Kinsey[7] pointed to oxygen therapy as the prime factor in RLF. By the 1960s, with oxygen restriction, the condition was exceedingly uncommon. This was accomplished by eliminating nonessential oxygen, and when oxygen was necessary, by restricting the concentration to 40%. The responsibility for the prevention of RLF then transferred to the pediatrician. In those cases in which oxygen was administered, monitoring of retinal vessels by direct ophthalmoscopy was advised.

The description of the condition at that time was well summarized by Duke-Elder,[8] who considered RLF an iatrogenic disease: "It is the usual biological (and human) response of a tissue refusing to struggle to develop when placed in a well intentioned but too luxurious environment and ridiculously overstriving when faced with the facts of life."

During the 1960s there was a marked reduction in the incidence of RLF and it became a distinct rarity. In the 1970s, however, cases began to reappear. By 1979 it was estimated that the annual number of infants blinded by ROP in the United States was 546, a figure comparable to that recorded during the peak years of the original epidemic, 1943–1953.[1]

A number of new and different factors were responsible for this change. Primarily, the emergence of neonatology as a pediatric subspecialty devoted to the care and treatment of premature infants markedly improved these infants' survival rates. At that time, the mortality rate of infants with birth weights below 1,500 gm was 70%. In the 1980s, however, the survival rate of infants weighing between 1,000 and 1,500 gm reached 80%.

Improved management of pediatric problems, including hyaline membrane disease, intraventricular cerebral hemorrhage, and infectious diseases, resulted in increased survival rates for extremely premature infants, with a concomitantly sharp increase in the incidence of retinopathy of prematurity. It was soon apparent that despite careful control of arterial oxygen levels, using the previously recommended criteria, cases of ROP were occurring with increasing frequency. Retinopathy of prematurity was now a disease not of oxygen excess, but a consequence of prematurity.

By the mid-1960s new ophthalmic techniques, unavailable in the 1950s, enabled clinicians to arrive at different interpretations and new therapeutic approaches to this problem. First and foremost was the development of binocular indirect ophthalmoscopy with scleral depression. Developed by Dr. Charles Schepens,[9] this technique revolutionized the examination of the retina. The indirect ophthalmoscope made it possible to identify and interpret the earliest stages of the disease in the extreme retinal periphery, a circumferential area previously not visualized using direct ophthalmoscopy.

Second, in 1948, Michaelson[10] postulated that the developing retina liberated a chemical substance that stimulated retinal neovascularization. In 1954, Ashton[4] theorized the release of the vasoformative factor from hypoxic retina. These two concepts were applied to interpreting the likely mechanism underlying the development of preretinal neovascularization in ROP.

Third, the development of fluorescein angiography identified the entity of capillary nonperfusion. Thus, all of the seemingly unrelated diseases such as diabetic retinopathy, sickle cell disease, and branch retinal vein occlusion were linked into a homogeneous pathologic group: they all showed capillary nonperfusion. Included in this category of proliferative retinopathy was ROP.[11]

Finally, in the 1960s the successful treatment of proliferative diabetic retinopathy began with the empiric spot treatment of abnormal new vessels using xenon arc photocoagulation. Subsequently in the 1970s, treatment of broad areas of nonperfused retina with laser and cryotherapy, without regard to location of neovascularization, resulted in striking involution and obliteration of the new vessels.

When the premature retina is examined using indirect ophthalmoscopy, it is apparent that starting at the ora serrata there is a peripheral avascular circumferential zone of varying width that indirectly correlates with the infant's birth weight and gestational age. The wider the avascular zone, the more likely it is that extensive preretinal neovascularization will develop.[13, 14]

ROP initially develops as a ridge that represents an arterio-venous shunt system at the posterior border of the avascular zone, accompanied by dilatation and tortuousity of the retinal vessels at the posterior pole. The undulating arterioles and widened retinal venules are often quite spectacular, in contrast to the quiet appearance of the broad, anteriorly located circumferential avascular zone, which is really the origin of the conflagration that often follows. It is this zone that presumably produces a chemical factor that stimulates new vessel growth.

Recognition of this condition, designated now as stage 3+ ROP[15] is crucial in the treatment of retinopathy of prematurity. Ablation of the avascular area only, with resultant rapid resolution of the untreated neovascularization, confirms the pathogenesis of the neovascularization in ROP. This is analogous to proliferative diabetic retinopathy, in which panretinal photocoagulation, in ablating the ischemic retina, causes involution of preretinal and disc neovascularization.

The history of the current therapeutic approach to ROP is similar to the treatment of retinal detachment. In both diseases a variety of surgical approaches in vogue at the time were tried with variable results. These surgical approaches represented misdirected attempts at treating retinal detachment and contained little specific therapeutic rationale for treating ROP. In the case of retinal detachment, sealing the retinal break resulted in reattachment of the retina in a once hopeless condition. With ROP, attempts at obliterating the neovascularization using the modalities of the time, including xenon arc, argon laser, and cryotherapy, met with varying degree of success, leading to great controversy.

It appears inevitable that in ophthalmology especially in retinal disorders, controversy will accompany every significant therapeutic advance. Consider the history of treatment of retinal detachment, age-related macular degeneration, and diabetic retinopathy.

With retinopathy of prematurity, controversy regarding the efficacy of cryotherapy was based on the conflicting results of treatment. These results depended on which stage was treated and whether or not the avascular zone was included in the treatment. Cryotherapy applied to the neovascular shunt has resulted in complications including hemorrhage and accelerated vitreous involvement with proliferative vitreoretinopathy. If the avascular zone was included in the treatment, the success rate improved. When a rational approach suggested that only the avascular zone required treatment, the success rate improved dramatically.[12–14]

Thus, in the 1970s Japanese investigators treated the demarcation line in stage 2, and the ridge in stage 3 with the immediately adjacent avascular zone.[16–18] Hindel and Leyton,[19] in Canada, treated the ridge, and the retina anterior and posterior to it. Direct treatment to the obvious neovascularization was the aim.

A different approach to treatment was suggested based on the rationale of McPherson, Hittner, and Kretzer,[20] who advocated treatment of the ridge and adjacent posterior avascular zone to obliterate the spindle cells, the presumed source of the angiogenic factor.

Ben Sira and Nissenkorn avoided treatment of the neovascular ridge and advocated treatment of the avascular zone only. Initially the technique was developed to prevent the complication of vitreous hemorrhage. However, in 1980[12] they considered ROP an ischemic retinopathy and stated that destruction of the avascular zone reduced the formation of a vasoformative substance, causing arrest of the disease.

Topilow and Ackerman[13] elaborated further on the similarity of ROP and proliferative diabetic retinopathy, emphasizing the width of the avascular zone as a prognostic factor and defining the role of cryotherapy in treatment.

With cryotherapy, it is important to use temperatures appropriate for premature infants. The tissue temperature required for retinal ablation is approximately −5° C. In adults it is necessary to use a cryoprobe with a tip temperature of −65° to −85° C in order to overcome the effects of the choroidal blood flow which acts as a heat sink. In the premature infant where the choroid is thin, we have found a probe temperature of −55° C to be ideal.

Lower temperatures can result in overtreatment, with possible complications such as hemorrhage, retinal tears, and freezing of the vitreous with subsequent condensation and traction.

Misconceptions have abounded regarding the efficacy of cryotherapy for proliferative ROP. The obvious aim of any treatment modality is to prevent retinal detachment. Cryotherapy reduces the incidence of retinal detachment by inducing regression of preretinal neovascularization. The criteria for success with cryotherapy is therefore resolution of neovascularization. If vitreous condensation has already occurred at the time of treatment, leading to eventual retinal detachment, then this new complication is more appropriately treated with scleral buckling[14] or vitrectomy techniques[21] designed to release vitreoretinal traction.

In keeping with the analogy to diabetic retinopathy, when treatment was directed to the avascular zone only, the success rate increased impressively. By eliminating the vasoformative factor, the untreated new vessels regressed, the tortuosity of the posterior pole vessels resolved, and the normal retinal vessels continued their growth to the periphery. As in diabetes, however, depending on the degree of vitreous involvement at the time of surgical ablation and the extent of preretinal neovascularization, cryotherapy did not completely prevent the proliferative changes from causing retinal detachment. In many cases this progression was managed successfully with conventional scleral buckling techniques,[13, 14] and in advanced cases, with open-sky vitrectomy.[21]

Despite the striking clinical findings of rapid resolution of vascular tortuosity and preretinal neovascularization following cryotherapy for stage 3+ ROP, convincing proof of the effectiveness of cryotherapy was required by those not versatile with indirect ophthalmoscopy. The requirement of statistical proof led to controlled clinical trials that compared treated and untreated cases.[22]

Although the actual angiogenic factor has not been isolated, its presumed presence has changed our thinking about ROP. Rather than incriminating oxygen and monitoring its use, observation of the peripheral retina is now essential. The wider the avascular zone, the worse the prognosis, and the more frequently these infants must be examined. In contrast to diabetic retinopathy, in ROP the progression from a developing shunt to florid neovascularization and subsequent retinal detachment can occur within a few weeks. In effect, advanced proliferative ROP acts like an accelerated diabetic retinopathy.

The responsibility for monitoring cases of ROP has returned to the ophthalmologist. It is essential to recognize the hazardous potential of a wide avascular zone. Prompt treatment of the avascular zone in eyes with stage 3+ disease and extensive preretinal neovascularization using cryotherapy result in resolution of neovascularization, usually with prevention of retinal detachment. These eyes retain the potential for excellent visual acuity.[23]

## REFERENCES


1. Ashton N: Retrolental fibroplasia now retinopathy of prematurity (editorial): *Br J Ophthalmol* 1984; 68:689.
2. Terry TL: Extreme prematurity and fibroplastic overgrowth of persistant vascular sheath behind each crystalline lens I. Preliminary report. *Am J Ophthalmol* 1942; 25:203–204.
3. Patz A, Eastham A, Higgenbotham DH, et al: Oxygen studies in retrolental fibroplasia: II: The production of the microscopic changes of retrolental fibroplasia in experimental animals. *Am J Ophthalmol* 1953; 36:1511.
4. Ashton N, Cook C: Direct observation of the effect of oxygen on developing vessels, Preliminary report, *Brit Ophthal*, 1954; 38:433–440, 1954; 38:291–308.
5. Campbell K: Intensive oxygen therapy as a possible cause of retrolental fibroplasia: A clinical approach. *Med J Aust* 1951; 2:48–50.
6. Lanman JT, Guy LP, Dancis J: Retrolental fibroplasia and oxygen therapy. *JAMA* 1954; 155:223–226.
7. Kinsey VE: Retrolental fibroplasia. Cooperative study of retrolental fibroplasia and the use of oxygen. *Arch Ophthalmol* 1956; 56:481–543.
8. Duke-Elder S: Retrolental fibroplasia. The retinopathy of prematurity. *Diseases of the Retina*. Vol 10, St. Louis, CV Mosby, 1967, pp 187–198.
9. Schepens CL: A new ophthalmoscope demonstration. *Trans Am, Acad Ophthalmol* 1947, 51:298.

10. Michaelson IC: *Retinal Circulation in Man and Animals*. Springfield, Ill, Charles C Thomas, Publisher, 1954.
11. Flynn JT: Fluorescein angiography in retrolental fibroplasia: Experience from 1969–1977. *Ophthalmology* 1974; 86:1700–1723.
12. Ben Sira I, Nissenkorn I, Grunwald E: Treatment of acute retrolental fibroplasia by cryopexy. *Br J Ophthalmol* 1980; 64:758–762.
13. Topilow HW, Ackerman AL, Wang FM: The treatment of advanced retinopathy of prematurity by cryotherapy and scleral buckling surgery. *Ophthalmology* 1985; 92:379–387.
14. Topilow HW, Ackerman AL, Wang F, et al: Successful treatment of advanced retinopathy of prematurity. *Ophthalmic Surg,* 1988; 19:781–785.
15. The Committee for Classification of Retinopathy of Prematurity: An international classification of retinopathy of prematurity. *Arch Ophthalmol* 1984; 102:1130–1134.
16. Nagata M: Treatment of acute proliferative retrolental fibroplasia with xenon arc photocoagulation: Its indications and limitations. *Jpn J Ophthalmol* 1977; 21:436–459.
17. Tamai M: Treatment of acute retinopathy of prematurity by cryotherapy and photocoagulation, in McPherson A, Hittner H, Kretzer F (eds): *Retinopathy of Prematurity: Current Concepts and Controversies*. Toronto, BC Decker, 1986, pp 151–159.
18. Majima A, Takahashi M, Hibino Y, Kamao N, Takai M: Clinical observation of photocoagulation on retinopathy of prematurity. *Jpn J Clin Ophthalmol* 1976; 30:93–97.
19. Hindle NW, Leyton J: Prevention of cicatricial retrolental fibroplasia by cryotherapy. *Can J Ophthalmol* 1978; 13:277–282.
20. McPherson A, Hittner H, Kretzer F (eds): *Current Concepts and Controversies. Retinopathy of Prematurity*. Toronto, BC Decker, pp 161–178.
21. Hirose T, Schepens CL: Open sky vitrectomy in retrolental fibroplasia. Presented at American Academy of Ophthalmology Annual Meeting, Atlanta, Nov 12, 1984.
22. Cryotherapy for Retinopathy of Prematurity Cooperative Group: Multicenter trial of cryotherapy for retinopathy of prematurity. *Arch Ophthalmol* 1988; 106:471–479.
23. Topilow HW, Ackerman AL: Cryotherapy for stage 3+ retinopathy of prematurity: Visual and anatomic results. (Presented at American Academy of Ophthalmology Annual Meeting, Las Vegas, Oct 11, 1988.) *Ophthalmic Surg,* in press.

Chapter 8

# Cryotherapy for Advanced Stage 3+ Retinopathy of Prematurity

Harvey W. Topilow, M.D.
Albert L. Ackerman, M.D.

With the advent of modern neonatal intensive care, the smallest, most immature preterm infants who are at greatest risk for developing severe retinopathy of prematurity (ROP), are surviving in increasing numbers.[1] With improved survival, the risk of blindness from sequelae of ROP, including macular distortion and traction retinal detachment, is also increasing. Over the past decade, studies indicating the effectiveness of cryotherapy for active ROP have varied in technique and rationale.[2–13] In 1982, we began treating both eyes of all infants with ROP who had severe arteriolar tortuousity, venous dilatation, peripheral elevated arteriovenous (AV) shunt formation at the posterior border of a wide avascular zone, and at least 180 degrees of preretinal neovascularization along the shunt.

We had found that this subset of eyes with advanced proliferative ROP, now classified as stage 3+,[14] would invariably progress to total traction retinal detachment without therapy.

We present our results of the treatment of 50 consecutive eyes of 25 very premature infants with stage 3+ ROP. The rationale for cryotherapy in this disorder, indications for surgical intervention, methods utilized, and anatomic and visual results are presented.

## RATIONALE FOR CRYOTHERAPY

Careful, indirect ophthalmoscopy of eyes with advanced proliferative

ROP, found to be at greatest risk for progression to traction detachment, revealed certain similarities to those adult eyes with diabetic retinopathy. In each situation, a factor unique to the disease process had either prevented vascularization of extensive areas of peripheral retina (ROP) or had destroyed preexisting capillary channels (proliferative diabetic retinopathy with capillary dropout). In each case, the disease process resulted in extensive areas of ischemic retina. These areas produced a presumed vasoproliferative factor hypothesized to cause neovascularization.

Cryotherapy, it was reasoned, by ablating the peripheral zone of avascular retina in proliferative ROP would destroy the source of the vasoproliferative factor that was causing the preretinal neovascularization, and the new vessels would secondarily regress. This was analogous to the situation in proliferative diabetic retinopathy in which panretinal photocoagulation therapy (PRP), in destroying the peripheral ischemic retina, represented an effective means for causing neovascular regression and control of the proliferative disease.

## PATIENT SELECTION

Patients who were referred with ROP stages 1 and 2 were examined at weekly intervals until normal retinal vascularization extended peripherally, anterior to the arteriovenous (AV) shunt, signifying disease resolution. In several of these eyes, however, even though ROP was diagnosed at an early stage of disease, the avascular zone was extremely wide, extending well posterior to the equator for 360 degrees. All these eyes progressed to stage 3+ disease over the course of several weeks and were treated if at least 180 degrees of preretinal neovascularization developed.

Between October 1982 and October 1987 a total of 25 premature infants (12 boys, 13 girls) with advanced stage 3+ ROP were referred to us for evaluation and treatment. Gestational age ranged between 23 and 29 weeks (mean 26 weeks) and birth weight between 624 and 1,610 gm (mean 925 gm).

Dilatation was obtained using two sets of $2^1/_2\%$ phenylephrine hydrochloride and 1% tropicamide drops one-half hour prior to examination. Topical anesthesia was obtained with 0.5% proparacaine hydrochloride. A neonatal wire or Sauer lid speculum was required for adequate exposure. Scleral depression to examine the peripheral retina was performed using a cotton-tipped applicator from which half of the cotton was removed. This instrument allowed gentle fixation and movement of the globe during indirect ophthalmoscopy.

Dilated fundus examination using indirect ophthalmoscopy and scleral

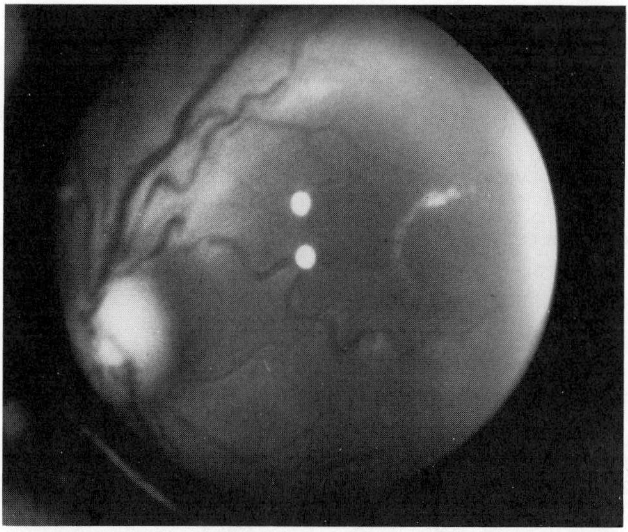

**FIG 8–1.**
Plus disease, with tortuous arterioles and dilated venules. Note bright red arteriolized blood in venules as a result of high flow rate through the peripheral AV shunt. See also Plate 1. *(From Topilow HW, Ackerman AL, Wang FM: Ophthalmology 1985; 92:379–387. Used by permission.)*

depression was usually performed when the infants were between 7 and 10 weeks of age. Detailed fundus drawings were made of each eye and the degree of ROP was classified stage 3+ according to the International Classification of Retinopathy of Prematurity (ICROP).[14] Cases seen prior to 1984 were reclassified using this protocol.

Each of these 50 eyes had marked arteriolar tortuousity and venous dilatation posteriorly and premature termination of the vascular arcades in a well-developed AV shunt (plus disease). In most eyes blood flow through the shunt was so rapid that bright red arteriolized oxygenated blood was noted in the major venous channels posteriorly (Fig 8–1; Plate 1). In three eyes, the shunt was located in zone 1, just outside the posterior pole; in 33 eyes the shunt was located in posterior zone 2, approximately 2 to 3 disk diameters posterior to the equator; and in 14 eyes the shunt was located in mid zone 2, at the equator.

Special emphasis was placed on accurate determination of the width and extent of the avascular zone. We have found a direct correlation between the size of the avascular zone and its posterior extent and the risk for progression to more advanced stages of the disease.[8, 13]

Two patients who were initially seen at stage 3+ in each eye with less than 180 degrees of contiguous preretinal neovascularization developed 180 degrees of new vessels within 2 to 3 weeks. The other 23 infants presented at stage 3+ with at least 180 degrees of neovascularization (Fig 8–2; Plate 2).

Of the 50 eyes treated, 10 met our minimal criteria for cryotherapy, having stage 3+ ROP with 180 degrees of contiguous preretinal neovascularization temporally. Two eyes had 200 degrees of preretinal neovascularization and 38 had 360 degrees of contiguous new vessels along the posterior border of the AV shunt.

## CRYOTHERAPY TECHNIQUE

All eyes examined during the course of this study that developed stage 3+ ROP with at least 180 degrees of contiguous preretinal neovascularization

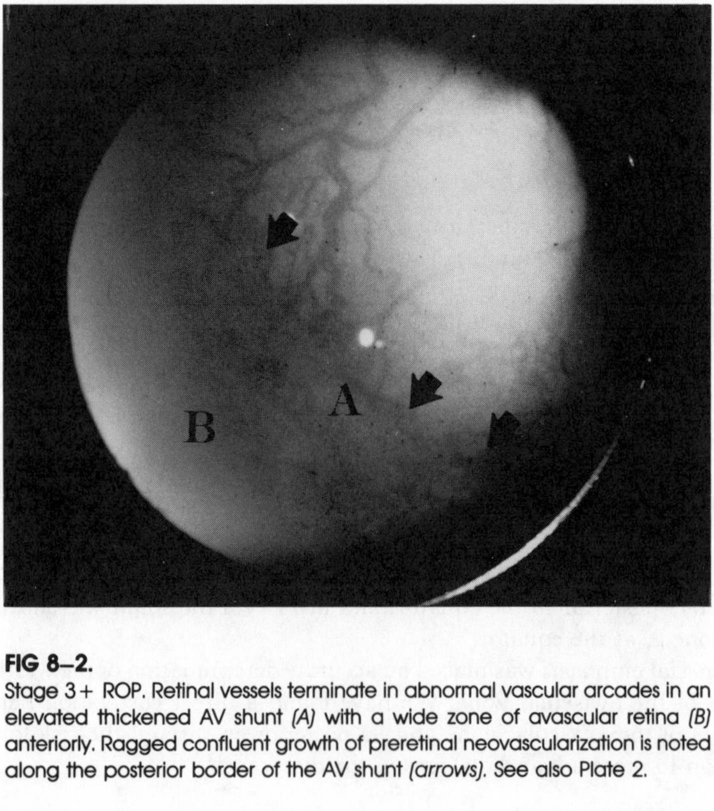


**FIG 8–2.**
Stage 3+ ROP. Retinal vessels terminate in abnormal vascular arcades in an elevated thickened AV shunt *(A)* with a wide zone of avascular retina *(B)* anteriorly. Ragged confluent growth of preretinal neovascularization is noted along the posterior border of the AV shunt *(arrows)*. See also Plate 2.

were included and treated with cryotherapy. Treatment was performed when the infants were between 7 and 20 weeks of age (mean 11 weeks) and under general anesthesia to avoid the severe respiratory alkalosis associated with hyperventilation when topical anesthetic alone is used.

Dilatation was obtained using two sets of $2^1/_2$% phenylephrine HCl and 1% cyclopentolate HCl drops 1 hour before surgery. A neonatal Sauer or Cook lid speculum with solid blades was used to retract the eyelids.

Using indirect ophthalmoscopic control, treatment was applied to the entire avascular zone anterior to the AV shunt up to the ora serrata. The Mira retinal and cataract cryo probes were used because (1) they are relatively thin and fit easily into the conjunctival fornices of these small eyes, (2) they thaw instantly, and (3) the temperature of the probes can be precisely regulated. A setting of −55° C was used routinely to produce a mild whitening of the avascular retina. Intense white retinal-vitreous freezing is not required and should be avoided. Occasionally, settings of −25° C are sufficient. Colder probe temperatures are not necessary and can easily produce severe freezing of the very thin sclera, choroid, retina, and overlying vitreous, predisposing to hemorrhage and vitreous contraction.

The avascular zone was treated in a stepwise subconfluent manner, leaving small untreated spaces between applications. No attempt was made to treat directly the AV shunt or preretinal neovascularization (Fig 8–3; Plate 3). Because of the low ocular perfusion pressure in these premature eyes, constant monitoring of the central retinal artery during treatment was essential to avoid occlusion from pressure by the cryo probe.

Even in cases in which treatment extended well posterior to the equator, it was not necessary to perform a conjunctival peritomy. Postoperatively, cyclopentolate HCl 1% and an antibiotic-steroid drop were used twice daily for 2 weeks. Eye patches were not used.

Of the 50 eyes treated, three had zone 1 involvement with 360 degrees of preretinal neovascularization, and all were treated for 360 degrees anterior to the AV shunt. Thirty-three eyes had posterior zone 2 involvement; 31 received 360 degrees of cryotherapy, and 2 were treated for 180 degrees, depending on the extent of preretinal new vessels. Of 14 eyes with mid zone 2 involvement, eight received 180 degrees of treatment, two required 200 degrees of cryotherapy, and four were treated for 360 degrees, depending on the extent of the preretinal neovascularization.

## RESULTS FOLLOWING CRYOTHERAPY

Fifty eyes of 25 preterm infants with stage 3+ ROP received 180 degrees to 360 degrees of cryotherapy to ablate the peripheral zone of avascular

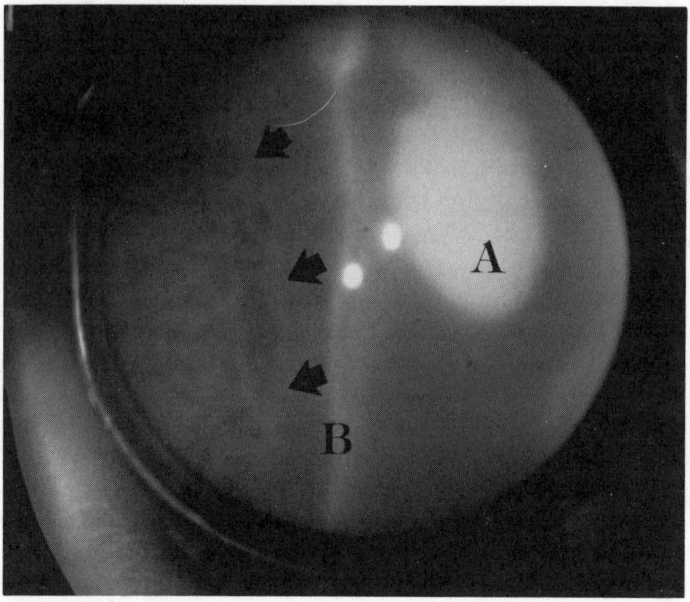


**FIG 8–3.**
Cryotherapy *(A)* is applied to the wide avascular zone anterior to the AV shunt *(B)*. Confluent preretinal neovascularization *(arrows)* is noted posterior to the AV shunt. See also Plate 3. *(From Topilow HW, Ackerman AL, Wang FM: Ophthalmology 1985; 92:379–387. Used by permission.)*

retina. Within 14 days following treatment the arteriolar tortuousity and venous dilatation (plus disease) had completely resolved in all cases. Preretinal neovascularization and the AV shunt regressed to fibrotic avascular remnants in 46 eyes (Fig 8–4; Plate 4). Additional cryotherapy was required in four eyes 3 weeks after initial treatment to achieve complete regression.

With resolution of the plus disease and regression of the neovascularization and shunt, the high flow state returned to normal, with restoration of the darker deoxygenated appearance to the venous channels.

Thirty-nine of these eyes had treatment to an avascular zone that extended from the ora serrata to either posterior zone 2 (25 eyes), or mid zone 2 (14 eyes). All of these cases showed complete and lasting regression of ROP without evidence of progression during a follow-up period that ranged from 6 to 70 months (mean 29 months).

Of these 39 eyes, the appearance of the optic nerve, macula, and major vascular arcades was normal in 27. Ten eyes had mild tractional straightening of the temporal vascular arcades, 1 had moderate temporal dragging with temporal macular heterotopia, and 1 had an idiopathic atrophic RPE defect in the fovea without serologic evidence of toxoplasmosis.

## PROGRESSION DESPITE CRYOTHERAPY

In 100% of cases, cryotherapy was successful in causing resolution of the neovascularization.

However, in a group of 11 eyes, vitreous traction to involuted fibrotic remnants of the neovascularization resulted in extensive traction retinal detachment 2 to 7 weeks (mean 4.4 weeks) following cryotherapy. The avascular zone in each of these 11 eyes was extremely wide, extending from the ora serrata to zone 1 in 3 eyes and to posterior zone 2 in 8 eyes. Prior to cryotherapy, these eyes had been characterized by fulminant, lush growths of

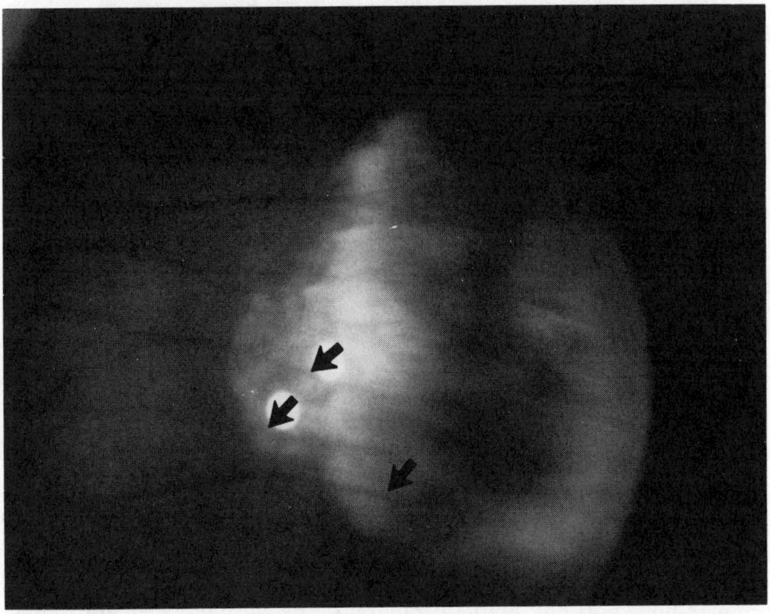

**FIG 8–4.**
Cryotherapy reaction 3 weeks after treatment, with complete resolution of the AV shunt and preretinal neovascularization previously located posterior to the area of treatment. Retinal vessels *(arrows)* now extend anteriorly into the zone of treatment, which had been avascular. See also Plate 4. *(From Topilow HW, Ackerman AL, Wang FM: Ophthalmology 1985; 92:379–387. Used by permission.)*

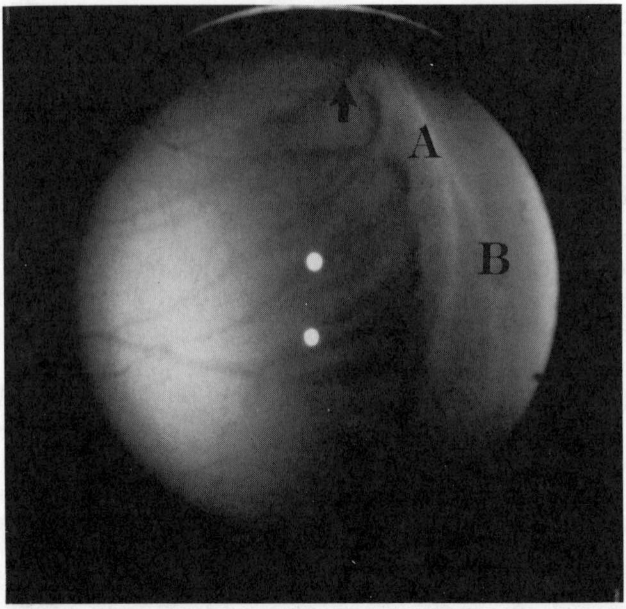


**FIG 8–5.**
Confluent preretinal neovascularization *(A)* covers the AV shunt. Wide zone of avascular retina *(B)* is present anteriorly. Vitreous traction causes elevation of preretinal neovascularization and retinal vessels *(arrows)*, which terminate in the underlying AV shunt. See also Plate 5.

confluent neovascularization extending into the vitreous for 360 degrees along the posterior border of the AV shunt (Fig 8–5; Plate 5).

The detachment was total in three eyes, was temporal, involving the fovea, in six eyes, and was temporal, extending posterior to the equator but sparing the fovea, in two eyes.

The distinctive features of these detachments were centripetal and anterior traction from condensed avascular vitreous bands firmly attached to the circumferential fibrotic remnants of the preretinal neovascularization. There was no remaining active proliferative neovascular element following cryotherapy. The areas of vitreous attachment were tented up, with the attenuated avascular retina anteriorly often folded posteriorly underneath the detached vascularized retina.

The usual configuration of these detachments consisted of marked elevation of the circumferential areas of vitreoretinal traction with the detached retina sloping posteriorly. No retinal tears were present in any of these 11 detachments, making them true tractional detachments.

The contour of these detachments differed significantly from exudative retinal detachments, which have shifting fluid not seen in the traction detachment. Also, exudative detachments do not have the classic configuration of wide areas of retina tented up by vitreous traction bands with a detached retina sloping away from the traction on either side. The exudative detachment is more likely to be a uniform, rounded, bullous formation. The traction detachments seen in our cases occurred on average more than 1 month following cryotherapy at a time when all proliferative neovascular activity had ceased.

## SCLERAL BUCKLING TECHNIQUE

Two of the 11 eyes that developed a traction detachment following cryotherapy had zone 1 involvement with retinal vascularization ending just outside the macula. One of these detachments was inoperable when first seen and the other could not be reattached following pars plicata vitrectomy. The other nine eyes with traction retinal detachment following cryotherapy were treated using scleral buckling techniques adapted to these small eyes which were often only 15 mm in length. Because cryotherapy had caused regression of the neovascularization in all cases, no additional cryo treatment was required.

Gentamicin drops were given every 6 hours the day prior to surgery. Preoperative drops included cyclopentolate HCl 1%, phenylephrine HCl 2.5%, and gentamicin every 15 minutes repeated three times during the 1 hour prior to surgery.

At the beginning of surgery, intravenous oxacillin, 25 mg/kg, was administered. With the infant under general endotracheal anesthesia, a neonatal Sauer or Cook lid speculum was used to expose the globe. Lid sutures were not required. The cornea was covered with Gelfoam soaked in balanced salt solution. A 360-degree conjunctival periotomy was performed at the limbus, with relaxing incisions at the 4-o'clock and 8-o'clock meridians. The four rectus muscles were secured with 4–0 black silk traction sutures. Indirect ophthalmoscopy and scleral depression with a diathermy probe and a blunt localizing tip were used to identify and mark all areas of circumferential vitreous traction to areas of regressed neovascularization in each quadrant. Mild localizing burns were placed on the areas of retinal traction and on the overlying sclera.

An encircling band 2.5 mm wide was placed circumferentially beneath the rectus muscles and anchored just posterior to the localizing marks; mattress sutures of 5–0 Dacron and microspatula needles were used. These needles are essential in preventing perforation of the extremely thin sclera in these premature eyes. Exposure was obtained using the rectus muscle traction sutures and a narrow, malleable retractor. The globe was softened using acetazolamide (5 mg/kg) in all cases and paracentesis in five. Subretinal fluid was drained in two eyes, with complete retinal reattachment accomplished in the operating room.

The band was tied superonasally with a clove hitch suture of 4–0 Mersilene and gently tightened to produce a moderate internal buckling effect that supported the areas of vitreoretinal traction. The external curvature of the globe was not distorted significantly by the encircling band, which produced only a minimal indentation of the sclera. The height of the buckle increased mildly within the first 24 hours postoperatively. An extremely high buckle is not required and should be avoided. It is essential to monitor the intraocular pressure immediately after tightening the band, and to observe the central retinal artery to be certain that the vessel remains patent and that adequate blood flow to the retina is maintained. Postoperatively, cyclopentolate HCl 1% and an antibiotic-steroid drop were administered twice daily for 8 weeks.

In the seven eyes in which subretinal fluid was not released, the retina completely reattached, with total absorption of subretinal fluid, within 1 week.

One patient developed a severe purulent otitis media 2 weeks postoperatively, with a secondary endogenous endophthalmitis. Pars plicata vitrectomy and intravitreous antibiotics were used, but phthisis bulbi developed.The retinas in the 8 other eyes have remained reattached, with follow-up ranging from 6 to 70 months (mean 31 months). Of these 8 eyes, 3 have marked temporal dragging of the vascular arcades and macula without falciform fold formation, 2 have moderate temporal macular heterotopia and vascular straightening, and 3 have mild vascular straightening only.

The encircling band was removed from 4 of these eyes between 7 and 10 months postoperatively (mean 8 months), to allow for ocular growth. Follow-up after band removal has ranged from 29 to 54 months (mean 43 months), without retinal redetachment or evidence of ongoing vitreous traction. In most cases a mild buckling effect persisted for several months after the band was removed.

## VISUAL RESULTS (TABLES 8–1 AND 8–2)

Sixteen eyes in 8 of these 25 children have been followed long enough to measure visual acuity using either Snellen letters or a picture chart. In the 12 eyes in this group that did not develop traction detachment, visual acuity measured 20/30 in 5 eyes, 20/40 in 3 eyes, 20/50 to 20/60 in 2 eyes,

**TABLE 8–1.**
Visual Acuity Following Cryotherapy for Stage 3+ ROP Without Retinal Detachment

| Visual Acuity | No. of Eyes |
|---|---|
| 20/30 | 5 |
| 20/40 | 3 |
| 20/50 | 1 |
| 20/60 | 1 |
| 20/100 | 1 |
| 18/400 | 1 |

20/100 in 1 eye and 18/400 in 1 eye. The 20/100 eye was esotropic and all others were orthophoric.

Of the four other eyes in which traction detachments did develop, visual acuity measured 20/60, 20/100, and 20/200 in three eyes in which the fovea had been detached. The fourth eye in which the fovea had not detached was amblyopic and the child was able to follow the movements of a small toy. One of these eyes was esotropic and two were exotropic and undergoing occlusion therapy.

In the group of 16 eyes in eight children old enough (4 to 5 years) at the last visit to have visual acuity measured, acuity was 20/30 to 20/60 in 11 (69%) eyes and 20/30 to 20/200 in 14 (87.5%). Every child in this group had acuity of at least 20/60 in the better eye.

One additional infant, with zone 1 involvement, developed bilateral inoperable retinal detachment.

The 16 remaining children were not old enough at their last visit to perform Snellen or picture acuity tests. Fourteen of these youngest children had orthophoria, one had esotropia with an RPE defect in the macula, and one had alternating exotropia. One of the 32 eyes in this group of 16 children too young to have visual acuity measured developed phthisis bulbi following endogenous endophthalmitis, and lost light perception. Thirty of the remaining 31 eyes in this group were able to hold fixation and follow the

**TABLE 8–2.**
Visual Acuity Following Cryotherapy and Scleral Buckling for Stage 3+ ROP With Secondary Traction Retinal Detachment

| Visual Acuity | No. of Eyes | Foveal Involvement |
|---|---|---|
| 20/60 | 1 | Yes |
| 20/100 | 1 | Yes |
| 20/200 | 1 | Yes |
| <20/400 | 1 | No |

movement of a light or a small toy. We expect the vast majority of these children will develop measurable acuity, comparable to that in the older children.

For the entire group of 50 eyes, two were lost because of inoperable detachments and one because of endogenous endophthalmitis.

Of the remaining 47 eyes, visual acuity in 16 could be measured accurately and ranged between 20/30 to 20/60 in 69% and 20/30 to 20/200 in 87.5%. Visual acuity in 30 of the remaining 31 eyes in the 16 children who were too young to test on Snellen or picture charts was normal for the children's age. One eye had reduced vision because of an idiopathic macular RPE defect.

## DISCUSSION

The exact causes for acute proliferative retinopathy of prematurity remain unknown more than 40 years after Terry's initial report.[15] What is known is that the smallest, most premature, and sickest infants who receive high concentrations of supplemental oxygen for the longest periods of time are at the greatest risk of developing ROP.

With modern neonatal intensive care, survival rates for the most premature infants at highest risk of developing ROP have improved dramatically over the past decade. With this improved survival has come an increase in the incidence of ROP.[1, 16, 17]

It is well recognized that early stages of ROP, with a narrow peripheral zone of avascular retina, often fail to progress. However, it is equally well known that more advanced stages of acute proliferative retinopathy of prematurity usually progress to total traction retinal detachment with disastrous visual results. These eyes are characterized by wide avascular zones of ischemic retina, extending posterior to the equator with extensive intravitreous neovascular formations for 180 to 360 degrees at their posterior borders. Posterior arteriolar tortuosity and venous engorgement are seen. Often there is such rapid flow of blood through the AV shunt that the posterior venous side of the circulation contains oxygenated arteriolized blood. It is extremely uncommon to see spontaneous involution of this advanced stage 3+ disease. It is, however, common to see rapid progression from this stage to total organized traction retinal detachment within a few weeks; therefore, extremely careful and frequent observation by experienced observers is required. It is our clinical impression that the normal adherence of the neurosensory retina to the pigment epithelium is underdeveloped in these premature eyes, which accounts for the rapid development of traction retinal detachment. This is in contrast to the adolescent situation, in which ongoing vitreous traction results in a retinal tear and rhegmatogenous detachment caused by the normal firm adherence of the neurosensory retina to the underlying pigment epithelium.

The increased incidence and survival of extremely high-risk premature infants dictated the need to recognize and treat ROP and its complications.

A direct analogy can be made between acute proliferative ROP and proliferative diabetic retinopathy or any other proliferative retinopathy. In each disorder a factor specific to the disease process results in capillary nonperfusion, with the development of wide zones of avascular ischemic retina. This retinal ischemia provides the stimulus for the presumed release of a vasoproliferative factor, which then directly causes the formation of intravitreous neovascular formations that bud from the closest remaining vascular bed capable of proliferating. In ROP, retinal vessels posterior to the AV shunt represent the closest remaining vascular bed capable of reacting to the vasoactive stimulus. It is the retinal ischemia, therefore, and not simply the supplemental oxygen therapy these infants receive, that is the cause for the intravitreous neovascularization. Retinal ischemia peripherally would also explain the posterior retinal vascular tortuousity and engorgement in terms of an autoregulatory response, increasing retinal blood flow in an attempt to deliver more oxygen to an ischemic peripheral retina.

In analyzing the current series of 50 eyes, it is our clinical impression that it is the width of the avascular zone that correlates most accurately with the potential severity of ROP. The wider the zone, the greater the probability of rapid progression from early to advanced stages of disease. These cases warrant frequent examination and prompt cryotherapy when indicated.

The concept that retinal ischemia from any etiology results in the release of a vasoproliferative substance from the retina, which in turn causes intravitreous neovascularization,[18] explains the effectiveness of laser photocoagulation in the treatment of proliferative diabetic retinopathy, as well as the effectiveness of xenon arc photocoagulation[19–26] and cryotherapy[2–13] in acute proliferative ROP. In each instance, the therapeutic modality, whether photocoagulation or cryotherapy, destroys the ischemic retina which presumably produces the vasoproliferative substance. The destruction of the avascular retina also eliminates the peripheral photoreceptor complexes which require a large oxygen supply. With their ablation, the retina's oxygen need is reduced. This results in a decrease in retinal blood flow, demonstrated by marked reduction in arteriolar tortuousity and venous engorgement seen in our patients in the days following cryotherapy and by the measured decrease in retinal blood flow when laser Doppler techniques were used following panretinal photocoagulation therapy in the treatment of proliferative diabetic retinopathy.[27] More recent studies suggest that RPE proliferation stimulated by cryotherapy may produce an antivasoproliferative factor as well.[28]

In all 50 eyes in our series with stage 3+ ROP treated with cryotherapy, rapid and predictable involution of the neovascularization and resolution of vascular tortuosity and dilatation occurred within 2 weeks following treatment. The retina's oxygen need peripherally was reduced, with secondary transformation from the clinically observed high-flow state (plus disease) to a more normal hemodynamic condition. There has been no evidence of progression in 39 of these eyes, with follow-up ranging between 6 to 70 months (mean 29 months).

In 11 eyes (22%) with the most extensive avascular zones and 360 degrees of preretinal neovascularization, ongoing vitreous traction to regressed fibrotic neovascular remnants resulted in traction detachment 2 to 7 weeks (mean 4.4 weeks) following cryotherapy, supporting our earlier conclusion that these eyes are most likely to progress.[8, 13] One zone 1 traction detachment was inoperable when diagnosed, and another could not be reattached following pars plicata vitrectomy. The other 9 detachments were successfully repaired by releasing the vitreoretinal traction with scleral buckling surgery, but one was eventually lost because of an endogenous endophthalmitis. The retina has remained attached in the 8 other eyes, with follow-up ranging between 6 to 70 months (mean 31 months). The analogy to proliferative diabetic retinopathy applies here as well.

It is well known that panretinal photocoagulation (PRP) therapy is effective in causing involution of intravitreous or disc neovascularization, but is ineffective in releasing vitreoretinal traction to fibrotic neovascular formations. Vitreous traction to these fibrotic remnants may progress. The late development of traction retinal detachment in diabetic retinopathy, despite successful PRP therapy to ablate neovascularization, can be seen. In much the same way, ongoing vitreous traction to fibrotic neovascular remnants caused the development of a traction retinal detachment in 11 of the 50 eyes in the current series, despite prior cryotherapy which was successful in causing involution of extensive preretinal neovascularization in these eyes with stage 3+ ROP.

That these eyes went on to develop a traction detachment despite prior cryotherapy should not be regarded as a failure of cryotherapy any more than a traction detachment following PRP for proliferative diabetic retinopathy represents a failure of PRP. The sole function of cryotherapy for ROP or PRP for proliferative diabetic retinopathy is to cause regression of preretinal neovascularization. If ongoing vitreous traction causes traction detachment, this new problem must then be addressed using methods that include scleral buckling surgery and vitrectomy techniques designed to release vitreous traction and allow retinal reattachment. It is essential to follow these patients carefully following cryotherapy so that if ongoing vitreous traction does result in the development of a traction retinal detachment, scleral buckling surgery can be used to release the traction, repair the retinal detachment, and prevent the development of a total, organized traction detachment. Once the detachment reaches this advanced stage of fibrotic organization, vitrectomy techniques must be utilized but are seldom successful in restoring useful visual acuity.

Early reports indicating no beneficial effect from cryotherapy in ROP must be reinterpreted in light of the concept indicating retinal ischemia as the cause for proliferative retinopathy in general and ROP in particular.

Cryotherapy was used by Keith[29] to treat 9 infants with advanced grade 3 disease and was not found to be beneficial. However, treatment was directed to the AV shunt and not the avascular retina anterior to it, and therefore no beneficial effect could be expected.

Kingham[30] treated 14 eyes of 12 infants with acute proliferative ROP and found a beneficial effect in only 1 or 2 of these cases. Treatment, however, was directed to the neovascular formation itself, and not the ischemic retina anteriorly. The cases treated with cryotherapy also included seven advanced cases with traction retinal detachment at the time of cryo treatment. This would be analogous to treating a diabetic traction detachment with additional PRP therapy. No beneficial effect would be expected. Scleral buckling surgery to release the vitreoretinal traction causing the detachment would be required.

The fact that 47 of the 50 (94%) stage 3+ eyes we treated remain attached at the last follow-up visit (mean 29 months postoperatively) is significant, considering that each of these eyes came from a group of infants at very high risk for developing traction detachment.

The final measure of any surgical procedure for ROP must be the resulting visual acuity. Eight children (16 eyes) were old enough at the last follow-up visit for measurement of visual acuity with a Snellen or picture chart. Twelve of these eyes never developed traction retinal detachment and visual acuity ranged between 20/30 (five eyes), 20/40 (three eyes), 20/50 to 20/60 (two eyes), 20/100 (one eye), and 18/400 (one eye). While the numbers are small, it seems significant that 10 of 12 eyes (83%) retain vision of at least 20/60.

Four of these eyes did eventually develop traction detachments that were successfully repaired with scleral buckling surgery. Three of the four detachments involved the macula, with resulting visual acuity postoperatively of 20/60, 20/100, and 20/200 respectively. The fourth detachment spared the macula but amblyopia has reduced vision to the ability to follow movements of a small toy. All children with amblyopia are being aggressively treated with occlusion therapy.

For the overall group of 16 eyes that could be accurately tested, 14 of 16 (87.5%), retain visual acuity of at least 20/200 in each eye. Another more useful way to view these acuity results is that every child in this group had acuity of at least 20/60 in the better eye.

Because 30 of the 31 remaining eyes in the younger infants exhibited normal following movements at the most recent evaluation, we expect that the vast majority will develop measurable acuities within a similar range.

These visual results are in contrast to those following closed vitrectomy for a series of eyes with stage 5 ROP.[31] In these eyes, in which the disease process had progressed to total organized detachment, 48% (41 of 85 eyes) were reattached. Twenty-six of these 41 developed at least light perception while 15 of 41, or 37%, of the successfully reattached group apparently never regained even light perception. If ROP progresses to total organized retinal detachment, even successful reattachment of the retina by vitrectomy techniques, which can be attained in only a minority of cases, results in an incidence of no light perception of approximately 37%.

The goal of therapy, therefore, should be to initiate cryotherapy at a relatively early stage in the proliferative process, at a time when it is unlikely that spontaneous regression will occur, but before massive intravitreous neovascular fronds have formed. Even if at a late proliferative stage cryotherapy is successful in causing involution of extensive neovascular formations, subsequent vitreous traction to the fibrotic remnants can cause traction retinal detachment and cicatricial dragging of the macula with severe visual loss.

Eyes most likely to benefit from cryotherapy and to progress without it are those that have rapidly advanced from early stages 1 and 2 to stage 3+ disease. These eyes have wide avascular zones of ischemic retina, well-developed AV shunts, and extensive intravitreous neovascularization. Engorgement of the posterior retinal venules and tortuosity of the retinal arterioles are present.

In this study, cryotherapy was performed on 50 eyes with advanced stage 3+ ROP to ablate avascular retina, and in all cases was successful in causing involution of extensive preretinal neovascular formations. These eyes with progressive ROP requiring treatment are analogous to eyes with proliferative diabetic retinopathy with extensive capillary nonperfusion that require panretinal photocoagulation therapy. If treatment is withheld from the diabetic eyes until evidence of massive neovascularization is present on the disc and retina, or until vitreous hemorrhage results, then a significant number of eyes will sustain permanent visual loss from traction retinal detachment and chronic vitreous hemorrhage that could have been prevented by timely administration of laser therapy.

Cryoablation of avascular retina in eyes with stage 3+ progressive ROP is extremely effective in causing involution of intravitreous neovascularization and in preventing late traction retinal detachment and cicatricial macular dragging. The retinal detachments that do develop as a result of ongoing vitreoretinal traction can be successfully repaired using scleral buckling techniques, with excellent visual results in most cases. The long-term follow-up of these 50 eyes has not uncovered any late onset complications related to cryosurgery when used at a temperature of −55° C.

Advanced stage 3+ ROP with extensive preretinal neovascularization is unlikely to regress spontaneously and usually progresses rapidly. Cryosurgery, if properly performed on appropriately selected patients, poses minimal risks and represents an effective means of preventing severe visual loss in this select group of patients with advanced proliferative ROP.

## REFERENCES

1. Campbell PB, Bull MJ, Ellis FD, et al: Incidence of retinopathy of prematurity in a tertiary newborn intensive care unit. *Arch Ophthalmol* 1983; 101:1686–1688.
2. Sasaki K, Yamashita Y, Maekawa T, et al: Treatment of retinopathy of prematurity in active stage by cryocautery. *Jpn J Ophthalmol* 1976; 20:384–395.
3. Hindle NW, Leyton J: Prevention of cicatricial retrolental fibroplasia by cryotherapy. *Can J Ophthalmol* 1978; 13:277–282.
4. Hindle NW: Cryotherapy for retinopathy of prematurity to prevent retrolental fibroplasia. *Can J Ophthalmol* 1982; 17:207–212.
5. Mousel DK, Hoyt CS: Cryotherapy for retinopathy of prematurity. *Ophthalmology*, 1980; 87:1121–1127.
6. Ben-Sira I, Nissenkorn I, Grunwald E, et al: Treatment of acute retrolental fibroplasia by cryopexy. *Br J Ophthalmol* 1980; 64:758–762.
7. Bert MD, Friedman MW, Ballard R: Combined cryosurgery and scleral buckling in acute proliferative retrolental fibroplasia. *J Pediatr Ophthalmol Strabismus* 1981; 18:9–12.
8. Topilow HW, Ackerman AL, Wang FM: The treatment of advanced retinopathy of prematurity by cryotherapy and scleral buckling surgery. *Ophthalmology* 1985; 92:379–387.
9. Tasman W: Management of retinopathy of prematurity. *Ophthalmology* 1985; 92:995–999.
10. Tasman W, Brown GC, Schaffer DB, et al: Cryotherapy for active retinopathy of prematurity. *Ophthalmology* 1986; 93:580–583.
11. Hindle NW: Cryotherapy for retinopathy of prematurity: Timing of intervention. *Br J Ophthalmol* 1986; 70:269–276.
12. Ben-Sira I, Nissenkorn I, Weinberger D, et al: Long-term results of cryotherapy for active stage of retinopathy of prematurity. *Ophthalmology* 1986; 93:1423–1428.
13. Topilow HW, Ackerman AL, Wang FM, et al: Successful treatment of advanced retinopathy of prematurity. *Ophthalmic Surg* 1988; 19:781–785.
14. The Committee for Classification of Retinopathy of Prematurity: An international classification of retinopathy of prematurity. *Arch Ophthalmol* 1984; 102:1130–1134.

15. Terry TL: Extreme prematurity and fibroplastic overgrowth of persistent vascular sheath behind each crystalline lens. I, Preliminary report. *Am J Ophthalmol* 1942; 25:203–204.
16. Kalina RE, Karr DJ: Retrolental fibroplasia: Experience over two decades in one institution. *Ophthalmology* 1982; 89:91–95.
17. Patz, A: Current therapy of retrolental fibroplasia: Retinopathy of prematurity. *Ophthalmology* 1983; 90:425–427.
18. Weiter JJ, Zuckerman R, Schepens CL: A model for the pathogenesis of retrolental fibroplasia based on the metabolic control of blood vessel development. *Ophthalmic Surg* 1982; 13:1013–1017.
19. Oshima K, Ikui H, Kana M, et al: Clinical study and photocoagulation of the retinopathy of prematurity. *Folia Opthalmol Jpn* 1971; 22:700–770.
20. Yamamoto M, Tabuchi A: Management of the retinopathy of prematurity. *Jpn J Ophthalmol* 1976; 20:372–383.
21. Nagata M, Tsuruoka Y: Treatment of acute retrolental fibroplasia with xenon arc photocoagulation. *Jpn J Ophthalmol* 1972; 16:131–143.
22. Uemura Y: Current status of retrolental fibroplasia: Report of the joint committee for the study of retrolental fibroplasia in Japan. *Jpn J Ophthalmol* 1977; 21:366–378.
23. Nagata M, Kobayashi Y, Fukuda H, et al: Photocoagulation for the treatment of retinopathy of prematurity. *Jpn J Clin Ophthalmol* 1968; 22:419–427.
24. Nagata, M, Kanenari S: Photocoagulation in the progressive cases of retinopathy of prematurity (report II). *Jpn J Clin Ophthalmol* 1970; 24:655–661.
25. Negata M, Tsuruoka Y, Yamamoto Y: Photocoagulation therapy of acute retrolental fibroplasia (third report). *Jpn J Clin Ophthalmol* 1972; 26:271–280.
26. Nagata M: Treatment of acute proliferative retrolental fibroplasia with Xenon arc photocoagulation: Its indications and limitations. *Jpn J Ophthalmol* 1977; 21:436–459.
27. Feke GT, Green GJ, Goger DG, et al: Laser doppler measurements of the effect of panretinal photocoagulation on retinal blood flow. *Ophthalmology* 1982; 89:757–762.
28. Glaser BM, Campochiaro PA, Davis JL, et al: Retinal pigment epithelial cells release inhibitors of neovascularization. *Ophthalmology* 1987; 94:780–784.
29. Keith CG: Visual outcome and effect of treatment in stage III developing retrolental fibroplasia. *Br J Ophthalmol* 1982; 66:446–449.
30. Kingham JD: Acute retrolental fibroplasia. II. Treatment by cryosurgery. *Arch Ophthalmol* 1978; 96:2049–2053.
31. Trese MT: Visual results and prognostic factors for vision following surgery for stage V retinopathy of prematurity. *Ophthalmology* 1986; 93:574–579.

Chapter 9

# The Cryo-ROP Study: A National Cooperative Study of Retinopathy of Prematurity

Rand Spencer, M.D.

## INTRODUCTION

The Cryo-ROP Study is an ongoing, prospective, randomized clinical trial of the use of cryotherapy in the treatment of retinopathy of prematurity (ROP). As a secondary objective, the study is also examining the natural history of ROP. Phase 1 of this study began recruitment of patients in January 1986. In January 1988, entries of new patients into the study and random assignment of cryotherapy ceased because the study's Data and Safety Monitoring Committee found that cryotherapy did reduce the incidence of adverse outcome from severe ROP by approximately 50% over the untreated (control) group. Phase 2 of the Cryo-ROP study began in June 1989. This phase is designed to monitor the long-term effects of cryotherapy on the eyes of the randomized group of patients during the first 6 years of life. In addition, some phase 1 study patients will be followed to gather information on the natural history of ocular and visual development in very low birth weight (VLBW) infants.

### Background of Study Development

The concept of the Cryo-ROP Study developed during a conference on ROP sponsored by Ross Laboratories, held in Washington, D.C., in December 1981 and attended by interested investigators from throughout the world.

It became apparent at this meeting that an internationally accepted classification system of ROP should exist. Responding to this need, in September 1982 Dr. Warren Hindle of Calgary, Canada, organized the first workshop to develop a classification system. An attendee at both the December 1981 and the September 1982 meetings was Dr. Earl A. Palmer of Portland, Oregon. Dr. Palmer noted a wide diversity of opinions and varying reports of successes, failures, and complications regarding therapy of ROP. While working with Dr. John Flynn of Miami on the committee from which the new International Classification of Retinopathy of Prematurity (ICROP) evolved, both investigators decided that a randomized study of cryotherapy for ROP was indicated. Palmer initially planned a northwest regional collaborative study; however, Dr. Flynn urged that this idea be expanded to a national level, with possible funding from the National Eye Institute (NEI). Palmer continued to correspond with ophthalmologists experienced in ROP cryotherapy throughout the world, collecting data on the criteria and techniques of treatment. By late 1983, Dr. Palmer had canvassed 29 institutions to determine their interest in a study of the use of cryotherapy, and had received an overwhelmingly positive response.[1]

From these responses were developed a Planning Committee and an Advisory Committee (Appendix 9A). From the work of the members of these two groups and after several meetings, the *Manual of Procedures for the Cryo-ROP Study* emerged in September 1985. By April 1985, support of the NEI for this project was obtained, and requests for proposals from clinical centers were sent to all those who were potentially interested. Sixty institutions made applications to become participants, and from these, 23 centers eventually received NEI funding and participated in the Cryo-ROP Study (Appendix 9B).

Funding for each of the 23 centers began in October 1985. In November 1985, all study center coordinators, representing each participating center, attended a training session in Houston. In December 1985, the principal investigators, photographers, and other coinvestigators from each center attended a training seminar in Portland. Patient recruitment into the study began on January 1, 1986.

## Historical Background of ROP

Over the past 40 years there has been a gradual move toward tiered care of newborns. Three different levels of care have been established. Level 1 nurseries are prepared to take care of healthy newborn infants. The level 2 nurseries are intermediate-care facilities capable of caring for some newborn problems and the larger premature infants. Level 3 neonatal intensive care units are staffed and equipped to care for the most difficult problems and for very low birth weight (VLBW) premature infants. Paralleling these levels of care has been the emergence of neonatology as a subspecialty of pediatrics. As a result, there has been a dramatic increase in the survival rate of VLBW infants. In 1950, a newborn weighing less than 1,000 gm at birth survived at a rate of 8%.[1] By 1980, this survival rate was reported as 35%.[2] By 1985, the survival rate of infants with birth weight less than 1,001 gm was reported as greater than 65% in some centers.[3] Paralleling this increased survival rate has been a corresponding increase in the incidence of ROP in the United States.[4, 5] Estimates are that 7,000 infants were blinded by ROP during the original epidemic four decades ago.[3] In 1981, it was estimated that approximately 550 infants per year in the United States were blinded by ROP[2] and that approximately 2,100 infants annually were affected by the cicatricial forms of the disease.[6] Thus, in the 1970s and 1980s, the impact of this vision-threatening disease has been similar in absolute numbers to the magnitude of the disease during the "epidemic" in the 1940s and early 1950s. From the time the current ROP epidemic began in the mid-1970s, it can be conservatively estimated, based on Phelps' data[2, 6] that more than 6,000 infants in the United States have been blinded by ROP and that the vision of tens of thousands more has been affected by its cicatricial changes.

Since the role of oxygenation in ROP (or retrolental fibroplasia, RLF) was first described in the early 1950s, the only prophylactic treatment that has been universally accepted has been to avoid excessive oxygenation in the premature infant.[7–16] Prophylactic therapy with antioxidants, such as vitamin E, has proved controversial. Despite initially encouraging reports from Hittner et al.[17] regarding vitamin E therapy, significant untoward effects occurred from the use of these high levels of vitamin E, and later reports seemed to contradict the initial successes.[18, 19]

## DESIGN OF THE STUDY

On January 1, 1986, patient recruitment into the Cryo-ROP Study began. Study design called for each infant who weighed less than 1,251 gm at birth at each participating hospital to be logged in as a potential study subject. Exclusion criteria were a fatal congenital anomaly, a major congenital eye anomaly, death within the first 28 days of life (or before the first eye examination), and/or lack of parental consent. The first eye examination on all surviving infants whose birth weight (BW) was less than 1,251 gm was performed between 28 and 42 days of life. After the initial examination, an information booklet, *About Premature Baby's Eyes*, and a consent form for study participation were left for the parents.

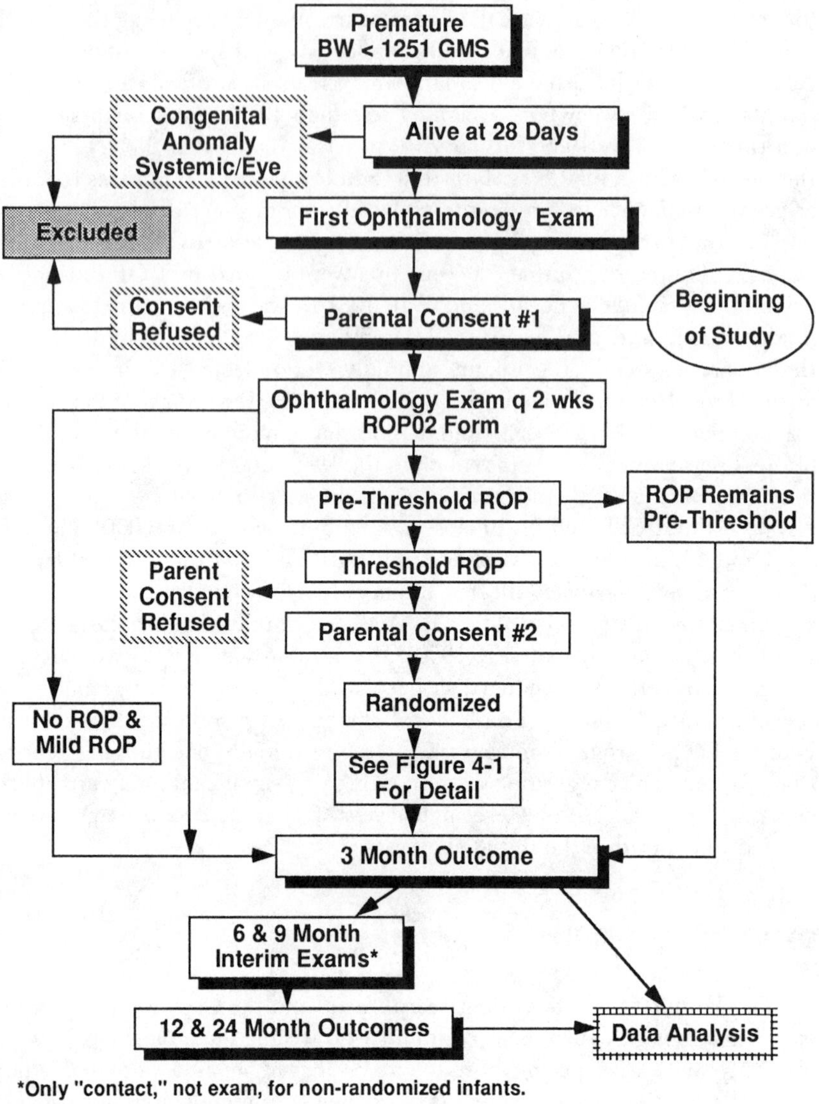


**FIG 9–1.**
Cryo-ROP study design.

## Study Groups Within the Cryo-ROP Study (Fig 9–1)

Once parental consent was obtained, all patients were entered into the *Natural History Group* of the study. Infants in this group were examined biweekly until either the retinas were completely vascularized or until significant progression of ROP occurred. ROP was graded according to ICROP, and data were recorded in a manner similar to that recommended by the classification committee.[20] After a child's retinas were fully vascularized, the child then received follow-up examinations at 3, 12, and 24 months after their original expected date of confinement (EDC). Those infants in whom retinopathy progressed to prethreshold ROP levels (any stage ROP in zone 1, stage 2 with plus disease in zone 2, stage 3 without plus disease in zone 2, or stage 2 with plus disease in zone 1 or 2 but less than five contiguous or less than eight cumulative clock hours of stage 3) were then followed at weekly intervals until there was regression of prethreshold disease, or until progression to threshold ROP occurred. Once a study subject developed threshold ROP, the child became eligible for entry into the *Randomized Study Group*.

The Randomized Study Group consisted of infants in whom threshold ROP (Fig 9–2) was reached in one or both eyes and in whom a further parental consent was obtained to randomize the infant for cryotherapy. Threshold ROP for the Randomized Study Group was defined as five or more contiguous or eight or more cumulative clock hours of stage 3 ROP in zone 1 or 2 with plus disease (Fig 9–3). The amounts of the stage 3 disease defining threshold ROP are arbitrary figures decided on by the study's de-

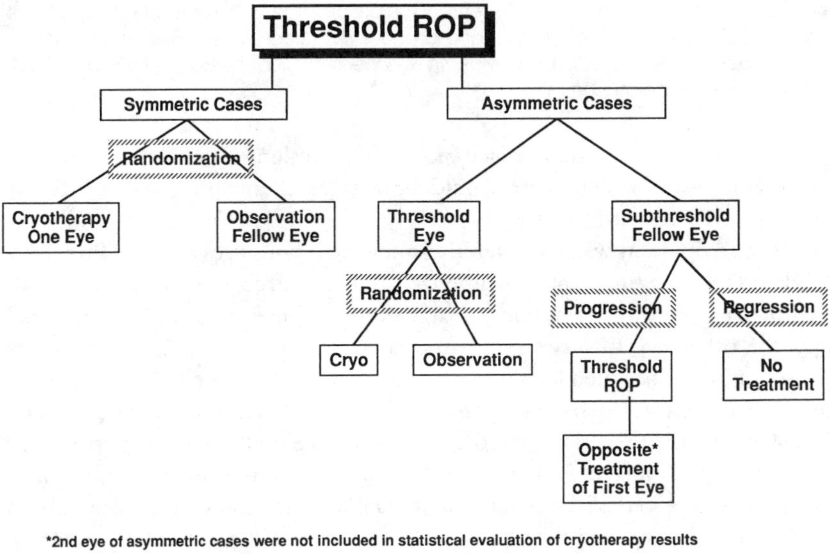


**FIG 9–2.**
Assignment of treatment of eyes reaching threshold ROP.

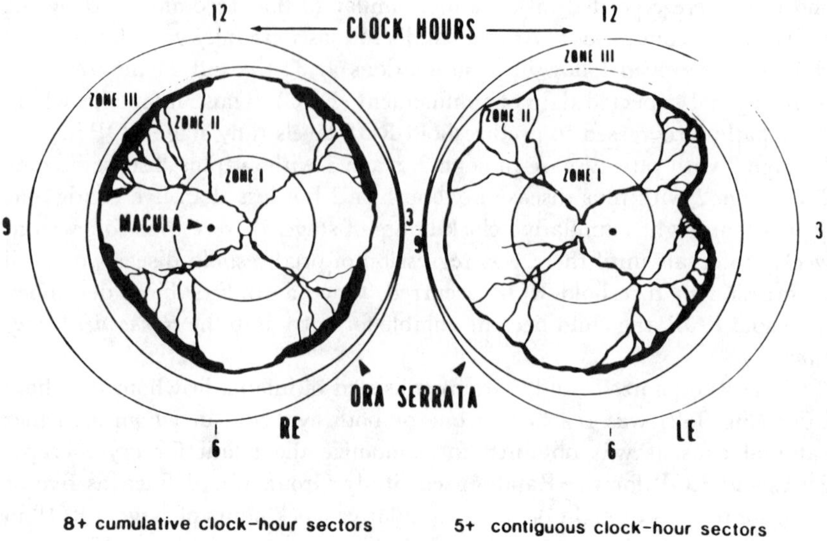


**FIG 9–3.**
Diagram of two representative eyes that have reached threshold ROP for randomization. Right eye *(RE)*: at least eight cumulative 30-degree sectors (clock hours) of stage 3. Left eye *(LE)*: at least five contiguous 30-degree sectors of stage 3. Thin line of retinopathy of prematurity represents stage 1 or 2, and broader sketched line signifies stage 3. *(From Cryotherapy for Retinopathy of Prematurity Cooperative Group: Arch Ophthalmol 1988; 106:472. Used by permission.)*

signers after many hours of discussion.[21] The design of threshold ROP was to be a point at which there would be a 50% chance of good or adverse outcome without cryotherapy.

A study patient was considered symmetric if both eyes reached threshold ROP at the same time, and asymmetric if only one eye had reached threshold. Symmetric cases were randomly assigned for one eye to receive cryotherapy and the other eye to serve as an untreated control. The asymmetric cases were randomly assigned for the eye at threshold to receive either cryotherapy or no treatment. If the second eye of an asymmetric, randomized case reached threshold ROP, then the second eye was to receive the opposite treatment from that randomized first eye. In this way no patient in the randomized group was deprived of the potentially beneficial effects of cryotherapy if both eyes eventually reached threshold ROP, or conversely, were spared exposure to conceivably harmful effects of cryo in both eyes. These second eyes of asymmetric cases were not included in the statistical evaluation of cryotherapy results in the Cryo-ROP Study.

## CRYOTHERAPY TECHNIQUES

### Timing of Cryotherapy

The efficacious results of cryotherapy for threshold ROP in the Cryo-ROP study are based on treatment being performed within 72 hours of the recognition of threshold disease. Part of the importance of this constraint within the study was the gathering of data on cryotherapy for a given degree of threshold ROP. Therefore, it was imperative that no change in ROP of a threshold eye occur before treatment. If stage 4 ROP (retinal detachment) developed between the time that threshold ROP was recognized and randomization occurred, that eye became ineligible for randomization and cryotherapy. From a clinical standpoint, timing is also important. The cryotherapist should perform the treatment as soon as possible after the recognition of threshold ROP, and if at all possible, within 72 hours. ROP in its very active phases (i.e., "rush" disease) can change significantly over a period of 5 to 7 days. This can result in stage 4 ROP, which probably significantly decreases the chance of a favorable outcome after cryotherapy.

### Anesthesia

For cryotherapy, general or local anesthesia can be used. This decision is left to the judgment of the cryotherapist and the infant's neonatologist. The decision on type of anesthesia is usually based on the infant's medical status, the availability of an anesthesiologist familiar with treating premature infants, and the cryosurgeon's experience. Generally, it is easier on the baby if local anesthesia is used, but easier on the treating ophthalmologist if general anesthesia is used. For a cryotherapist's first few cases, it may be advisable to use general anesthesia when medically possible, to facilitate application of cryotherapy.

#### *Local or Topical Anesthesia*

Local or topical anesthesia is usually performed in the neonatal intensive care unit (NICU), with assistance from the infant's nurse and with a neonatologist present in the unit. It should be noted that some cryotherapists in the Cryo-ROP study reported performing treatment with only topical anesthesia. The infants were observed to tolerate the treatment under topical anesthesia quite well and with no apparent pain.

Topical proparacaine 0.5% solution is instilled in the eye to be treated twice at 5-minute intervals. A lid speculum is inserted and then lidocaine is infiltrated subconjunctivally in each quadrant with a 3-ml syringe and a short 25- or 27-gauge needle. The injection is made between the rectus muscles in each quadrant, with the amount of infiltration about 0.25 ml per quadrant. The bevel of the needle should be kept toward the globe, with the angle of the needle tangential to the surface of the eye. After injection of the local anesthetic agent, the lid speculum is removed and the surgical team waits 5 to 10 minutes before proceeding with the cryotherapy.

Approximately 30 minutes prior to cryotherapy with the patient under local anesthesia, the neonatologist may administer sedation with chloral hydrate (25 to 50 mg/kg). This may help the infant's overall tolerance of the procedure.

### *General Anesthesia*

General anesthesia can be administered in an operating room or in the NICU, and should be given only by an anesthesiologist familiar with general anesthesia for premature babies. It is important before the child is anesthetized that all necessary equipment and personnel be readied so that there are no delays once the child is asleep. This will help minimize the time, and amount of anesthesia.

## Conjunctival Incisions

These are made only as necessary to reach the more posterior areas of the retina to be treated. Small, scissors incisions of 1 to 2 mm are made between the rectus muscles in each quadrant. If a conjunctival incision is made, then the field is kept sterile. Usually these small incisions do not require closure by suturing.

## Techniques

The objective of treatment is contiguous, but not overlapping, freezes of the entire avascular retina. The posterior extent of cryotherapy is the anterior edge of the fibrovascular ridge. The anterior extent of the zone of cryotherapy is the ora serrata. Attempts should be made to avoid treating directly under or posterior to the fibrovascular ridge (Fig 9–4). The preferred technique of cryotherapy is to start by applying treatment in a row just behind the ora serrata. Then gradually, row by row, the cryo applications are extended posteriorly to cover the entire vascular retina to the anterior margin of the fibrovascular ridge. Starting the treatment anteriorly allows for gradual softening of the globe, making the more posterior areas that require treatment more easily accessible and minimizing the need for conjunctival incisions.[22]

In the Cryo-ROP Study, cryotherapists were allowed to use a standard retina probe, a pediatric probe, or a cataract probe. I have used the standard retinal probes made by MIRA, Keeler (Amoils), and Frigitronics (Fig 9–5). Of the three, the MIRA standard retinal probe seems to be the easiest

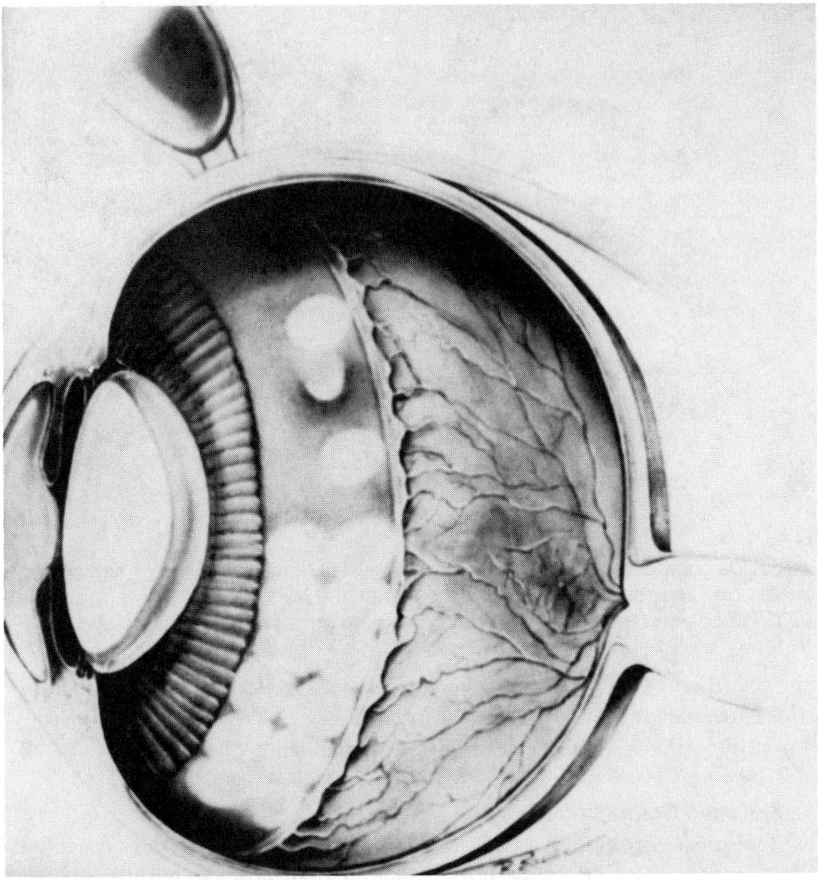

**FIG 9–4.**
An artist's conception of contiguous, nonoverlapping cryo applications between the anterior edge of the fibrovascular ridge and the ora serrata.

to use. This probe is slightly smaller in size, and because it requires no insulating boot, it is easier to manipulate around the small eye and orbit of the premature infant. The recently introduced "hammerhead" pediatric probes made by Frigitronics and MIRA seem to have great promise because they allow treatment of larger areas with each cryo application.

## Complications of Cryotherapy in the Cryo-ROP Study

In the study, complications associated with cryotherapy were recorded by ophthalmologists at the time of treatment and by pediatricians 3 days

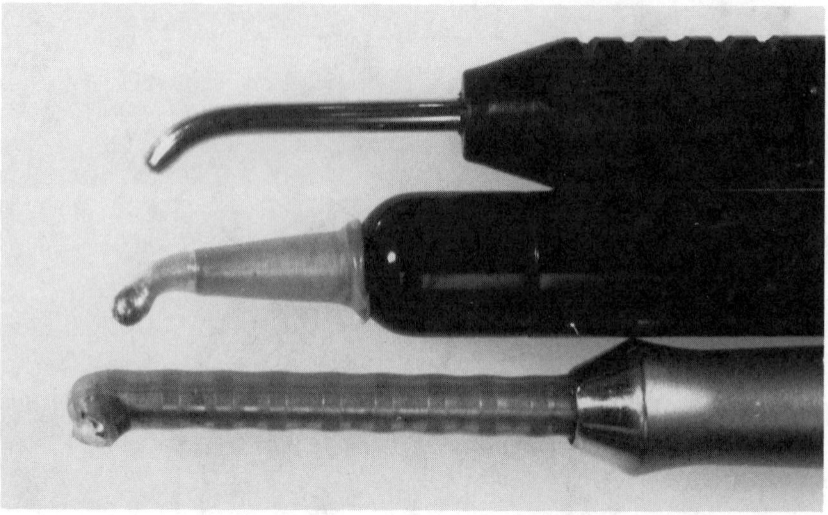

**FIG 9–5.**
Side-by-side comparison of standard retinal cryoprobes made by MIRA *(top),* Keeler/Amoils *(middle),* and Frigitronics *(bottom).* Of these three, the MIRA robe is smaller, requires no insulating boot, and is well suited for use around the small premature globe and orbit.

after cryotherapy. There were very few serious systemic or ocular complications from the cryotherapy in the treated eye (Table 9–1). In the study, no infant deaths were associated with sequelae from cryotherapy.

### *Systemic Complications*

The most common systemic complication from cryotherapy on infants in the Cryo-ROP Study was significant bradycardia or arrhythmias during or immediately after treatment. This complication, which occurred in 8.9% of cryo-treatments performed, underlines the importance of cardiac monitoring during the procedure, especially when it is performed under local anesthesia in the NICU. In the study, when one of these complications occurred during treatment, it was managed by temporarily stopping the cryo application and allowing spontaneous recovery of the heart rate. If spontaneous recovery of heart rate did not occur within a few seconds, then the bradycardic infant was gently stimulated by manual manipulation of the body. In my experience, of 19 cryotherapies performed at our center during the study (all under local anesthesia in the NICU), in no instance were resuscitative efforts or cardiac drugs necessary to counteract an episode of bradycardia or an arrhythmia that occurred during cryotherapy.

Acquired or increased cyanosis occurred in 1.4% of the 157 eyes that received cryotherapy in the Cryo-ROP Study. This usually resulted from

**TABLE 9–1.**
Intraoperative Complications During Cryotherapy (As Reported by Cryo-ROP Study in 157 Eyes)

| Complication | % |
|---|---|
| Ocular | |
| Hemorrhage: retinal, preretinal, vitreous | 19.1 |
| Conjunctival hematoma | 10.2 |
| Conjunctival laceration, unintended | 5.1 |
| Other | 1.3 |
| Systemic | |
| Bradycardia or arrhythmias | 8.9 |
| Other | 2.5 |
| Acquired or increased cyanosis | 1.9 |

apnea and/or bradycardia during the procedure. When local anesthesia was used, this was usually managed by temporarily stopping cryotherapy, manually stimulating the infant to breathe, and by increasing the level of inspired oxygen. In our center's experience, in no instance was it necessary to assist breathing during cryotherapy by using an Ambu bag or by intubation and mechanical ventilation. In one case at our center, however, approximately 2 hours after the cryotherapy the patient developed profound apnea and required intubation and mechanical ventilation for two days.

In general, cryotherapy as performed by the Cryo-ROP Study seems to be a systemically safe and relatively uncomplicated procedure. As more statistical information on the systemic complications of cryotherapy during the Cryo-ROP Study becomes available, more in-depth analysis of complications and risks will be made. Of particular interest will be the comparison of systemic risks between those infants treated under general anesthesia vs. those treated under local.

#### *Ocular Complications*

In the Cryo-ROP Study the most commonly observed complication was intraocular hemorrhage which occurred in 19.1% of the cases. This complication included large retinal, preretinal, or vitreous hemorrhages. These complications are significant not only because of the effects on visual development, but also because a large hemorrhage during a procedure may prevent adequate visualization for completion of the cryotherapy. In addition, the presence of vitreous hemorrhage may tend to exacerbate vitreous contraction and lead to retinal elevation. Further statistical analysis of these complications by the Cryo-ROP Study Group will yield more information about the long-term visual and anatomic sequelae. In an effort to avoid these intraocular hemorrhages, it is necessary to keep in mind several caveats. The first is to use very gentle techniques when manipulating these small globes during cryotherapy. Next, it is important to avoid excessive pressure on the eye with the cryoprobe and especially any movement of the probe during a freeze. It is also believed that refreezing previously treated areas may make hemorrhage more likely, particularly when these areas are located on the anterior skirt of an area of stage 3 ROP. Finally, avoiding treatment directly under areas of stage 3 or stage 2 fibrovascular proliferation will help minimize the possibility of intraocular hemorrhage.

The second most common ocular complication observed was the development of conjunctival hematoma in 10.2% of cases. The term conjunctival hematoma is intended to mean more than just subconjunctival hemorrhage that occurs during essentially all cryotherapy procedures. The implication of hematoma is that a tumorous hemorrhage has occurred. It is not felt that this is likely to be a visually threatening complication.

Unintended conjunctival lacerations occurred in 5.1% of cases, presumably from excessive pressure of the cryoprobe into the conjunctival cul-de-sac while an attempt was made to reach posterior areas requiring treatment. If these lacerations are small, they can be managed as small stab incisions made intentionally, and allowed to heal without suturing. If larger rips occur, and particularly if they leave areas of the globe uncovered by conjunctiva, then suturing is advisable.

Prior to the performance of the Cryo-ROP Study, many putative as well as observed ocular complications of cryotherapy were addressed by the study's developers. Fortunately, many of the most serious theoretical complications of cryo, such as fracturing the wall of the globe or inadvertently freezing the optic nerve, were not observed in any of the 157 cases initially reported by the study. However, these potentially severe complications cannot be excluded as future possibilities.

## DISCUSSION OF RESULTS

The Cryo-ROP Study data indicate that cryotherapy is a safe and efficacious means of reducing the chance of an unfavorable anatomic outcome (i.e., retinal detachment involving zone 1 of the posterior pole, a retinal fold involving the macula, or retrolental tissue or "mass") from severe ROP. The preliminary 3-month outcome data of the study have shown that when applied at the point of threshold ROP, cryotherapy will reduce the incidence of unfavorable outcome by approximately 50% compared with untreated eyes. Based on photographic data 3 months following cryotherapy, the untreated eyes had an unfavorable outcome in 43% of cases, compared with an unfavorable outcome in only 21.8% of the treated eyes. These numbers

**TABLE 9–2.**
Outcome Data (3 Months after Cryotherapy)

| | Percent Treated Eyes (n = 156) | Percent Untreated Eyes (n = 149) |
|---|---|---|
| Photographic outcome | | |
| Favorable | 78.2 | 57.0 |
| Unfavorable* | 21.8 | 43.0 |
| | P = <0.00001 | |
| Ophthalmoscopic outcome | | |
| Favorable | 76.5 | 54.4 |
| Unfavorable* | 23.5 | 45.6 |
| | P = <0.00001 | |

**Defined as a retinal detachment involving zone 1 of the posterior pole, a retinal fold involving the macula, or retrolental tissue or "mass."*

also closely reflect the 3-month follow-up data in the same eyes, based on ophthalmoscopy (Table 9–2).

From a statistical standpoint, it is the examination of the discordant pairs of eyes that provides the most compelling evidence of the effectiveness of cryotherapy for treating threshold ROP[23] (Fig 9–6). Discordant pairs represent eyes in which the treated eye and the untreated eye of a patient had different outcomes. This is distinguished from concordant pairs, in which both eyes (treated and untreated) had a similar outcome. Thus, in concordant pairs of eyes, both eyes of that study subject ended with either favorable or unfavorable outcomes. Of the discordant pairs, there are two groups: (1) those in which the treated eye had a favorable outcome and the untreated eye had an unfavorable outcome, and (2) those in which the treated eye had an unfavorable outcome but the untreated eye had a favorable outcome. When the ratio of these two groups of discordant pairs is calculated, it is 12:1 (graded ophthalmoscopically). Statistical analysis of this comparison gives a highly significant Chi-square value of 27.92. When judged photographically, the ratio of these discordant pairs was 34:6 with a Chi-square value of 19.6.[24] Thus, the statistical analysis of the Cryo-ROP Study data strongly support the efficacy of cryotherapy for reducing the incidence of anatomically adverse outcome from threshold ROP.

## Unanswered Questions From Current Cryo-ROP Results

### *Are Anatomic Results Equivalent to Visual Results?*

The primary outcome variable initially evaluated by the Cryo-ROP Study[24] is anatomical. It was assumed that the presence of a macular fold, a retrolental mass, or posterior retinal detachment would equate with a poor visual outcome, and conversely, that the absence of these findings would yield a good visual outcome. No one disputes that the adverse outcome criteria produce a poor visual result. What is less certain is the effect on vision of a severely dragged macula without a fold, or a retrolental membrane that does not reach the visual axis, or a temporary serous macular detachment which reattaches spontaneously after one month, or cryotherapy scars that come within 1 to 2 disk diameters (DD) of the macula after treating threshold ROP in zone 1. Many other similar situations have arisen that do not constitute an anatomically adverse outcome but that may yield a visual adverse outcome.

In an effort to correlate visual and anatomical results, in late 1987 the Cryo-ROP Study began visual acuity testing on all infants in the randomized portion of the study, and on all the natural history study subjects at four of the 23 centers involved in the study. The Visual Acuity Testing (VAT) program was started on the randomized cohort at the 1-year follow-up examination. The testing is performed at all 23 centers on a rotating basis by one of the four itinerant certified VAT testers. Testing is performed using Teller Acuity Cards, as described by Dobson et al.[25] As further data are

| | Treated Eye Favorable | Treated Eye Unfavorable |
|---|---|---|
| Untreated Eye Favorable | 67 | 3 |
| Untreated Eye Unfavorable | 36 | 28 |

Discordant Pairs (shaded cells)

$\text{Chi}^2 = 27.92$

**FIG 9–6.**
Evaluation of paired outcome in 134 symmetric cases, based on ophthalmoscopy.

collected by the VAT portion of the study, a more definitive correlation will be made between visual and anatomical results.

### *What Are the Risks of Cryotherapy to Visual Development?*

Indications are that the short-term ocular and systemic effects of cryotherapy seem to be relatively safe, compared with the short-term effects of a retinal detachment in zone 1, a macular fold, or retrolental tissue development. Cryotherapy appears to be particularly safe systemically when performed under local anesthesia in the NICU, because the potential risks involved with general anesthesia can be avoided. What we do not know are the long-term complications of cryotherapy on vision, or the efficacy of cryotherapy in subthreshold eyes, which may have a much greater than usual chance of spontaneous regression. The potential adverse long-term effects of cryotherapy may dissuade the surgeon from its use in *all* threshold ROP. In addition, certain variations of what is currently defined as threshold ROP may have as good a chance of regression (with good vision) spontaneously as they would if cryotherapy were applied. Some of the potential long-term untoward effects of cryotherapy for ROP are reduction of peripheral visual field, higher incidence of retinal break formation, reduction of central vision, increased incidence of strabismus, and creation of high refractive errors. Thus far, none of these untoward effects has surfaced from the Cryo-ROP study data, but some may appear in future analysis.

There seems to be little argument that cryotherapy will diminish peripheral visual field in eyes that receive treatment. Phase 2 of the Cryo-ROP study will evaluate this possibility in these treated infants by formally measuring the peripheral extent of visual field when these children are 5 and 6 years old. This information will provide objective evidence of the destructive effects of cryotherapy on peripheral vision.

As mentioned by Tasman,[26] the formation of retinal breaks and rhegmatogenous retinal detachment have been observed in infants after cryotherapy. Often the retinal breaks have occurred at the margins of the cryo scars. This is not totally unexpected because these eyes have considerable centripetal vitreoretinal traction at the sites of extraretinal proliferation, and cryotherapy creates firm chorioretinal adhesions at the peripheral margins of these areas of traction. Furthermore, as these eyes grow, a tangential component of traction on the retina may be created.

This author (R.S.) has seen one eye of a patient (not in the Cryo-ROP study) develop a definite rhegmatogenous detachment after cryotherapy for threshold ROP. The patient received bilateral cryotherapy for symmetric threshold ROP in August 1988. Six weeks later, the left eye was found to have a total, open funnel retinal detachment. A scleral buckle was performed, and at the time of surgery two slit-like retinal breaks at the posterior margin of the cryotherapy were identified. The buckling procedure was successful in reattaching the retina, although by November 1988, tractional elevation of the macula occurred as a result of a vitreous strand to that area. A vitrectomy was performed, which was successful in flattening the macular area; however, it was necessary to remove the lens because of the peripheral redundancy of the retina. Thus it was necessary that the vitrectomy instruments and infusion terminal be introduced through the ciliary body to prevent peripheral retinal damage. Consequently this child is now unilaterally aphakic in the eye where the macula was detached twice. An additional procedure (in 6 to 12 months) to cut the encircling No. 240 band will be necessary to allow for ocular growth in the future. The parents and pediatric ophthalmologist now face the very difficult tasks of helping the child to overcome amblyopia and to cope with aphakia. The visual prognosis for this type of eye is for moderate amblyopia at best. It is not known whether cryotherapy played a role in the development of retinal detachment in this child. It is known from the Cryo-ROP study that this eye would have had approximately a 53% chance of *not* having had an adverse outcome without cryotherapy, and a 76.5% chance of no adverse outcome with cryo. However, future data collection from Cryo-ROP study subjects should provide risk characteristics beyond the current definition of threshold ROP; this may help identify eyes at greater and lesser risk of adverse visual outcome.

Correlations have been made between the ischemic pathogenesis of retinal vascular proliferation in ROP with those of diabetic retinopathy and sickle cell retinopathy.[27, 28] Thus, the rationale for the use of ablative therapy in ROP has stemmed from experience with photocoagulation in diabetic retinopathy. Initial efforts at ablative ROP treatment in the U.S. and Japan involved the use of photocoagulation.[29–34] It is known from the results of the National Cooperative Diabetic Retinopathy Study that from one to five lines of central vision were lost in some patients who underwent peripheral scatter retinal photocoagulation for proliferative diabetic retinopathy unrelated to direct macular damage from photocoagulation.[35] Often this visual loss occurs from severe cystoid macular edema after panretinal photocoagulation. Therefore it may be reasonable to expect that some central visual loss may accompany cryotherapy for ROP. This is still an unrecognized long-term complication, but one that must be considered as a possibility.

Similarly, the effects of cryotherapy on the development of strabismus or on the production of higher than usual refractive errors may also represent potential long-term untoward effects of cryo. Certainly a considerable amount of cryotherapy must be received by the rectus muscles in and around their tendinous insertions when it is applied in the manner performed by the Cryo-ROP protocol.[36] This may produce some temporary or permanent muscular paresis that may exacerbate strabismus. Loss of accommodation from pe-

paresis that may exacerbate strabismus. Loss of accommodation from periphery retinal cryotherapy or panretinal photocoagulation is a well-recognized complication of these treatments in adults.[37, 38] Although usually transient (lasting from 1 to 6 months), this type of complication may have a more profound effect on vision during the first few months of visual development. The Cryo-ROP study data may help to answer some of these possibilities.

### *Should Cryotherapy Be Applied Bilaterally in Symmetric Cases?*

Another primary unanswered question from the preliminary report of the study has been whether or not cryotherapy should be applied to both eyes of an infant who has bilateral threshold ROP. The preliminary report of the Cryo-ROP Study takes the position that this question should be left to the clinical judgment of the ophthalmologist and based on current knowledge.[24] As further long-term experience with the effects of cryotherapy on retinal function and ocular function accumulates, the Cryo-ROP study data will be able to shed more light on this important question. The answers will come both from long-term study of cryo-treated eyes as well as from further analysis of the risk factors for treatment intervention. This information will allow us to fine-tune the current criteria for "threshold ROP." In the meantime, the cryosurgeon is charged with making the decision of whether to treat both eyes when at threshold ROP. The ophthalmologist alone must determine the risk-benefit ratio of performing cryotherapy bilaterally.[38a]

A clinical impression that seems to be widely accepted within the Cryo-ROP Study Group is that threshold eyes with zone 1 disease have a worse prognosis than do eyes with peripheral zone 2 disease. Also, it seems to follow that eyes at threshold ROP with severe stage 3 disease have a worse prognosis than those with mild or moderate ROP. Using these clinical impressions, this author has developed an algorithmic approach to cryotherapy for ROP to serve as a guide for when to treat one eye, or both eyes (Fig 9–7); this approach is intended to serve until such a decision can be based upon objective data. The recommendations of this treatment schema are as follows:

1. Cryotherapy should be applied to the more severely affected eye first, if such exists.
2. Cryotherapy should be applied to the second (fellow) eye whenever:
   a. There is any stage 3 ROP in zone 1.
   b. Stage 3 ROP in zone 2 is posterior to vortex vein ampullae in any quadrant.
   c. Stage 3 ROP in zone 2 is severe (in any area) and anterior to vortex vein ampullae.

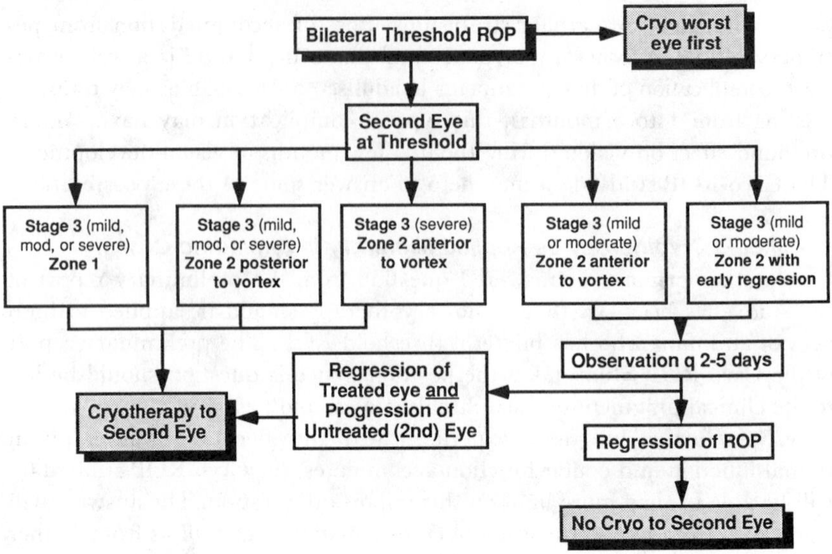


**FIG 9–7.**
Algorithm for cryotherapy to second eye in a patient with bilateral threshold ROP.

3. The second eye should be followed with frequent examinations (every 2 to 5 days) if:
   a. All stage 3 ROP is mild or moderate and anterior to vortex ampullae in all quadrants.
   b. All stage 3 ROP is mild or moderate and in zone 2 and if there are early indications of regression, i.e., a widening white zone peripheral to the shunt, or buds of retinal vessels that extend through the shunt into the avascular retina (Fig 9–8, A and B; Plates 6 and 7).
4. Cryotherapy should be applied to an observed second eye at threshold ROP when there has been regression of ROP in the treated eye and any progression of threshold ROP in the untreated eye.

This rationale for treatment can apply to either symmetric or asymmetric cases of threshold ROP in which the first eye reaches the threshold level three or more days before the second eye.

### *Is There a Better Technique of Cryotherapy Than That Used in the Cryo-ROP Study?*

The Cryo-ROP protocol called for contiguous, nonoverlapping cryo applications to be applied to the avascular retina, peripheral to the demarcation

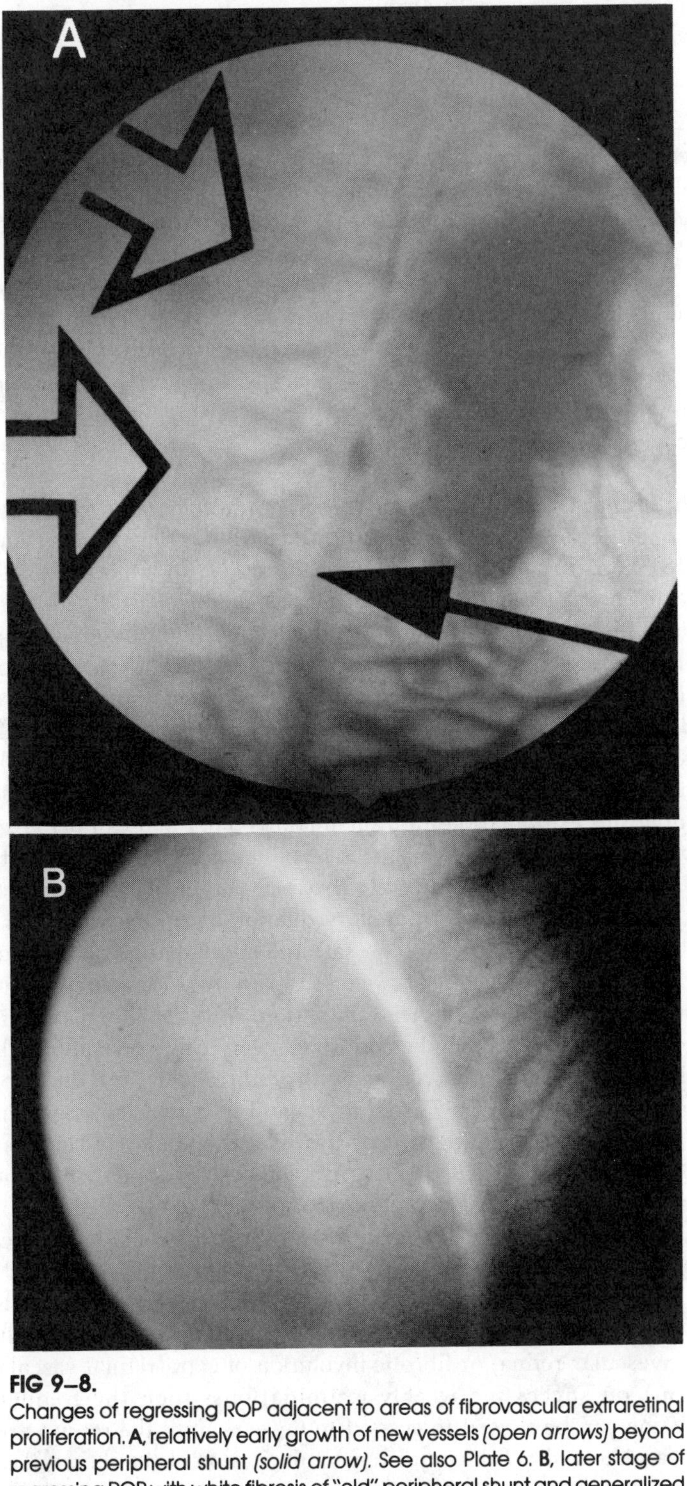


**FIG 9–8.**

Changes of regressing ROP adjacent to areas of fibrovascular extraretinal proliferation. **A**, relatively early growth of new vessels *(open arrows)* beyond previous peripheral shunt *(solid arrow)*. See also Plate 6. **B**, later stage of regressing ROP with white fibrosis of "old" peripheral shunt and generalized attenuation of vessel caliber. See also Plate 7.

between vascularized and avascular retina (see Fig 9–4). Is this perhaps more extensive cryotherapy than is necessary to cause regression? Should the cryo applications overlap so that no untreated areas between cryo spots exist? Should cryotherapy be performed directly beneath areas of stages 2 and 3? Would laser photocoagulation, perhaps, be more effective and produce fewer side effects than cryotherapy? These are some of the important questions to which answers will be sought by future investigational studies as this ablative modality of interdictive therapy is refined. At this time, no technique differing from that used by the Cryo-ROP Study has proved to be efficacious.

### *What Is the Optimal Timing for Screening Examinations for ROP?*

A major legacy of the Cryo-ROP Study will be the extensive data collected by the natural history portion of the study. In addition to affirming the effectiveness of the International Classification of ROP, the screening protocol of the study has been found to be effective, and will serve as a proven model for the screening of ROP in the future (Fig 9–9). According to study data, the earliest time of threshold ROP development was at 6.57 weeks of life and the average time of threshold development was 11.33 weeks (±2.40).[24] Therefore, if current criteria for cryotherapy intervention are used, the first eye examination should be performed before 6.57 weeks of life. Because postponing this examination until the infant is older and can better tolerate the examination is advantageous, it is recommended that the exam be performed during the sixth week of life (between 35 and 42 days of age). Cyclomydril which was used for pupillary dilation in eye examinations in the Cryo-ROP Study, was shown to be a safe and effective mydriatic agent when 1 drop was instilled in each eye twice (10 to 15 minutes apart) about 60 to 90 minutes before the time of the examination. After the initial examination, eye examinations should then be performed every two weeks until either the retina is completely vascularized or until prethreshold ROP develops (any stage ROP in zone 1, stage 2 plus, or stage 3 in zone 2 or stage 3 plus in zone 2 but less than 5 contiguous or less than 8 cumulative clock hours of stage 3). Once prethreshold ROP is present, eye examinations should be performed weekly until either progression to threshold ROP occurs or until there is evidence of regressing ROP in zone 3. Once threshold ROP is reached, cryotherapy should be performed according to the procedures outlined above and in Figure 9–7. Once there is definite evidence of regressing ROP in zone 3 (loss of previously present plus disease, growth of retinal vessels into previously avascular retina, or fibrotic involution of extra-retinal vascular proliferation) on successive weekly examinations, then the frequency of examination can be slowed to every 4 to 6 weeks until the retinas are completely vascularized. With complete vascularization of the retina, the infant

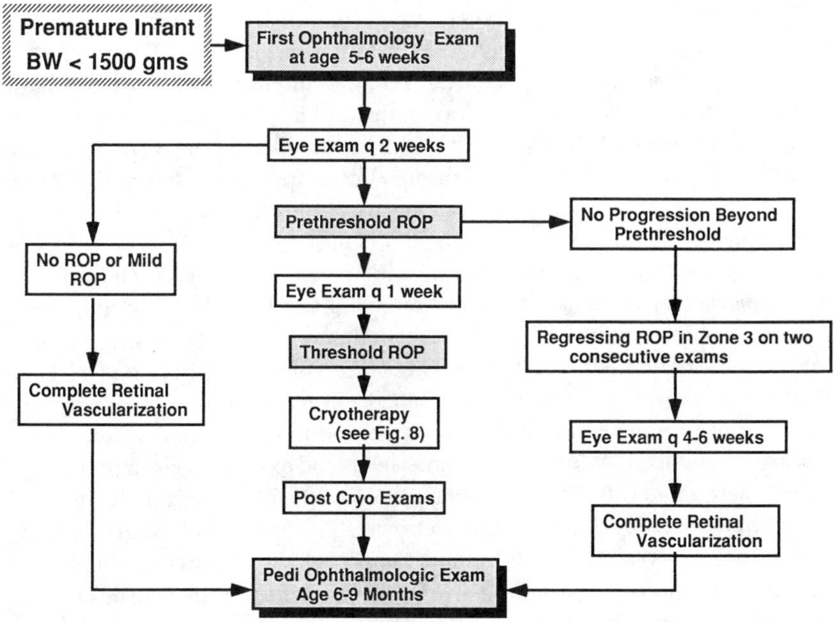


**FIG 9–9.**
ROP screening protocol based on Cryo-ROP study experience.

is referred for a pediatric ophthalmologic follow-up examination at age 6 to 9 months. Parents are cautioned to schedule this examination sooner should they notice a constant strabismus.

### *What Are the Directions for Future Investigative Work in ROP?*

With the results of the Cryo-ROP Study, there are now two proved therapies for ROP: control of amount of supplemental oxygen, which is preventative, and cryotherapy, which is interdictive. In reattaching the very difficult retinal detachments associated with cicatricial ROP, corrective therapies such as vitrectomy and scleral buckling have met with limited anatomic success and with very discouraging visual success. Although surgical techniques and timing of retinal reattachment are likely to improve, the visual results will probably continue to be poor because of the rapid amblyopia that develops in the infant's visual system. Therefore, at this time, the prophylactic and interdictive therapies seem to hold the most promise of saving vision.

The two prophylactic investigational modalities of therapy that look encouraging are antioxidants and light reduction. Although initial work with a vitamin E system has been controversial,[17–19] ongoing work is being done with other antioxidants (penicillamine, ceruloplasmin, apotransferrin, deferoxamine) which are more potent than vitamin E and can enter the developing retina at earlier stages of development than can vitamin E.[39–42] Provocative work by Glass et al.[43] has renewed interest in the idea that light exposure may exacerbate ROP development. This thesis was originally explored almost four decades ago,[44, 45] but the results did not support a role for light as a cause of ROP at that time. These original studies on light and ROP were performed before the role of oxygen in exacerbating this disease was appreciated, and at a time when lights in the nursery were perhaps not as intense as they are at present. A randomized, prospective, clinical trial will be necessary to answer the question of light and ROP more definitively.

Areas of interest involving interdictive therapies include oxygen therapy, the use of attenuated cryotherapy, and laser photocoagulation. Dr. Dale Phelps has shown in kittens that if blood oxygen saturation levels are increased during the healing phase of oxygen-induced retinopathy, less severe disease is produced.[46–48] Actually increasing blood oxygen levels in premature infants with moderate ROP may possibly alter the course of the disease and prevent more severe changes from occurring. This method of oxygen therapy needs further investigation in humans, and probably will require a clinical trial at multiple centers. Likewise, the use of an attenuated form of cryotherapy or laser therapy in lieu of cryotherapy deserves further clinical investigation as interdictive treatment for ROP in the future.

## APPENDIX 9A

### Cryo-ROP Planning Committee (Dec 1983)

Earl A. Palmer, M.D. (Chairman), Portland, Ore.
John T. Flynn, M.D., Miami, Fla.
Robert J. Hardy, Ph.D. (Biometrist), Houston
Arthur L. Rosenbaum, M.D., Los Angeles
David B. Schaffer, M.D., Philadelphia

### Cryo-ROP Advisory Committee (Dec 1983)

Albert W. Biglan, M.D., Pittsburgh
Israel Goldberg, Ph.D. (Ex-officio), National Eye Institute
N. Warren Hindle, M.D., Calgary, Alta., Canada
James D. Kingham, M.D., Sarasota, Fla.
Andrew Q. McCormick, M.D., Vancouver, B.C., Canada
Dale L. Phelps, M.D., Los Angeles
William S. Tasman, M.D., Philadelphia

## APPENDIX 9B

### Cryo-ROP Study Group

#### *Study Headquarters*

Oregon Health Sciences University, Portland
Study Chairman: Earl A. Palmer, M.D.

#### *Coordinating Center*

Coordinating Center for Clinical Trials
School of Public Health
The University of Texas Health Science Center at Houston
Principal Investigator: Robert J. Hardy, Ph.D.

#### *Clinical Study Centers and Principal Investigators*

Baltimore: Serge de Bustros, M.D.
Birmingham, Ala.: Frederick J. Elsas, M.D.
Charleston, S.C.: Richard A. Saunders, M.D.
Chicago: Marilyn T. Miller, M.D.
Cincinnati: Miles J. Burke, M.D.
Columbus, Ohio: Gary L. Rogers, M.D.
Dallas: Rand Spencer, M.D.
Durham, N.C.: Edward Buckley, M.D.
Indianapolis: Forrest D. Ellis, M.D.
Louisville: Charles C. Barr, M.D.
Miami: John T. Flynn, M.D.
Minneapolis: Robert C. Ramsay, M.D.
Nashville: Stephen S. Feman, M.D.
New Orleans: Robert A. Gordon, M.D.
Philadelphia: David B. Schaffer, M.D.
Pittsburgh: Albert W. Biglan, M.D.
Portland: Earl A. Palmer, M.D.
Upstate New York (Rochester): Dale L. Phelps, M.D.
Detroit: Michael T. Trese, M.D.
Sacramento, Calif.: Alan M. Roth, M.D.
Salt Lake City: Jane D. Kivlin, M.D.
San Antonio: W.A.J. van Heuven, M.D.
Washington, D.C.: William S. Gilbert, M.D.

#### *Fundus Photograph Reading Center*

Oregon Health Sciences University, Portland
Principal Investigator: Robert Watzke, M.D.

## REFERENCES


1. Multicenter Trial of Cryotherapy for Retinopathy of Prematurity: *Manual of Procedures.* 1985, p 1–2.
2. Phelps DL: Vision loss due to retinopathy of prematurity. *Lancet* 1981; 1:606.
3. Hittner H, Kretzer F: Retinopathy of prematurity: Pathogenesis, prevention and treatment, in Chiswick ML (ed): *Recent Advances in Perinatal Medicine.* New York, Churchill Livingstone 1985; pp 145–163.
4. Patz A: Retrolental fibroplasia (retinopathy of prematurity). *Am J Ophthalmol* 1982; 94:552–554.
5. Palmer EA: Optimal timing of examination for acute retrolental fibroplasia. *Ophthalmology* 1981; 88:662–668.
6. Phelps DL: Retinopathy of prematurity: An estimate of vision loss in the United States—1979. *Pediatrics* 1981; 67:924–925.
7. Patz A, Hoeck LE, De La Cruz E: Studies on the effect of high oxygen administration in retrolental fibroplasia. Nursery observation. *Am J Ophthalmol* 1952; 27:1248–1253.
8. Lanman JT, Guy LP, Dancis J: Retrolental fibroplasia and oxygen therapy. *JAMA* 1985; 155:223–226.
9. Kinsey VE: Retrolental fibroplasia: Cooperative study of retrolental fibroplasia and the use of oxygen. *Arch Ophthalmol* 1956; 56:481–543.
10. Gyllensten LF, Hellstrom BE: Retrolental fibroplasia: Animal experiments. The effects of intermittently administered oxygen on the post natal development of the eyes of full term mice: A preliminary report. *Acta Paediatr Scand* 1985; 41:577–582.
11. Ashton N, Ward B, Serpell G: Role of oxygen in the genesis of retrolental fibroplasia: Preliminary report. *Br J Ophthalmol* 1953; 37:513–520.
12. Ashton N, Cook C: Direct observation of the effect of oxygen on developing vessels. Preliminary report. *Br J Ophthalmol* 1954; 38:433–440.
13. Patz A, Eastham A, Higginbotham DH, et al: Oxygen studies in retrolental fibroplasia. II: The production of microscopic changes of retrolental fibroplasia in experimental animals. *Am J Ophthalmol* 1953; 36:1511–1522.
14. Gyllensten LF, Hellstrom BE: Experimental approach to the pathogenesis of retrolental fibroplasia. Changes of the eye induced by exposure of newborn mice to concentrated oxygen. *Acta Paediatr Scand [Suppl]* 1954; 100:131–148.
15. Gesschman R, Nadig PW, Snell AC Jr. et al: Effect of high oxygen concentrations on the eyes of newborn mice. *Am J Physiol* 1954; 179:115–118.
16. Michaelson IC, Herz N, Lewkowitz E, et al: Effect of increased oxygen on the development of the retinal vessels. An experimental study. *Br J Ophthalmol* 1954; 38:577–587.
17. Hittner HM, Godio LB, Rudolph AV, et al: Retrolental fibroplasia: Efficacy of vitamin E in a double-blind clinical study of preterm infants. *N Engl J Med* 1981; 305:1365–1371.
18. Finer NN, Schindler RF, Grant G et al: Effect of intramuscular vitamin E on frequency and severity of retrolental fibroplasia. *Lancet* 1982; 1:1087–1091.
19. Phelps DL, Rosenbaum AL, Isenberg SJ, et al: Tocopherol efficacy and safety

for preventing retinopathy of prematurity: A randomized controlled double-masked clinical trial. *Pediatrics* 1987; 79:489.

20. Committee for the Classification of Retinopathy of Prematurity: An international classification of retinopathy of prematurity. *Arch Ophthalmol* 1984; 102:1130–1134.
21. Palmer EA: Personal communication, March 1987.
22. Tasman WS: Personal communication, Dec 1985.
23. Hardy R: Personal communication, March 1988.
24. Cryotherapy of Retinopathy of Prematurity Cooperative Groups: Multicenter trial of cryotherapy for retinopathy of prematurity: Preliminary results. *Arch Ophthalmol* 1988; 106:471–479.
25. Dobson V, Schwartz TL, Sandstrom DJ, et al: Binocular visual acuity in neonates: The acuity card procedure. *Dev Med Child Neurol* 1987; 29:199–206.
26. Tasman W: Multicenter trial of cryotherapy for retinopathy of prematurity (editorial). *Arch Ophthalmol* 1988; 106:463–464.
27. Multicenter Trial of Cryotherapy for Retinopathy of Prematurity: *Manual of Procedures*, 1985, Chap 2.
28. Ashton N: The pathogenesis of retrolental fibroplasia. *Ophthalmology* 1979; 86:1695–1699.
29. Patz A, Maumenee AE, Ryan SJ: Argon laser photocoagulation advantages and limitations. *Trans Am Acad Ophthalmol Otolaryngol* 1971; 75:569–579.
30. Tanabe Y, Ikema M: Retinopathy of prematurity and photocoagulation therapy, *Acta Soc Ophthalmol Jpn* 1972; 76:269–276.
31. Nagata M, Kanenaris: Light-coagulation in cases of progressive retinopathy of prematurity. Report II. *Rinsho Ganka* 1970; 24:655–661.
32. Oshima K, Ikae H, Kano M, et al: Clinical study and photocoagulation of retinopathy of prematurity. *Folia Ophthalmol Jpn* 1971; 22:700–707.
33. Nagata M, Isuruoka Y: Treatment of acute retrolental fibroplasia with xenon arc photocoagulation. *Jpn J Ophthalmol* 1972; 16:181–243.
34. Payne JW, Patz A: Treatment of acute proliferative retrolental fibroplasia. *Trans Am Acad Ophthalmol Otolaryngol* 1972; 76:1234–1241.
35. Diabetic Retinopathy Research Group: Preliminary report on effects of photocoagulation therapy. *Am J Ophthalmol* 1976; 81:383–396.
36. Multicenter Trial of Cryotherapy for Retinopathy of Prematurity: *Manual of Procedures*, 1985, Chap 7.
37. Lerner BC, Lakhanpal V, Schocket SS: Transient myopia and accommodative paresis following retinal cryotherapy and panretinal photocoagulation. *Am J Ophthalmol* 1984; 97:704–708.
38. Pruett RC: Internal ophthalmoplegia after panretinal therapy. *Arch Ophthalmol* 1979; 97:2212.

38a. Phelps DL, Phelps CE: Cryotherapy in infants with retinopathy of prematurity: A decision model for treating one or both eyes. *JAMA* 1989; 261:1751–1756.

39. Lakatos L, Lakotos Z, Hatvami I, et al: Controlled trial of use of D-penicillamine to prevent retinopathy of prematurity in very low-birth-weight infants, in Stern L, Oh W, Friis-Hansen B (eds). *Physiologic Foundations of Perinatal Care*, vol. 2. New York, Elsevier, 1986, pp 9–23.
40. Sullivan JL: Retinopathy of prematurity and iron: A modification of the oxygen hypothesis. (Letter to editor) *Pediatrics* 1986; 78:1171–1172.

41. Sullivan JL, Newton RF: Serum antioxidant activity in neonates. *Arch Dis Child* 1988; 63:748–750.
42. Sullivan JF: Iron, plasma, antioxidants and "oxygen-radical disease of prematurity." *Am J Dis Child* 1988; 142:1341–1344.
43. Glass P, Avery GB, Subramanian KNS, et al: Effects of bright light in the hospital nursery on the incidence of retinopathy of prematurity. *N Engl J Med* 1985; 313:401–404.
44. Hepner WR, Krause AC, Davis ME: Retrolental fibroplasia and light. *Pediatrics* 1949; 3:824–828.
45. Locke JC, Reese AB: Retrolental fibroplasia. *Arch Ophthalmol* 1952; 48:44–47.
46. Phelps DL, Rosenbaum AL: Effects of marginal hypoxemia on recovery from oxygen-induced retinopathy in the kitten model. *Pediatrics* 1985; 73:1–10.
47. Phelps DL, Rosenbaum AL: Effects of variable oxygenation and gradual withdrawal of oxygen during the recovery phase in oxygen induced retinopathy: Kitten model. *Pediatr Res* 1987; 22:297–301.
48. Phelps DL: Reduced severity of oxygen-induced retinopathy in kittens recovered in 28% oxygen. *Pediatr Res* 1988; 24:106–109.

Chapter 10

# Vitrectomy in the Treatment of Retinopathy of Prematurity Stages 4 and 5

Rainer N. Mittl, M.D.

The pioneering efforts of Charles, Hirose, Machemer, and Schepens have formed the basis for the surgical approach to the late stages of retinopathy of prematurity (ROP). Initial attempts to approach these desperate cases go back as far as the early 1970s. The first vitrectomy for ROP was performed by Machemer in 1972.[1, 2]

Treister et al. used vitrectomy for grade 3 to 5 retrolental fibroplasia (RLF) and for RLF-simulating diseases.[2] Charles mentioned he had performed surgery for this indication since the mid-1970s.[3] Other reports of successful reattachment of the retina followed.[4–15] From the onset, two surgical approaches were pursued: closed vitrectomy and open-sky vitrectomy. The vast majority of vitrectomies in adults is performed via pars plana. In the infant eye, the size of the anterior segment and the location of the retrolental plate suggested that open-sky vitrectomy was a valid alternative. Easy access to the anterior loop is probably the main reason why open-sky vitrectomy is still widely used to treat these cases.

ROP had been dormant for years. The disease has regained significance, and a recent resurgence has assumed near-epidemic proportions. Therefore, the number of cases eligible for surgery has actually increased.

The surgical options were quite limited initially, because only vitreous cutters were available.[1, 2]

Membrane peeling or stripping has little or, at best, limited value in the surgical approach to stage 5 ROP.[3, 6] The turning point arrived with the introduction of intravitreal scissors.[3] The basis for surgery in ROP remains sharp dissection.

## INDICATIONS

Initially, it was believed that "grade 5 RLF" was not amenable to surgical treatment.[2, 6, 7, 16] Grade 3 or 4 detachments were sometimes successfully reattached by scleral buckling and/or vitrectomy.[2] Now there is general agreement that vitreous surgery should be reserved for stages 4B and 5, when the detachment is too severe to be relieved by scleral buckling alone.[14] Vitrectomy can be successful in cases where both cryotherapy and scleral buckling have failed. Extensive bilateral near-total or total traction, or sometimes rhegmatogenous retinal detachments, or a recent history of rapid progression to complete detachment, are surgical prerequisites.[8, 14] The macula lutea must be detached or threatened.[16] Exudative detachments are not considered for surgery unless they are combined with a traction detachment.[9, 10]

Because the infants are at a significant anesthetic risk,[9] all detachments must be irreversible. Total retinal detachments do not reattach spontaneously.[8] They are always funnel shaped. Unilateral total retinal detachments should be considered for surgery only if there is a high likelihood that the retina of the fellow eye will also detach.[10] Charles believed that because of the certainty of severe amblyopia, most unilateral cases should not undergo surgery.[3] Eyes should be excluded from surgery if total destruction of the retina can be assumed.[8] Eyes with severe subretinal membranes, exudate, or blood may need to be judged "inoperable."

The moral implications of subjecting very sick infants to eye surgery are severe. Although proper case selection is imperative, it is difficult to accomplish. Therefore, eyes will come to surgery that have no evidence of light perception and little or no chance for successful treatment.[14] The issue is confounded by the fact that accurate determination of visual acuity is frequently not possible, neither before surgery, nor later.[14] One of the reasons is that these infants are developmentally delayed.[14] The reversibility of optic nerve and retinal damage is unknown, however. Therefore, a reasonable attempt at surgical reattachment should be made.[14] As Kalina pointed out in discussing Trese's paper, an attached retina holds visual potential; a detached retina does not.[10] Functional improvement remains highly uncertain, however, even if successful reattachment is achieved.

## PROGNOSTIC FACTORS

Clues exist for better visual results. Larger dilated pupils preoperatively, and deeper anterior chambers, are favorable signs.[13] Children with shallow detachments of the macula lutea tend to have better visual results.[10] The single most important morphologic feature, however, is funnel configuration.[22] A wide funnel is more likely to be associated with anatomic and functional success than is a narrow funnel.[13, 17] This may suggest that the infants should undergo surgery before the funnel contracts. Multiple adverse circumstances, most notably associated health problems, may interfere with the performance of eye surgery at the most favorable time. Should eyes containing narrow funnels then be condemned preoperatively? This is impossible for one simple reason: It is difficult to determine the accurate configuration of the funnel with certainty. Ultrasonography is helpful but of limited value.[18, 19] Funnels may be narrow anteriorly and wide open posteriorly. On the other hand, a demonstrated narrow funnel, combined with a flat anterior chamber, posterior synechiae, increased intraocular pressure, enlarged cornea, and subretinal bleeding, severely limits postoperative expectations.[14] However, none of these are absolute exclusion criteria.[15]

Another prognostic factor is the surgical anatomy of the membranes. They are so closely associated with the retina that blunt separation is usually impossible. Large amounts of proliferative tissue may have to be left behind. The result is inadequate release of traction and reproliferation.

Beyond pathoanatomic considerations, surgical skill plays a greater than usual role in the outcome of ROP surgery. There is no other eye condition in which iatrogenic retinal tears are as detrimental as they are in ROP.[13] However, sharp membrane dissection, the surgical technique of choice, is prone to producing retinal breaks.

## TIMING OF SURGERY

The age range for surgery is from a few months to 2 or more years of age. Chong et al. have operated on children as young as 3 months.[13] It is the pathology of the eye, not the age of the patient, that should determine when to perform surgery.[8, 9] The retina should be reattached as soon as possible after the detachment has occurred to assure optimal visual results.[8, 9] The dramatic difference in success rates between open and closed funnel detachments certainly suggests early surgery.[9] In Trese's series, children with shape recognition had surgery at an average age of 4.8 months. Shape recognition included the grasping of brightly colored objects or the stacking of rings, head turning or grasping of a pen light, or identification of targets at arm's length. On the other hand, children who had retinal reattachment without light perception were operated on at an average age of 6.3 months.[10] Eyes coming to surgery earlier because of regression of vascularity, however, may have a milder form of ROP.[10]

McPherson et al. based the timing of surgery on ultrastructural studies of membranes removed from eyes with retrolental fibroplasia.[12] In these investigators' experience, the duration of the retinal detachment correlated best with potential restoration of vision. Pathological specimens obtained at 4 to 5 months postnatal age consisted almost exclusively of red blood cells and myofibroblasts arranged in sheets. They considered this the optimal time to perform vitrectomy. Membranes removed during the sixth postnatal month contained plasma cells, polymorphonuclear leukocytes, macrophages, and retinal pigment epithelial cells. They considered this still an appropriate time to place the pliable retina back into position. In children from 7 to 16 months of age, retrolental membranes included ghost vessels, lysed cellular material, and autolytic macrophages. The cell remnants were interspersed between fibrillary material condensed into sheets. As a result, because of extensive necrosis of retinal neurons, the retina appeared to be less viable. These findings were in part confirmed by de Juan et al.[20]

Although emphasis has frequently been placed on early surgery, sometimes there may be merit in delay.[3] Dilated iris and retinal vessels, as well as subretinal exudates, indicate plus disease and are relative contraindications to surgery.[10] In these active cases, the reproliferation rate is higher. Another advantage of delaying surgery is the reduction of the anesthetic risk in an older infant with greater body weight and better pulmonary function.[3]

Obviously, a compromise has to be reached between a multitude of factors. The primary objective is to preserve the infant's life; preserving the infant's eye is second. This is particularly true because the visual prognosis is usually uncertain.

## PATHOANATOMY

Stage 5 surgery has yielded dynamic details of the mechanisms of retinal detachments in advanced cases, which had not been available from histopathologic examination.[17] Following are some conclusions derived from surgical observations.

Proliferation along the anterior hyaloid face creates the retrolental membrane. The majority of vessels at this interface are retinal vessels translocated centrally.[3] As the retina and the ora serrata are pulled anteriorly and medially by circumferential traction, they are almost in contact with the lens.[3, 6] Ultimately, the retrolental plate consists of the following layers: anterior hyaloid, posterior hyaloid, and retina.[3] The retrolenticular space may be occupied by heavily vascularized tissue in active cases, or by white tissue with few blood vessels in others.[21]

Stage 5 ROP produces dragging of the retinal vessels and even of the entire optic disc, also retinal folds, proliferation of the retinal pigment epithelium, chorioretinal scarring, vitreous membranes and traction, or even rhegmatogenous retinal detachments.[6] The retinal detachment is the end of a sequence initiated by immature angioblastic cells leaving the retina from the ridge of proliferative tissue.[22] They migrate anteriorly and posteriorly along fine, collagenous strands in the vitreous.[22] As they interact with these collagens, they produce new fibers. The strands become oriented along traction lines, and traction in itself promotes proliferation.[22] Retinal detachment is the end result.

Early membranes contain branching vessels that resemble retinal vessels.[22] There is no anatomic plane between the membranes and the retina. Tissue can only be removed at the risk of making at least partial-thickness retinal cuts. Bleeding is unavoidable.[22]

Machemer described the mechanisms operative in the late stages of ROP: contraction of the shunt with retinal stretching, contraction of proliferative tissue with retinal elevation, and finally, proliferation within the vitreous.[17] Contraction produces traction on the retina. Avascular and vascular retina respond differently to the forces of stretching. The areas between the major vessels and the avascular periphery thin out without detaching. Vessels, on the other hand, stretch until they are straight. Once their limit of tolerance has been reached, the retina detaches.[17]

Machemer considered the location of the shunt to be a factor of utmost importance. Because the shunt is typically located in the temporal periphery, the major vessels are reoriented temporally. With continued traction, the temporal retina will become elevated. When the shunt involves the entire circumference, traction is exerted equally and major displacement of vessels will not occur.[17]

The more premature the baby, the more posterior the location of the shunt.[17] Anterior shunts are associated with high detachments of the anterior retina and shallow detachments of the posterior retina. Proliferation posterior to the equator drags the retina anteriorly and centrally. The posterior retina is vascularized, however, and cannot stretch. Therefore, a high retinal detachment and a narrow funnel are the result. The opposite occurs in the anterior portions. The avascular retina stretches and may even remain attached. It folds over anteriorly toward the contracting ring, producing a deep circumferential trough.[17]

With very posterior location of the shunt, the proliferative tissue does not gain access to the anterior vitreous cavity. The retina may remain attached between disc and temporal vascular arcades. But highly detached retina surrounds the posterior pole. In another scenario, the retina appears to be attached, with the exception of a posterior, whitish mound. The entire peripheral retina is avascular. The mound consists of connective tissue and collapsed retinal folds.[17]

Total retinal detachments are necessarily funnel-shaped.[21] The funnel may be open or narrow, with any number of possible combinations. The most frequent configuration is a funnel open in both anterior and posterior portions.[21] Open funnel detachments have an orange reflex.[8] The more visible the posterior retina, the smaller the degree of anterior fibrosis and the better the prognosis. In these cases, the detachment is concave and extends to the optic disc.[21] The second most common funnel is closed anteriorly and posteriorly, and the detached retina is located immediately behind the lens.[6, 21] Other less common configurations are funnels open anteriorly but narrow posteriorly, and finally funnels narrow anteriorly and open posteriorly.[18, 21] In the Jabbour et al. series, 49% of all funnels were closed or narrow, 23% were closed posteriorly, 3% were closed anteriorly, and 21% were open.[23]

Another mechanism in the pathogenesis of retinal detachments is contraction of proliferative tissue. If only a few clock hours are involved, the effects are not noticeable. With extension to most or all quadrants, however, the shunt acts as a contracting ring. In extreme cases, the retina may be detached anterior and posterior to the shunt.[17] Sometimes a red reflex may be retained, even though there is a shallow detachment.

The third component in the formation of detachments is intravitreal proliferation. It is found only in the most severe cases.[17] Usually all four quadrants are involved. The new tissue invades the anterior vitreous primarily. The hyaloid surface eventually turns white as a result of collagen deposition.

Photoreceptor development is incomplete in the immature retina. In addition, outer retinal degeneration with intraretinal gliosis and subretinal membrane formation are common. In severe cases, subretinal blood and pigment proliferation may be prominent.[22]

Regressed ROP may leave severe sequelae such as distortion of the foveal architecture, displacement of major retinal vessels, dragging of the retina over the disc, traction and rhegmatogenous, and rarely, exudative detachments.[21] Other changes include prominent areas of retinal avascularity, abnormal branching of vessels, and formation of arcades and telangiectatic vessels. Pigmentary changes may be subtle or conspicuous and clearly visible through the avascular retina.[21] Other sequelae of regression include myopia, anisometropia, strabismus, and amblyopia.[21]

Anterior segment changes, when severe, are secondary to retinal detachments. Corneal edema may signify elevated intraocular pressure or hypotony. Iris atrophy, posterior synechiae, or ectropion uveae may occur.[21]

Glaucoma is caused by contraction of peripheral intravitreal proliferations and forward movement of the lens.[7, 17, 21] The anterior chamber becomes increasingly shallow and angle closure may result. Glaucoma only develops with retrolental proliferation.

## PREOPERATIVE EVALUATION

For office evaluation, observation of eye movements without physical restraint or lid retraction is the best method.[3] Indirect ophthalmoscopy and hand-held biomicroscopy may be used.[10] Sedation should be avoided because of the risk of cardiac or respiratory arrest.[3] Light perception can be determined by the child's blinking or head movements in response to light.

Prior to surgery, the iris should be examined for neovascularization and extensive synechiae along the pupillary border. Flat anterior chamber, glaucoma, and the amount of neovascular activity in the retrolental region are prognostic signs. Many patients are said to have iris neovascularization when in fact they have a persistent tunica vasculosa lentis.[3]

Jabbour et al. evaluated morphologic features of eyes undergoing surgery and combined these features with postoperative results.[23] The following factors were considered: corneal clarity, anterior chamber depth, posterior synechiae, pupillary dilation, anterior membranes, status of the lens, blood vessel content and opaqueness of retrolental membranes, configuration of the funnel, location of the circumferential ridge, retinal vascularization, folds, displacement, persistence of the hyaloid artery, subretinal membranes, and blood. The most significant prognostic anterior segment features were posterior synechiae, pupillary membranes, and a shallow or flat anterior chamber.[23] These characteristics correlated closely with partially or totally closed or narrow funnels and preretinal membranes, which in turn are poor prognostic posterior segment features. Unfavorable anatomic outcome was associated with posterior extension of retrolental membranes as preretinal membranes, vascularization of retrolental membranes, subretinal organization or blood, persistent hyaloid artery, retinal folds, retinoschisis, and retinal dragging.[23]

These investigators also found that it is rather difficult to assess the vascularity of the retrolental membrane preoperatively.[23] Of all operated eyes, 30% had vascular connections between retina and membrane. It was almost impossible to clarify preoperatively if those were extensions of preretinal membranes, or retinal vessels.

Elevated intraocular pressure, found in 31% of operated eyes, was prognostically less significant.[23] Most corneas and lenses were clear preoperatively. Corneal edema developed with cornea-iris contact caused by pupillary block.

In the advanced stages of ROP, the value of ultrasonography is limited. It is considered important by some authors, and equivocal or misleading by others.[3, 19] Nevertheless, an attempt should be made to interpret the findings and to incorporate them into surgical decision-making. Ultrasonography is significant if the cornea or the retrolental plate are totally opaque,[3] and provides indirect clues. In the Shapiro et al. series, ultrasound characteristics of ROP presenting with leucocoria included increased corneal thickness, shallow anterior chamber, malpositioned lens, cataract, fibrous proliferation in the anterior vitreous, retinal detachment, choroidal thickening, and acoustic shadowing of orbital fat in advanced cases.[18] de Juan et al. considered ultrasonography particularly useful in eyes with posterior synechiae, dense retrolental membranes, and vitreous hemorrhage.[19] It was possible to discover traction retinal detachments early or before severe visual deficits developed. The configuration of these detachments was concave, as compared with convex exudative detachments.[19] More sophisticated examination with high-resolution contact B-mode scans also allowed determination of the severity and progression of the retinal detachment, fibrovascular proliferation in the vitreous cavity, location and extent of the peripheral trough, and subretinal or choroidal hemorrhages.[19] Funnel configuration and retinal folds could be outlined. Even unusual detachments were sometimes appreciated, for example a funnel narrow anteriorly but open posteriorly.[9, 19] Usually, anterior narrowing preceded posterior narrowing. Eyes with open posterior configuration had a better prognosis than eyes with closed posterior funnels.[19] Ultrasound was sometimes misleading in closed funnel detachments: The detached retina was easily misinterpreted as a "stalk."[3]

Jabbour et al. found ultrasonography the single most important tool in preoperative evaluation.[23] They thought it provided invaluable information about the retrolental membrane, the funnel, the circumferential fold, subretinal organization, the persistence of the hyaloid system, retinal dragging, retinal folds, traction, and retinoschisis.

The electroretinogram is always nonrecordable in total retinal detachments.[3] It may fail to demonstrate any retinal function. This is not unexpected in the presence of dense anterior scar tissue and a thinned-out and stretched anterior retina. No clear evidence exists that the visual evoked potential is of any significant predictive value.[3, 10, 13]

## SURGICAL TECHNIQUE

The goal of ROP surgery is "complete" removal of preretinal tissue with release of traction.[1, 14] Vitrectomy makes it possible to sever fibrovascular traction both anteriorly and posteriorly, allowing the retina to fall back into place.[3] It is essential to avoid iatrogenic retinal breaks and hemorrhage.[14]

Intraocular instruments may include the vitreous cutter, the fiberoptic light pipe, the infusion cannula, tissue forceps, and intraocular scissors. Blunt or sharp bent needles are of limited value in membrane dissection. The "manipulator" is sometimes of value if suction and illumination are required simultaneously.

## Closed Vitrectomy

### *Entry Sites*

The location of the entry sites is in part the preference of the surgeon. The eye has to be entered anterior to the pars plana. The remainder is a trade-off. Pars plicata, ciliary body, corneo-scleral limbus, and cornea have all been used as entry sites.[8–10] The closer the incision to the limbus, the more instrument manipulation is impaired. The farther the incision is moved posteriorly, the greater the risk of producing iatrogenic retinal tears.

de Juan et al. entered the anterior chamber at the posterior limbus, 0.5 mm behind the conjunctival insertion.[1] Instruments entered via limbus may distort the cornea during surgical manipulation and interfere with contact lens placement.[8] Therefore, a small contact lens should be used, which is not displaced during surgery.[3, 6] Limbal entry may be associated with striate keratopathy, localized or progressive corneal edema, and poor access to pre-equatorial traction.[3]

Charles considers entry through ciliary body or iris root, 0.5 mm behind the limbus, the safest approach.[3] Ciliary body entry, however, can result in retinal tears because peripheral retrolental scar tissue may be pulled anteriorly when the instrument is inserted.[1] Irrigation fluid may then seep under the retina. Trese enters the eye via pars plicata, but this approach, too, may result in a break in the detached pars plana epithelium.[9, 10, 22]

Pars plana entry brings the instruments into the subretinal space and creates an obligatory dialysis.[1, 3] The pars plana in infants is incompletely developed and the peripheral retina is pulled anteriorly to a position near or even in contact with the posterior lens capsule.[2, 6]

### *Number of Ports*

Closed vitrectomy can be performed using two or three ports.[1, 13] de Juan et al. use three entry sites immediately posterior to the limbus, with small conjunctival flaps.[1] Most vitrectomies for ROP will require three ports for greater flexibility in exchanging instruments. Posterior dissection is sometimes more difficult without the fiberoptic light pipe.[1] Frequently, however, coaxial illumination will suffice because of the short axial length. Charles feels it is adequate because of the anterior location of the retinal disease process.[3]

### *Infusion Cannulas*

The use of intraocular scissors requires a separate infusion cannula. A small elbow-shaped metallic infusion tube, attached to a flexible plastic line, is entered through an inferior incision.[1] The metal tube is attached to the limbus with a single suture to prevent movement. Infusion can also be supplied with a 30-degree, bent, blunt-tipped infusion cannula.[3] Trese believes that infusion cannulas sutured to the limbus distort the cornea. All instruments, including infusion cannulas, should be placed anterior to the iris to avoid tears in the delicate pars plana epithelium.[22] Posterior to the iris, infusion cannulas cannot be used because of instability and the anterior location of the pars plana.[24] Charles maintains that infusion cannulas are prone to rotate into the subretinal space.[3] The problems with infusion cannulas were bypassed by Trese, who used sodium hyaluronate infusion to maintain the volume of the vitreous cavity.[24] Frequent washout is necessary, however, as blood mixes with the sodium hyaluronate.[1]

### *Iridectomy*

The question of an iridectomy is largely dependent on the location of the entry site. In closed vitrectomy, the iridectomy is necessary for visualization of the retinal periphery and dissection of anterior loop traction.[3, 13] Limbal or ciliary body entry frequently requires a sector iridectomy or passage anterior to the iris.[3, 8] Chong et al. needed a large superior iridectomy in 64% of their cases.[13] In the presence of posterior synechiae, a superior sphincterotomy or iridectomy will need to be performed.[1] Prolapse of the iris is then prevented during surgical manipulation, particularly during exchange of instruments. Sometimes, when the anterior chamber fails to deepen, even with infusion, perforation of the iris may be necessary. Failure to do so may result in disinsertion of the iris, traction on the retina, and hemorrhage.[1] Charles presses the iris diaphragm back with a micro-iris spatula in the presence of peripheral anterior synechiae or a flat anterior chamber.[3] This maneuver may, however, cause disinsertion at the iris base, traction on the peripheral retina, or rupture of blood vessels.[1]

If the pupil can be dilated adequately, an iridectomy is unnecessary.[1, 9] The anterior chamber should be deep enough, however, or the vitreous cutter will pull on the iris root.[1] The more posterior the port, the less likely that an iridotomy or iridectomy will be required.

### *Intraocular Infusion Fluid*

Balanced salt solution (BSS Plus) is the most suitable infusion fluid.[1] Low-pressure infusion is essential to avoid compromising the cornea. The systolic blood pressure in these patients is in the range of 80 to 90 mm Hg and the blood supply can easily be compromised.[1] Once the infusion has been placed, the anterior chamber should deepen and further manipulations will be easier.

### *Lens Removal*

Although the lens is usually clear, it should be removed because proliferation is heaviest in the anterior portion of the vitreous, adherent to the lens capsule.[6,8] All cortex should be aspirated using scleral depression for visualization of the periphery.[3] Retained lens material will proliferate rapidly. Capsule remnants should be removed by gentle traction. This harbors the risk of creating retinal tears, because the lens capsule may be adherent to peripheral fibrous tissue and the ciliary body.[1]

In an infant, it is easily possible to remove the clear lens with the vitreous cutter. The vitrectomy instrument may, however, become clogged and dulled while a combination of aspiration and cutting is used.[7] Charles considers vitrectomy instruments too slow for lensectomy and uses continuous ultrasonic fragmentation and aspiration.[3] Trese also prefers fragmatome lensectomy.[9] Ultrasound however, may contribute to endothelial damage. de Juan et al. believe ultrasonic fragmentation is too traumatic.[1]

A sclerotome may be guided through the root of the iris into the clear lens.[8] A myringotomy knife, a 1.4 mm lancet tip microvitreoretinal (MVR) blade, or a ruby knife may be used alternately.[1,3,11]

### Retrolental Plate

Depending on the size of the funnel, the retina may not be in contact with the posterior lens capsule throughout. It is important to recognize the difference in appearance of the retrolental plate vs. the retina. The retina is shiny and pale yellow, whereas the retrolental plate is of a matte finish and white.[3] The retrolental tissue should be slightly elevated with forceps prior to incision.[1] If the membrane is so taut that it cannot be grasped, the initial opening can be punctured with two sharp opposing needles. The incision may also be made with the Charles modified Sutherland scissors.[3] Another possibility is using a disposable 21- or 22-gauge needle.[1,9] A myringotomy knife is equally suitable for a slit-like cut in the tissue.[8] Vitrectomy instruments, on the other hand, are frequently inadequate in initially cutting retrolental tissue.[8]

de Juan et al. and Trese use MPC scissors after the central cut has been obtained.[1,9] The edge of the hole is held with forceps, while the opening is enlarged toward the superior and inferior periphery.[1] The retrolental tissue should not be moved horizontally ("zero displacement" cutting), because this will create large dialyses that may include the retinal pigment epithelium and choroid.[3]

Although the sharp tips of the scissors are required for the initial incision, 45-degree or 90-degree scissors with blunt tips will need to be used later on.[3] Multiple radial incisions originating at the center are extended toward the pre-equatorial region, creating a stellate appearance.[3,6,9] The cuts should include the posterior lens capsule as well as the anterior and posterior hyaloid, allowing for visualization of the retinal surface.[3] Alternately, the initial incision can be made circumferentially. In this case, radial cuts are directed toward the center from the pre-equatorial region.[3] The membranes are dissected up to the ridge of the anteriorly dragged retina. Bleeding is common at this stage because the membranes have diffuse fibrous and vascular connections to the retinal surface.[1] Ciliary body and peripheral retina are frequently incorporated into contracting vitreous.[12]

### Membranes

Proliferations are difficult to remove because they originate in the retina and therefore cannot easily be peeled away from its surface. Segmentation leaves too much epiretinal membrane and structural rigidity. Delamination is the best method for removal of the posterior hyaloid face and epiretinal membranes.[3, 9] This is accomplished with modified Sutherland scissors, with the blades parallel to the retinal surface.[3] The posterior fibrous proliferatious are tightly adherent to the retina. Nevertheless, epiretinal membranes should be cut as closely as possible to the retinal surface.[6] On the other hand, any cut into the retina during dissection jeopardizes the success of surgery. The flared tissue is removed with the vitrectomy instrument. Peripheral proliferative tissue that is impossible to remove must be cut radially and thinned out near the retinal surface.[8] Because the vitreous is so intimately connected to the retina, sharp dissection with scissors should be done in small steps, with the goal of separating the tight retinal folds.[1] Peeling places too much stress on the thin tissues.

Remnants of the hyaloid system, drawn temporally, are frequently present.[8, 25] Recognition of a large, persistent, hyaloid artery has important prognostic value. The vessel may be adherent to the retina and retrolental membrane, complicating surgery.[25]

The demands on surgical skill are greatest when it comes to dissection of the stalk from the retina near the optic nerve.[1] Blunt dissection may be necessary, and even with this technique, retinal holes may be created.

For maximum mobility of the retina, posterior membranes should be removed. Eyes in which these membranes cannot be removed have a poorer visual prognosis.[13] The difficulties are directly related to the status of the funnel. Open funnels provide more accessibility and visibility than do narrow or closed funnels. Surgery near the optic nerve requires an expanded funnel. This is the one situation in which closed and open-sky vitrectomy present a similar problem. The use of sodium hyaluronate is a logical solution, but it mixes with blood, frequently reducing visibility.[24]

### Peripheral Trough

In most cases of total retinal detachment, the peripheral retina is folded into a trough anterior to the retinal ridge.[17] This adds unique problems. Troughs may be open and easily visualized or be hidden behind opaque fibrous tissue.[1] They are entered in a quadrant where fibrous tissue is either transparent or less white.[1] Narrow folds are opened by dissecting dense fibrous tissue from the crest toward the periphery.[11] Traction should be avoided at all costs when working on the trough because the retina is extremely thin. It is necessary to open the trough for mobilization, although attempts to separate all folds may result in disaster. The goal is to remove as much membrane as possible without jeopardizing the final outcome. In the Chong et al. series, the extent to which the trough was opened had no influence on surgical results.[13]

### *Subretinal Fluid Drainage*

If adequate apposition cannot be achieved because of retinal shortening, subretinal fluid drainage may aid in reattachment.[1] Frequently, thick, yellow-brown material is found in the subretinal space. In late cases, it may have been replaced by honeycomb-like plaques, dendritic structures, and cholesterol crystals.[3] Subretinal fluid drainage is usually not necessary because the detachment is nonrhegmatogenous.[8] External drainage can lead to posterior retinal tears because deep troughs may extend unexpectedly far posteriorly.[1] Also, a thin retina may tear during drainage as the vitreous cavity expands.[8, 10] Internal drainage should be avoided because the structural rigidity of the retina often prevents complete reattachment, and subretinal air or gas may follow the needle into the subretinal space.[3] It is advisable to avoid retinotomies. Proliferation from these sites may determine the fate of the eye.[1] Charles performs external drainage of subretinal fluid in cases with retinal breaks and high detachments, using a 25-gauge needle.[3] Drainage is terminated when the fluid stops flowing, to avoid tears of the retina.[3] Trese drains through a capillary tube placed into the subretinal space via a well-diathermized sclerostomy.[9, 10]

### *Scleral Buckling*

Charles believes scleral buckling is unnecessary if delamination of the retrolental plate combined with pre-equatorial dissection and release of anterior loop traction are adequate.[3] He suggests circumferential segmental buckles only occasionally for retinal breaks. An apparent disadvantage of scleral buckling is the increased chance of iris-retinal adherence. Also, scleral intrusion of the buckle is possible.[3, 8] If sufficient relaxation of all concentric contraction cannot be achieved, an encircling band is placed in an attempt to support the posterior border of the area of proliferation that has been delaminated and segmented.[8–10] Bands of 2 mm silicone have been used in some cases.[15] Tight encircling bands may have to be cut later.[7] Machemer routinely leaves bands in place, but concedes that erosion into the eye necessitates removal.[8] Prophylactic encircling bands are not necessary.[13]

### *Vitreous Replacement*

Vitreous substitution is not considered necessary in an eye that harbors a traction retinal detachment without retinal breaks. However, vitreous replacement is necessary in case of retinal breaks, or if the subretinal space communicates with a cleft under the nonpigmented epithelium anteriorly through the entry sites of the instruments.[3] Other indications are postoperative expansion of the retina, intraocular bleeding, and volume replacement after drainage.[15] Infusion fluid (BSS plus), hyaluronic acid, air, sulfur hexafluoride and air (30:70), or perfluoropropane in a nonexpansible 15% concentration, as well as silicone oil, have been used.

Because of a lack of surface tension, infusion fluid enters through retinal breaks, causing a bullous retinal detachment.[3] Similarly, hyaluronic acid, having minimal surface tension, easily reaches the subretinal space. It also raises the intraocular pressure temporarily and promotes reproliferation.[3] Air is routinely injected to separate the retinal surfaces temporarily until fibrinous exudation subsides.[1, 9] This is particularly important in cases of extensive membrane dissection and surface bleeding.[13] Air injection may dislodge the retina from its anterior insertion.[7] With intraocular air, the child has to be placed in a special crib in face-down position for 24 to 48 hours.[9] Air-gas mixtures can cause postoperative iris-retina adherence and play a part in reproliferation.[3] Machemer is not convinced that expanding gas mixtures are necessary in the absence of retinal breaks.[8] Silicone oil may be a good alternative, but will have to be removed within three to six months because it causes glaucoma and corneal changes.

### *Complications*

**Iatrogenic Retinal Breaks.**—Retinal breaks are associated with a high rate of surgical failure. In the Chong et al. series, 19 of 24 eyes with iatrogenic breaks progressed to failure, whereas only 18 of 32 cases without tears were unsuccessful.[13] The retina is shrunken irregularly and cannot be reattached with conventional techniques.[1] Characteristically, the tears occur in thin anterior portions of the retina or in detached pars plana epithelium.[1] Often this delicate tissue consists only of one or two layers and communicates with the subretinal space.[22] Tears may occur at the posterior edge of the ciliary body; they may be very small and covered by heavy fibrous tissue.[22] Frequently, they cannot be found. Even entering the eye through the pars plicata may cause a break in the detached pars plana. Also, deepening the anterior chamber with movement of the lens-iris diaphragm may cause strain on the pars plana, followed by a retinal break.[22]

Another mechanism for creating iatrogenic retinal breaks is the direct cutting of the retina with scissors. Finally, retinal rupture may occur as a result of expansion of the vitreous cavity during subretinal fluid drainage or vitreous replacement.[1] Expanding gases are particularly dangerous because the retina is not pliable.

The management of retinal breaks remains largely an unresolved issue. Cryopexy is unsatisfactory and should be used in association with an encircling band.[1] Inadvertent cyclocryotherapy may occur, and therefore the lesions are placed closer to the equator. Nonexpanding gas mixtures such as 20% sulfur hexafluoride or 15% perfluoropropane may be helpful for internal tamponade.[1] Expanding gas mixtures, though more effective, frequently result in corneal clouding or may tear the retina.[1] Intraocular pressures are difficult to determine postoperatively.

Cyanoacrylate glue injection is probably the most promising method for closing posterior retinal tears permanently.[3] Retinochoroidal dialysis is usually associated with loss of the eye. A desperate attempt to resolve the situation can be made by placing a through-and-through retinal-choroidal-scleral suture.

**Hemorrhage.**—Bleeding from retinal blood vessels should be avoided at all costs.[1] Diathermy is useful for both prevention and treatment of hemorrhages. Intraocular infusion and temporary elevation of the infusion bottle may contain the bleeding and at the same time wash out the blood.[1] Sodium hyaluronate delineates the bleeding site but rapidly mixes with blood, leading to loss of visibility in the operative field.[24]

Infusion of thrombin has been found to be successful in reducing bleeding without severe side effects in one report.[26] However, thrombin should be used only as a last resort, and then only temporarily, because it is associated with increased postoperative inflammation and reproliferation. It also makes surgery more difficult by increasing the amount of clotted blood and fibrin within the eye.[1]

**Corneal Clouding.**—The corneal endothelium in infants is very vulnerable. The cornea may cloud as a result of intraocular infusion pressure to a point where continuation of the procedure is impossible.[1] Permanent corneal opacification necessitates open-sky vitrectomy.

**Reproliferation.**—Recurrent proliferation occurs in 30% to 40% of cases.[3] In both closed and open-sky vitrectomy, a significant number of cases will redetach as a result. Factors that play a significant role in reproliferation include lens material, blood, surgical disruption of the internal limiting membrane, the amount of dissection, diathermy, and surface tension agents.[3] Iris-retinal adherence is a frequent problem and is caused by surgical trauma to the iris and peripheral retina.[3]

The basis for reproliferation is incomplete removal of scar tissue. Membranes used to be cut from the retinal surface, leaving extensive residual collagen. This tissue may serve as a matrix for further membrane formation and contraction.[1] Another mechanism is shrinkage of newly formed preretinal tissue.[1] Reproliferation may be rampant and associated with immediate as well as late failure occurring months or even years following surgery.[8] Substances such as 5-fluorouracil have been used without measurable success to suppress reproliferation.[3] Polypeptide-blocking receptors, by which glial cells attach to collagen, fibrin, and elastin, may prove more useful.

**Failure.**—Complications in unsuccessful cases include development of pupillary membranes, glaucoma, corneal blood staining, and phthisis bulbi.[13] Postoperative hyphema and vitreous hemorrhage often lead to pupillary membranes.[13]

## Open-Sky Vitrectomy

Open-sky vitrectomy is preferred by some surgeons.[4, 5, 12, 15] It is a truly bimanual technique. One problem is the prolonged hypotony, another the increased operating time because corneal surgery is involved. The advantages include easier access to peripheral tissues.[1] The position of the instruments can be changed readily. Anterior fundus structures are more visible and more easily accessible, but posterior dissection is limited.[1, 5] It is dangerous to perform excision of membranes too close to the vitreous base because extensive detachment of the nonpigmented epithelium of the pars plana, followed by detachment of the ora serrata, may occur. During the course of excision, the vitreous base and even the detached nonpigmented epithelium may be torn, causing a giant retinal break.[5] In most eyes, the adhesion of the vitreous base to the retina extends more posteriorly than the ora serrata, sometimes as far back as the equator.[5] Therefore, removal of vitreous anterior to the equator should be performed with great care.

Open-sky vitrectomy in infants requires unique surgical techniques and instruments. Collapse of the globe should be prevented by a Flieringa ring or a scleral supporter.[5, 15] All instruments must fit under a surgical microscope with a focal length of 125 mm. Therefore, handles need to be shorter than 100 mm and angulated to keep the surgeon's hand out of the operative field.[5] Because the instruments are used in a surgical field located 17 to 25 mm behind the pupillary opening, they must have long shafts.

Special instruments include modified Colibri forceps, miniaturized deWecker scissors, and blunt or sharp disposable aluminum spatulas.[5] Liquid is removed from the vitreous cavity with a suction spatula. When bulging retinal folds must be moved, a tiny retractor is used. To explore the area of the optic disc or macula, a gold or plastic ring is placed over the posterior pole.[5]

The cornea is opened with a trephine.[15] Clear cornea measuring 1 to 1.5 mm should be left near the limbus.[12] The corneal button is removed and stored in McCarey-Kaufman medium.[15] Posterior synechiae are lysed with a cyclodialysis spatula. Underwater diathermy is performed on iris vessels. Keyhole iridotomies are performed at the 6 o'clock and 12 o'clock positions,[12, 15] and should be closed later with 10-0 Prolene or nylon sutures.[15]

Bleeding is a major problem. A shielded electrode adapted for underwater use prevents or stops intraocular bleeding. Small blood vessels in infants should be cauterized before excessive traction is placed on membranes, causing hemorrhage. Underwater diathermy can weaken the retina and produce tears.[12] Older infants lack open vessels. Heparinized BSS plus is used to push back retinal folds, visualize adhesions, and minimize tissue edema. The retinas of infants under seven months old are more pliable than those of older infants and can sustain more expansion without bleeding or tearing.[12]

Hyaluronic acid is used on the iris surface to prevent angle closure caused by adhesion between the iris surface and the scleral edge of the corneal incision.[5] In the vitreous cavity, hyaluronic acid opens the funnel.[15] It also is injected to offset problems caused by the accumulation of transudative fluid in the suprachoroidal and subretinal spaces. Epiretinal surgery is carried out beneath the surface of this clear viscous solution.[5, 15] Hyaluronic acid tends to form a convex meniscus at the air-fluid interface as a result of surface tension. This may cause severe distortion that interferes with precise dissection of preretinal membranes. Therefore, the eye is filled with hyaluronic acid to the edge of the corneal incision. Now a convex meniscus is formed that acts optically like an artificial cornea. Because visualization through the surgical microscope is subsequently impossible, a small, flat, contact lens mounted on a tripod of fine metallic wire is placed over the convex meniscus of hyaluronic acid.[5] This contact lens rests on the scleral surface so that instruments can be introduced into the vitreous cavity through a space between the lens and the scleral edge of corneal incision.[5] Alternately, a small, round, Corning glass cover can be placed over the corneal opening.[12]

The lens is removed by cryoextraction.[15] The retrolental membrane is then incised, dissected, and excised. Tasman et al. begin membrane removal at the ora serrata.[15] All of these maneuvers are easier to perform through the open-sky than the closed vitrectomy technique because exposure is better and bimanual manipulation is possible. Tasman et al. suggest that open-sky vitrectomy eliminates the problems encountered in opening the peripheral trough and removing anterior loop traction.[15]

Frequently, the retina will not be completely flat following the first open-sky procedure. The infant will have to return to the operating room several weeks or months later for further evaluation. More membranectomies may need to be performed. This follow-up surgery is essential because phthisis bulbi may ensue if traction results in ciliary body detachment.[12] Additional vitrectomy, sodium hyaluronic acid injection, and subretinal fluid drainage may be required to flatten the retina.[12]

### Complications

Open-sky vitrectomy requires corneal incision, which may have disadvantages. Corneal transparency may be compromised and iridotomies may be required.[5] Peripheral anterior synechiae, sometimes with closure of the anterior chamber angle, may occur. Therefore a 170-degree scleral incision over the pars plana has been suggested.[5] In this situation, cornea and iris remain intact. Peripheral anterior synechiae are less likely to form and there is no tendency for angle closure. The wound opening is larger and the distance between the incision and the posterior pole is shortened by 4 mm. With this approach, ischemia of the iris and ciliary body will occur in some cases, but massive necrosis has never been observed.[5]

Besides corneal complications, rubeosis iridis, ectropion uveae, and cyclitic membranes are unique to open-sky vitrectomy. The membranes may shrink so much that they cause adhesion of the retina to the pupillary border.[5] In rare cases, a neovascularized preretinal membrane seems to originate from conjunctival vessels and grow under the corneal epithelium through the tightly closed corneal wound. An intraocular membrane may form that continues its growth on both iris surfaces, the ciliary processes, the unexcised portions of the vitreous base, and the entire inner retinal surface.[5]

Complications in unsuccessful eyes include the development of pupillary membranes and glaucoma.[12] Eyes with glaucoma may develop corneal blood staining or phthisis. Eyes with iatrogenic retinal breaks tend to progress to failure.[12]

## Overall Results

Surgical results following closed and open-sky vitrectomy are comparable (Table 10–1). The anatomic reattachment rates overall were between 25% and 45%. Complete zone 1 reattachment should be the anatomic criterion for success.[14] Partial attachments in zone 1 should be recorded but not considered a success. The minimum follow-up period should be 6 months.[13, 14]

Charles has by far the largest series of closed vitrectomy cases. His overall reattachment rate in 586 cases in 1986 was 46%. The remainder failed as a result of reproliferation. Anatomic reattachment was defined as attachment of the posterior pole.

In the Lightfoot et al. series of five cases, three retinas were reattached successfully.[6] The severity of the fibrovascular proliferative tissue at the

**TABLE 10–1.**
Results After Closed and Open-Sky Vitrectomy

| Author (Year) | No. of Eyes | No. of Children | Birth weight (gm) | Age at Surgery | ROP Stage 4–5 | Additional Surgery: Before Vitrectomy | Additional Surgery: At Vitrectomy | Additional Surgery: After Vitrectomy |
|---|---|---|---|---|---|---|---|---|
| **A. History** | | | | | | | | |
| Treister et al[2] (1977) | 5 | | 1, 1,360, 1, Term | 6 mo–28 yr | 2, c Exudative RLF<br>2, Grade 3 | | Cryotherapy, intraocular gas, scleral buckle | |
| Charles[3] (1986) | 586 | | | | | | | |
| Lightfoot et al[6] (1982) | 5 | | 794–1,100 1, Term | 4 mo–4 yr | 2, Total detachment and dialysis<br>1, Retina drawn into circumferential ring of traction<br>1, Detached except on buckle<br>1, Detached except small area between disc and macula | Peripheral cryoablation<br>Encircling scleral buckle | Encircling band, cryopexy, gas-fluid exchange, drainage | Vitrectomy, air injection |
| Merritt et al[7] | 13 | 9 | 800–1,560 | $3^1/_2$–18 mo | 13 | | Cryotherapy, 2 mm silicone band, scleral buckling | |
| Machemer[8] (1983) | 15 | | 810–1,359 | 5–24 mo | 15 | | $SF_6$ and air | |
| Trese[10] (1986) | 85 | 45 | 640–1,400 | 3–24 mo | 85 | | 53, Scleral buckle<br>20 Drainage of subretinal fluid | |
| McPherson et al[12] (1986) | 47 | 32 | 560–1,400 | | 47 | | | 21, Additional vitrectomy<br>Scleral buckle or Healon<br>12, Donor corneas |

*(Continued.)*

**TABLE 10–1 (cont.).**
Results After Closed and Open-Sky Vitrectomy

| Author (Year) | No. of Eyes | No. of Children | Birth weight (gm) | Age at Surgery | ROP Stage 4–5 | Additional Surgery: Before Vitrectomy | Additional Surgery: At Vitrectomy | Additional Surgery: After Vitrectomy |
|---|---|---|---|---|---|---|---|---|
| Chong et al[13] (1986) | 58 | 46 | 483–1,450 (avg 911) | 6.7 mo (avg) | 58 | | 11, External drainage,<br>Several, prophylactic encircling bands<br>22, Air<br>14, $SF_6$<br>1, $C_3F_8$<br>9, Sodium hyaluronate<br>3, Silicone oil | 1, Elective removal of silicone oil<br>8, Additional vitrectomies |
| Tasman et al[15] (1987) | 23 | 18 | 539–1,950 (avg 1,038 mean 980) | (avg 12) | 23 | 2, Scleral buckle<br>1, Lensectomy/ vitrectomy | 6, External drainage attempted<br>3, Successful | |
| Jabbour et al[23] (1987) | 260 | 150 | 996 | | 260 | | | |

| Author (Year) | Vitrectomy: Open-Sky | Vitrectomy: Closed | Anatomical Outcome: Attached Funnel: Wide | Anatomical Outcome: Attached Funnel: Narrow | Anatomical Outcome: Failure or Considered Inoperable | Follow-Up | Visual Outcome: NLP | Visual Outcome: LP Funnel: Wide | Visual Outcome: LP Funnel: Narrow | Visual Outcome: Fix/Follow Funnel: Wide | Visual Outcome: Fix/Follow Funnel: Narrow | Visual Outcome: Identify Targets | Visual Outcome: Visual Acuity |
|---|---|---|---|---|---|---|---|---|---|---|---|---|---|
| **B. Surgical Outcome** | | | | | | | | | | | | | |
| Treister et al[2] (1977) | | 5 | | 1 | 1 | 13–36 mo (median 20) | 1 | | | | | | 20/30–6/300 |
| Charles[3] (1986) | | 586 (46%) | | | | | | | | | | | 20/200 |
| Lightfoot et al[6] (1982) | | 5 | 3 | | 2 | 18 mo–4$^1/_2$ yr | 1 | | | | 1 | | |
| Merritt et al[7] | | 13 | | | 13 | Up to 3 yr | 18 | | | | 1 | | |
| Machemer[8] (1983) | | 15 | | 8 | | 3–34 mo | | | | 8 | | | |

| | | | | | | | | | | | | |
|---|---|---|---|---|---|---|---|---|---|---|---|---|
| Trese[10] (1986) | | 85 (48%) | | | | 6–36 mo | Overall 26 (31%) | | | 18 | 10, Grasp brightly colored objects or stacked rings<br>15, Turn head or grasp pen light<br>6, Identify lighted targets at arm's length | |
| McPherson et al[12] (1986) | 47 | | 2 (22%), 4(11%) Low residual detachment Overall 42% | | | | | | | | | |
| Chong et al[13] (1986) | | 58 | 10 (83%) | 15 (33%) | | 6–40 mo (avg 14.3) | 5 | 2<br>7 | 6<br>4 | | | 20/800 |
| Tasman et al[15] (1987) | 23 | | | | 8 (34.7%) | | | | | | | |
| Jabbour et al[23] (1987) | 260 | | 81% | 19% | 2 | | | | | | | |

| Author (Year) | ROP Grade | Funnel | | Vitrectomy | |
|---|---|---|---|---|---|
| | | Wide | Narrow | Open-sky | Closed |
| C. | | | | | |
| Treister et al[12] (1977) | | | | 260 | |
| Machemer[17] (1985) | | | 47% Total<br>25% Closed posteriorly | | |
| Shapiro and Stone[18] (1985) | V | 31 | 20 | 20 (87%) Primary procedure<br>3 (13%) Secondary procedure | |
| | V | | 10, Vascularly active process | | 10 |

posterior pole was considered the determining factor for success or failure of surgery. In the Merritt et al. study of 17 cases, surgical intervention in infants with stage 5 ROP was uniformly unsuccessful.[7]

Machemer had an overall anatomic reattachment rate of 8 of 15 cases, but believed that the functional results were probably poorer.[8] The retina was considered attached if it was flat posterior to the buckle. Sometimes there were ragged dry folds or vessels. When Machemer's results were evaluated in more detail, it was found that 60% were attached in the operating room and 45% 6 months later.

In 1984, Trese was able to demonstrate a 45% attachment rate in 40 consecutive cases with 6-month follow-up.[9] Eyes with an open or partially closed funnel were attached in 63% vs. 26% in those with a closed funnel.[9] By 1986, Trese had operated on 85 eyes of 45 children. The retina was reattached in 48%.[10] This rate was further improved by his two-step technique. Ten of more than 250 eyes received cryotherapy first, followed by lensectomy, vitrectomy, and membranectomy.[11] The anatomic reattachment rate of zone 1 increased to an astonishing 80%.[11]

Chong et al. reviewed the results in 58 eyes.[13] Successful reattachment was defined as at least total repositioning of the macula lutea.[13] Ten (83%) of 12 eyes with partial detachments were successfully reattached; of the 46 eyes with total detachments, only 15 (33%) were attached.

Success rates in open-sky vitrectomies were similar. In the McPherson et al. series of 47 eyes in 32 infants with a follow-up of 9.7 months, successful reattachment was achieved in six (13%) of 38 eyes with closed funnels.[12] Success was defined as the ability to open the funnel with or without anatomic reattachment of the retina, along with maintenance of a clear cornea. Of nine eyes with partially open funnels, two were anatomically reattached.

Jabbour et al. combined evaluation of vision with the number of detached quadrants, and vascularity and pigmentation of the reattached retina.[23] They found through statistical analysis that the most important prognostic factor was the configuration of the funnel. Open funnels had an 81% attachment of one or more quadrants, and the anatomic failure rate was lower. Eyes with totally closed funnels had a 19% reattachment rate.[23] Other factors statistically related to poor prognosis were, in decreasing order of significance, posterior extension of retrolental membranes to the retinal surface, vascularization of retrolental membranes, subretinal organization or blood, persistence of the hyaloid artery, retinal folds, retinoschisis, and dragging of the retina. Radial retinal folds correlated closely with failure to reattach the same quadrant where the fold was located.[23]

Posterior location of the circumferential fold in zone 1 resulted in reduction of the four-quadrant reattachment by 19%. It also increased the risk of total failure by 3%. Poor visual prognosis was closely associated with a zone 1 circumferential fold. Visual progress was directly proportional to vascularization of the retina and inversely proportional to subretinal pigmentation.[23]

Successful surgical outcomes were associated with larger dilated pupils preoperatively, deeper anterior chambers, open configuration of the funnel, and more posterior membranectomies.[1] Anatomic success was more frequent in eyes with wide anterior funnels than in eyes with narrow anterior funnels.[23] Retinal reattachment was rare in eyes with closed anterior funnels.

Anterior membrane dissection was less difficult than posterior membrane removal with relief of posterior traction. Successful reattachment was highly dependent on adequate posterior membranectomy.[1] A persistent hyaloid artery was associated with more prominent vascularization of the membrane and increased intraoperative bleeding.[26]

## Visual Outcome

While it is true that some eyes will develop an electroretinographic response following surgery, the majority of closed funnel cases will not. Visual function is based on successful retinal reattachment, which is difficult to achieve. Moreover, even after successful reattachment, the retina may be so stretched and thinned out that it is barely functional.

In order to avoid amblyopia, it is crucial to fit the child with corrective glasses within 2 months after surgery.[1, 10] Rapid postoperative refraction and aggressive teaching of visually stimulating tasks has resulted in higher visual success rates.[9] Accurate retinoscopy is frequently not possible and the child's world is focused as well as possible at arm's length.[10] Prolonged visual deprivation and stretching of the retina contribute to decreased visual function.[10]

The effects of the retinal detachment and of visual deprivation on visual pathway development may be limiting factors. Retinal attachment without light perception was associated with large preoperative amounts of subretinal fluid.[10] Children with lower iron content of the subretinal fluid tended to have better visual results.[10]

Overall, visual success rates were about 10% lower than anatomic reattachment rates. Vision is more difficult to assess and standardize than are anatomic results. Visual acuity may be established by light perception, blinking in response to light, fixing and following, fixation of a light source on a moving hand, and tracking of a 20/200 or smaller target at various distances.[1, 10] Clues such as the ability to ambulate are subject to bias.[14] In addition, the infants may use other sensory clues.[1] Electrophysiologic or psychophysical tests should be used for nonverbal infants.[14]

In Charles' series of 586 cases with an anatomic reattachment rate of 46%, a functional result was achieved in 36%.[3] Machemer was able to reattach the retina in 15 cases. At 6 months, 30% of the children were able to follow lights and grasp objects. Trese operated on 85 eyes with a reattachment rate of 48% and found visual function in 31%.[10] With the two-step techniques, using cryotherapy first, the reattachment rate increased to 80%, with visual function in 70%.[11]

Finally, in the Chong et al. series, fixing and following was achieved in six of ten eyes with partial retinal detachments, two continued to have light perception, and two were anatomical failures.[13] Fixing and following resulted in four eyes with total detachments; seven had light perception, and three had no light perception. One eye achieved a visual acuity of 20/800.

The evaluation of visual results requires a minimum 2-year follow-up. The ultimate evaluation should be performed at age 6 years, when verbal responses and visual acuity or equivalents can be obtained.[1, 14]

## REFERENCES

1. de Juan E Jr, Machemer R: Retinopathy of prematurity. Surgical technique. *Retina* 1987; 7:63–69.
2. Treister G, Machemer R: Results of vitrectomy for rare proliferative and hemorrhagic diseases. *Am J Ophthalmol* 1977; 84:394–412.
3. Charles S: Vitrectomy with ciliary body entry for retrolental fibroplasia, in McPherson AR, Hittner HM, Kretzer FL (eds): *Retinopathy of Prematurity*, Toronto: BC Decker, Inc, 1986, pp 225–234.
4. Hirose T, Schepens CL: Complications in open-sky vitrectomy, in Freeman HM, Hirose T, and Schepens CL (eds): *Vitreous Surgery and Advances in Fundus Diagnosis and Treatment.* p 479. New York: Appleton-Century-Crofts, 1977, p 479.
5. Schepens CL: Clinical and research aspects of subtotal open-sky vitrectomy. *Am J Ophthalmol* 1981; 91:143–171.
6. Lightfoot D, Irvine AR: Vitrectomy in infants and children with retinal detachments caused by cicatricial retrolental fibroplasia. *Am J Ophthalmol* 1982; 94:305–312.
7. Merritt JC, Lawson EE, Sprague DH, Eifrig DE: Lensectomy-vitrectomy for stage V cicatricial retrolental fibroplasia. *Ophthalmic Surg* 1982; 13:300–306.
8. Machemer R: Closed vitrectomy for severe retrolental fibroplasia in the infant. *Ophthalmology* 1983; 90:436–441.
9. Trese MT: Surgical results of stage V retrolental fibroplasia and timing of surgical repair. *Ophthalmology* 1984; 91:461–466.
10. Trese MT: Visual results and prognostic factors of vision following surgery for stage V retinopathy of prematurity. *Ophthalmology* 1986; 93:574.
11. Trese MT: Surgical therapy for stage V retinopathy of prematurity. A two-step approach. *Graefes Arch Clin Exp Ophthalmol* 1987; 225:266–268.
12. McPherson AR, Hittner HM, Moura RA, et al: Treatment of retrolental fibro-

plasia with open-sky vitrectomy, in McPherson AR, Hittner HM, Kretzer FL (eds): *Retinopathy of Prematurity,* Toronto: BC Decker, Inc, 1986, pp 193–208.

13. Chong LP, Machemer R, de Juan E: Vitrectomy for advanced stages of retinopathy of prematurity. *Am J Ophthalmol* 1986; 102:710–716.
14. de Juan E Jr, Machemer R, Charles ST, et al: Surgery for stage 5 retinopathy of prematurity (letter). *Arch Ophthalmol* 1987; 105:21.
15. Tasman W, Borrone RN, Bolling J: Open sky vitrectomy for total retinal detachment in retinopathy of prematurity. *Ophthalmology* 1987; 94:449–452.
16. Tasman W: Late complications of retrolental fibroplasia. *Trans Am Acad Ophthalmol Otolaryngol* 1979; 86:1724–1740.
17. Machemer R: Description and pathogenesis of late stages of retinopathy of prematurity. *Ophthalmol* 1985; 92:1000–1004.
18. Shapiro D, Stone RD: Ultrasonic characteristics of retinopathy of prematurity presenting with leucocoria. *Arch Ophthalmol* 1985; 103:1690–1692.
19. de Juan E Jr, Shields S, Machemer R: The role of ultrasound in the management of retinopathy of prematurity. *Ophthalmology* 1988; 95:884–888.
20. de Juan E Jr, Gritz DC, Machemer R: Ultrastructure characteristics of proliferative tissue in retinopathy of prematurity. *Am J Ophthalmol* 1987; 104:149–156.
21. An international classification of retinopathy of prematurity. II: The classification of retinal detachment. The International Committee for Classification of the Late Stages of Retinopathy of Prematurity. *Arch Ophthalmol* 1987; 105:906–912.
22. de Juan E Jr, Machemer R, Flynn JT, et al: Surgical pathoanatomy in stage 5 retinopathy of prematurity, in Flynn JT, Phelps DL (eds): *Retinopathy of Prematurity: Problem and Challenge,* New York, Alan R Liss, Inc, 1988, pp 281–286.
23. Jabbour NM, Eller AE, Hirose T, et al: Stage 5 retinopathy of prematurity. Prognostic value of morphologic findings. *Ophthalmology* 1987; 94:1640–1646.
24. Trese MT: Two-hand dissection technique during closed vitrectomy for retinopathy of prematurity. *Am J Ophthalmol* 1986; 101:251–252.
25. Eller AW, Jabbour NM, Hirose T, et al: Retinopathy of prematurity: The association of a persistent hyaloid artery. *Ophthalmology* 1987; 94:444–448.
26. Blacharski PA, Charles ST: Thrombin infusion to control bleeding during vitrectomy for Stage V retinopathy of prematurity. *Arch Ophthalmol* 1987; 105:203–205.

Chapter 11

# Scleral Buckling in Acute Retinopathy of Prematurity Stages 4 and 5

Juan Orellana, M.D.

When discussing retinal detachments in patients with active retinopathy of prematurity (ROP), a distinction must be made between those cases that result from a rhegmatogenous break, those caused by exudation, and those caused by tractional forces. Rhegmatogenous detachments are not a common occurrence and most likely result from iatrogenic causes. Over the last 4 years, I have treated rhegmatogenous detachments in children who had previously received ardent cryotherapy to their ridge/arteriovenous shunt. These rhegmatogenous detachments were the result of temporal traction on a region that had received intensive treatment, eventually resulting in a retinal tear and detachment.

Plasma leakage from shunt neovascularization causes the accumulation of subretinal fluid in patients with an exudative detachment. Over time, the continued leakage from the neovascular tissue and possibly from the choroidal or retinal vessels results in both subretinal yellow precipitates and fluid. Invariably, treatment of these cases increases vessel permeability and also the extent of the detachment. Exudative detachments have shifting fluid and demonstrate a convex bullous elevation, in contrast to the tented elevation of a tractional detachment. In this chapter, I address the entity of traction retinal detachments in patients with active stages 4a, 4b, and 5 ROP.

Deviation from the normal development of the retinal vasculature system forms the basis for the retinal detachments seen in ROP. Normally, the

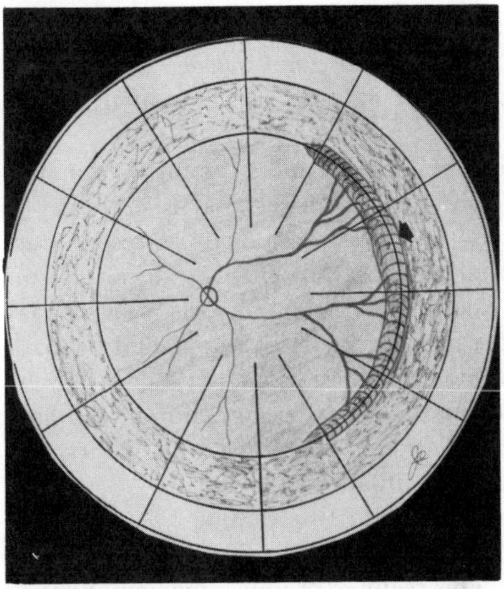

**FIG 11–1.**
The transformation of the vascular mesenchymal cells from a vasoformative role to a vasoproliferative role initiates the formation of the temporal ridge. The *arrow* indicates the ridge which may thicken and elevate. There is evidence that the peripheral vessels leading to and from the ridge are dilated and tortuous; that is, plus disease is present.

vascularization of the human retina proceeds from the optic disc to the ora serrata.[1] It arrives at the nasal ora serrata at 8 months gestation, and at the temporal ora serrata at birth (nine months).[2] Mesenchymal precursors of the vascular system travel within the nerve fiber layer to reach the ora serrata.[3] If these mesenchymal cells, destined to be the vascular system, deviate from their plan, they undergo metamorphosis from a vasoformative role to one of vasoproliferation. Because the temporal retina is larger than the nasal retina, the neovascular process begins in the temporal quadrants (Fig 11–1). In time, this collection of neovascular tissue composed of mesenchymal and endothelial cells, and arteries and veins, attains both height and width in the temporal quadrants and becomes the arteriovenous shunt/ridge. If resolution does not occur, the shunt line begins to thicken and expand circumferentially (Fig 11–2). Contracture of the shunt as it both thickens and increases in height detaches the retina (Fig 11–3,A and B). As the neovascular tissue bleeds, there is an interaction with the vitreous and the formation of early membranes. This may aid in stimulating further contraction of the shunt and increase the retinal detachment. If, as in most cases, the active phase—the progression of the arteriovenous shunt and further intraretinal and extraretinal neovascularization—slows down, we see a regression of the shunt and the ultimate resolution of the retinal detachment without therapy. On the other hand, if the shunt continues to thicken and elevate, the detachment proceeds to involve the posterior pole (Fig 11–3B). Thus, the eye may harbor a detachment that is localized to the periphery or may have a detachment that has entered the macular region. Although encountered infrequently, there is a period in which the retina can be totally detached in a funnel configuration yet be very pliable and amenable to surgical correction by means of a conventional scleral buckle. These retinas seem to have very little shunt activity, or may represent shunt regression after the retina has detached.

Preoperative assessment of these children requires careful examination of the anterior segment either in the office or nursery.[4] It is necessary to determine whether or not a persistent tunica vasculosa lentis is present. Care must be taken not to produce excessive ocular movement or to contuse the globe in any manner during the examination or surgery, as a vessel may bleed, producing a hyphema. In the nursery, pediatricians should be made aware of a child with a persistent tunica vasculosa lentis, in order to prevent overzealous placement of respirator masks. I have seen children who have sustained a hyphema because the pediatrician compressed the globes with the edge of the breathing mask during ventilation.

Dilation for surgery is accomplished with tropicamide 1% and phenylephrine 2.5% ophthalmic solution in both eyes every 20 minutes, repeated three times 2 hours before surgery. This regimen produces maximal dilation in neonates without the risk of convulsions associated with the use of cyclopentolate. To avoid needless waste of operating room time and to decrease anesthesia time, the pediatrician should start the intravenous line in the nursery with an angiocatheter. The line should be placed securely in an extremity and not in a scalp vein.

Over the last 4 years, I have followed up a group of nine premature infants (13 eyes) with stage 4a, 4b, or early stage 5 ROP. Five children (nine

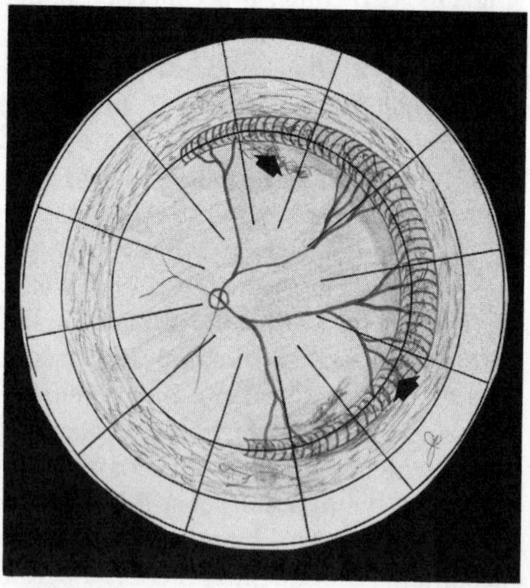

**FIG 11–2.**
If the ridge grows, it will continue to thicken and elevate. The ridge/shunt has extended into the nasal quadrants and demonstrates extraretinal fibrovascular proliferation *(arrows)*. There are more dilated vessels.

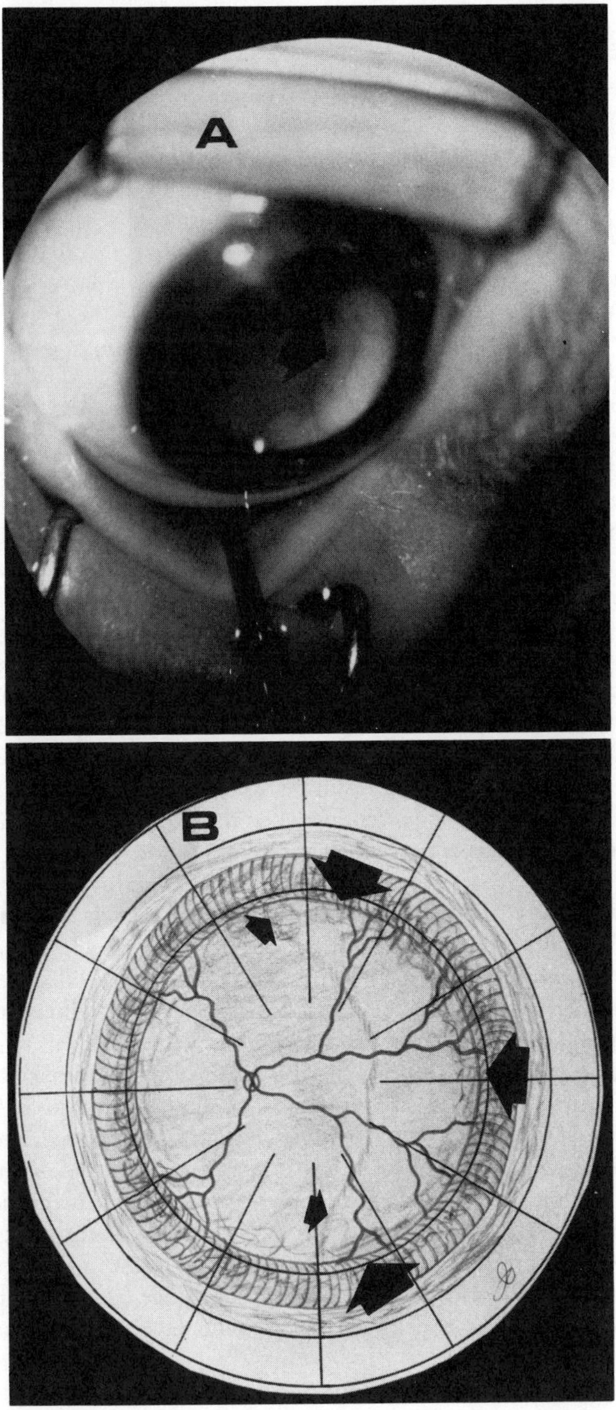


**FIG 11–3.**

**A and B**, the ridge has progressed to form a complete active ring of extraretinal fibrovascular tissue, and forms the leading edge for the retinal detachment *(large arrows)*. If the detachment continues into the macula *(small arrows)* a scleral buckling procedure should be performed.

eyes) had detachments that did not initially involve the posterior pole. These detachments were located posterior to the shunt but did not enter the posterior pole in any quadrant. Of these, two children (four eyes) developed a retinal detachment that ultimately involved the macula. Five eyes (three children) resolved without therapy. Two eyes (two children) had an exudative detachment with extensive exudation. Both of these eyes did not receive any therapy and settled within 2 months. Two eyes (two children) demonstrated a total detachment with detached macula. The retina was freely mobile in an open funnel configuration. Although the shunt region was visible in all cases, it exhibited only minimal neovascular activity in the totally detached cases. No breaks were found in any of the cases, indicating that they all were tractional detachments.

Confronted with a detachment at the posterior pole, I have treated with scleral buckling with cryopexy. A detachment that includes the macula may settle over a period of time, but the retina will not possess much function. Light micrographs of postmortem retinal tissue removed from both successful and unsuccessful scleral buckling cases have demonstrated the necrosis of retinal elements in longstanding detached retinas. The successfully reattached retinas demonstrated an organized retinal architecture.[5] I believe that anatomical success attained after the retina has been detached for a long time will not yield a good visual result because of the deterioration of retinal elements. Prompt surgical intervention when the detachment has entered the posterior pole will at least preserve the retinal architecture at the posterior pole and provide a reasonable basis for a functional outcome.

Six eyes with retinal detachments involving the macula were treated by scleral buckling procedures. A pediatric Cook or Sauer speculum was placed. I avoided lid sutures because they produce unnecessary lid trauma. The conjunctiva was opened over 360 degrees with two relaxing incisions placed in opposing oblique quadrants. This technique helps hide the scars under the upper and lower lids (Fig 11–4) (Plate 8). Although the orbit in these infants may appear to hinder exposure, I have preferred to avoid a lateral canthotomy. The horizontal and vertical muscles are isolated and tagged with 5-0 silk sutures (Fig 11–5). It is important to proceed with caution when isolating muscles in an infant. I prefer to use small pediatric muscle tenotomy hooks to gently isolate the four rectus muscles. As in adults, muscle isolation can also produce a bradycardia. It is important to keep the cornea clear. I bathe the cornea with a viscoelastic substance (e.g., Healon or Amvisc), although other surgeons prefer to use Gelfoam soaked in balanced salt solution.

With an indirect ophthalmoscope, the areas of vitreo-retinal traction are marked on the scleral surface with carefully applied diathermy. A 30 diopter lens enables the surgeon to view a greater area (albeit not as magnified as

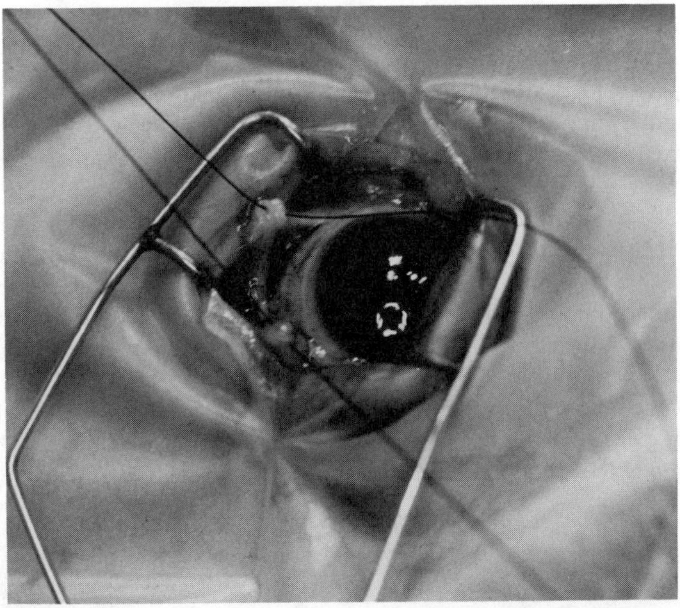

**FIG 11–4.**
Relaxing incisions are made in the conjunctiva in oblique quadrants and the edges are tagged with black silk to facilitate reapposition at the end of the procedure. See also Plate 8.

with a 20 diopter lens). A pediatric carbon dioxide cryoprobe is used to treat the avascular retina. I do not advise treatment of the shunt itself, and am careful to avoid premature removal of the cryoprobe from the scleral surface. Cryopexy must be applied under direct visualization to avoid iatrogenic damage such as fracturing the choroid, freezing the ridge/shunt, or applying cryopexy to a temporally displaced macula (Fig 11–6). Excessive cryopexy will cause dispersion of retinal pigment epithelium, as seen in Fig 11–6. Even though the child may have active ROP, there may be many elements of cicatricial disease. In each quadrant, a 6-0 Mersilene suture is used to anchor either a no. 40 (2 mm wide) or no. 240 (2.5 mm wide) solid silicone band to the sclera (Figs 11–7 to 11–9) (Plate 9). The distance between the superior and inferior scleral bites should not be more than 1 mm wider than the band. Care must be taken to gently pass the band beneath all four rectus muscles. The tie is made in the inferior temporal quadrant with a 6-0 Mersilene suture. I avoid any other method of tying off the band, such as use of a sleeve. Because of the thin sclera in these infants, I am concerned about erosion. The band must not be pulled too tight, or the buckle will be very high and the intraocular pressure difficult to control. In these children, a high buckle will easily move the iris-lens plane forward, causing a glaucoma.

I prefer to drain the eyes of these children posterior to the buckle. Although it may not be necessary to drain subretinal fluid in every case, attachment is aided by apposing the pigment epithelium to the detached retina. The sclerotomy site is closed with a 6-0 Mersilene mattress suture. Care must be taken to create a small drainage site to ensure that the choroid does not prolapse through the sclerotomy site or the subretinal fluid drain too quickly. Prompt and copious drainage may inadvertently create a tear should there be an area of enhanced vitreoretinal traction. Because of the thin nature of the sclera in these children, I do not advise scleral imbrication or scleral dissection.

The central retina artery is examined before closing to ensure that the artery is perfusing the retina. The band and sclera are cultured. The area is lavaged with a polymixin B-neomycin-bacitracin solution. The conjunctiva

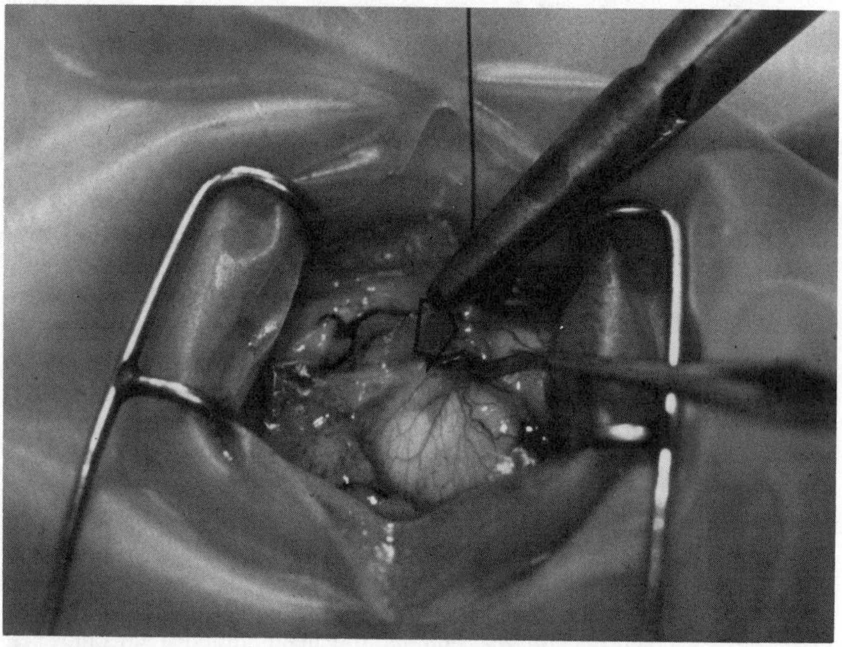

**FIG 11–5.**
The horizontal and vertical muscles are gently isolated with a pediatric tenotomy hook. A 5-0 black silk suture is passed beneath the belly of the muscle for traction and exposure during the procedure *(arrowhead)*. Care must be taken not to pull excessively on the muscles, because they can avulse or be cheese-wired by the silk sutures.

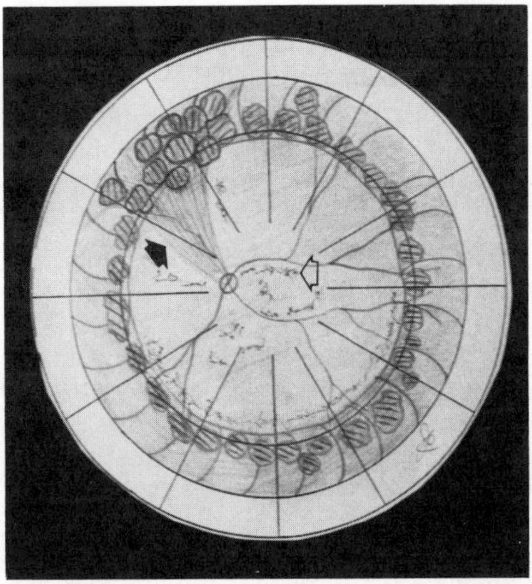

**FIG 11–6.**
Inadvertent shunt cryopexy in this case produced a retinal fold *(arrow)* extending from the disc to the periphery. Because the remaining shunt was well supported on the buckle, the fold did not cause the remaining retina to detach. The *open arrow* indicates dispersed pigment secondary to cryopexy.

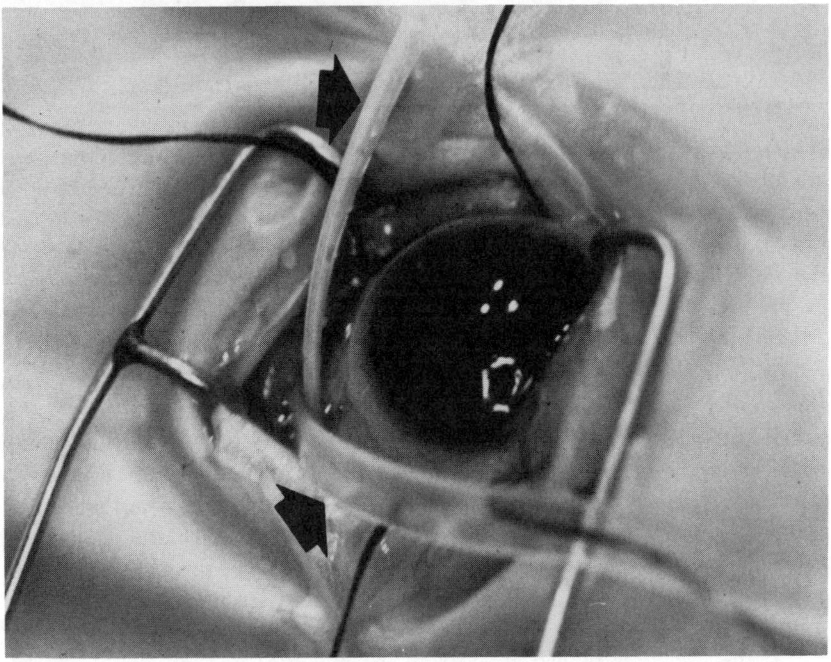

**FIG 11–7.**
A No. 240 solid silicone band serves as the buckle in this case *(arrows)*. It is carefully passed beneath all the horizontal and vertical muscles and tied with a Mersilene suture. To avoid erosion, clips are not used.

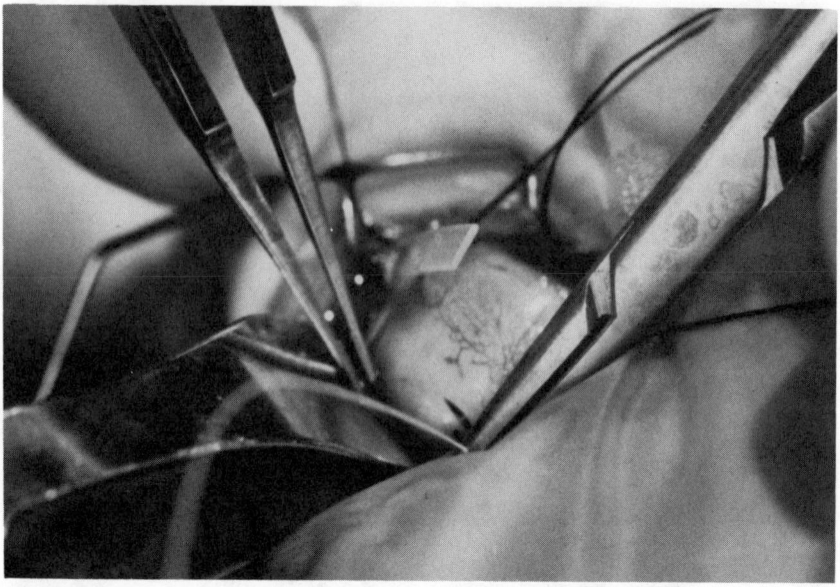

**FIG 11–8.**
A 5-0 Mersilene suture is used to anchor the band into position as an exoplant.

is closed with either 6-0 or 7-0 plain catgut sutures. Indirect ophthalmoscopy should reveal a low to moderately elevated buckle supporting the shunt, a pink optic nerve head, and buckle sutures not visible internally. A low buckle does not necessarily require more constriction. One or 2 days after surgery, the buckle will appear significantly higher than at the end of surgery.

Acetazolamide (5 mg/kg) can be given in lieu of drainage to soften the globe. Should hypotony develop after drainage, an intraocular injection of balanced salt solution through a 30-gauge needle inserted 2 to 2.5 mm from the limbus, corresponding to the pars plana, will increase the intraocular pressure to normalcy. Postoperatively, the child's intraocular pressure should be monitored with a pneumotonometer (Tonopen). Because there can be a fair amount of lid edema after surgery, a Schiotz tonometer can add more trauma to the globe. Care should be taken to follow corneal abrasions, as a corneal ulcer can easily result. The child should receive 1 drop of tropicamide 1% three times per day and 1 drop of an antibiotic-steroid combination every 6 hours for 3 weeks after surgery.

If the buckle is placed away from the maximal traction sites, or is left too low, vitreous traction incited by the cryopexy will further stimulate ridge contraction. This will cause an accelerated redetachment or a retinal break. Ultimately, an open-sky or closed vitrectomy approach may then be required.

However, buckle revision can be attempted, especially if the buckle was placed too far from the ridge.

Transection of the band is performed 3 to 6 months after the scleral buckling procedure, using general anesthesia. This is done to safeguard against erosion into the globe. The band should certainly be transected before the child is 1 year old, or growth will be restricted.

Postoperatively, the six eyes that underwent a scleral buckling procedure have been followed from 17 to 40 months. All the children are able to fixate and follow with the treated eye. One child has visual acuity of 20/100 and 20/400 (both with compound myopic corrections). Table 11–1 shows the postoperative results. Of the six eyes, only one demonstrated a large retinal fold produced by aggressive cryopexy (Fig 11–6). The dark arrow in Figure 11–6 demonstrates peripheral cryocoagulation which caused a retinal fold from the periphery to the disc. One eye has residual mild macular heterotopia, and the remaining four eyes demonstrate mild to moderate vessel straightening. Excessive cryotherapy, especially in the temporal quadrants, will cause increased retinal traction and can be the principal cause of macular displacement.

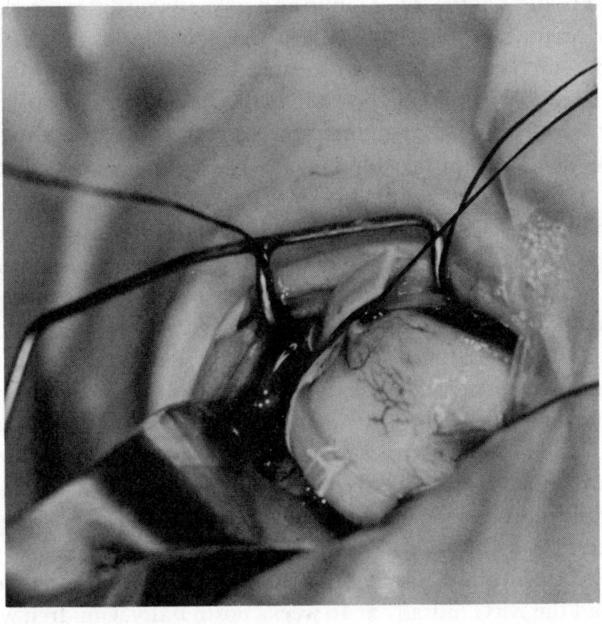

**FIG 11–9.**
The band is now in position and the excessive strip of solid silicone has been trimmed. The buckle will support areas of vitreoretinal traction.

**TABLE 11–1.**
Eyes With Scleral Buckling Procedure

| Birth Weight (gm) | Gestational Age at Birth (wk) | Procedure | Follow-up (mo) | Results at Follow-up |
|---|---|---|---|---|
| 1,050 | 30 | Buckle + cryo, OS | 17 | Fixates, superior fold |
| 1,200 | 31 | Buckle + cryo | 26 | Fixates |
| 940 | 30 | Buckle + cryo, OD | 30 | Fixates |
| 940 | 30 | Buckle + cryo, OS | 30 | Fixates, alt. exotropia |
| 1,100 | 29 | Buckle + cryo, OD | 40 | 20/400 |
| 1,100 | 29 | Buckle + cryo, OS | 40 | 20/100 |

Electroretinography (ERG) may have value in the preoperative and postoperative care of these children. However, using ERG successfully in children is laden with pitfalls. In addition to the great amount of patience needed to carry out the test, its correct interpretation can be difficult. Hollyfield and coworkers[6] have shown that the retina of a full-term infant with hydrocephaly has significant maturation of the neurotransmitter system which occurs after birth. Anatomically, the foveal photoreceptors are less dense in the human infant than in the adult.[7] The mass response in infants must be interpreted in light of these anatomic and physiologic differences. In essence, ERG in a premature child will be less developed than that seen in a full-term child, which is less than that seen in the adult. If we consider that rods greatly outnumber cones in the retina, the best hope of obtaining a mass response such as an ERG in an immature retina would be the scotopic ERG. In a nursery, this is not feasible and therefore the photopic ERG has been evaluated.

The stimulus threshold of the newborn retina is often greatly raised, producing responses with small amplitudes and prolonged implicit times, even with greatly augmented light stimuli. At times, it is possible to produce an ERG without a demonstrable a wave.[8] Even with these difficulties, the ERG may still serve a purpose when used in conjunction with the clinical picture and when repeated under similar conditions in the same child over a period of time.

Five of the aforementioned nine infants with active ROP detachments have been studied. Three children were initially seen with stage 4a disease and two children had stage 5 disease. The gestational age of these children ranged from 29 to 31 weeks and included four boys and one girl. Three children had the initial ERG at 12 weeks postnatally, whereas the other two children had the ERG initially at 16 weeks postnatally. Children were studied either in the neonatal intensive care unit (NICU) or in the physician's office. All children had been off the respirator for at least 1 week.

A Cadwell 5200 machine was used because it is compact and easily portable. The children's pupils were dilated with 1% tropicamide and 2.5%

phenylephrine. The retinas had not been bleached by light for at least 30 minutes prior to ERG testing. The stimulus was a strobe light, similar to a timing light used for engine tuning, which produced a bright-flash study. Because it is difficult to place an infant at the Ganzfield stimulator, the ERG must be done with the strobe stimulus. After the instillation of a topical anesthetic, an ERG-Jet corneal contact lens was placed on the cornea. This contact lens served as the active electrode. The ground and reference electrodes were placed as shown in Figure 11–10. The ERGs were recorded monocularly. The light intensity in the ICU or office was reduced 30 minutes before the test was performed in order to avoid too-bright ambient light. Phototherapy, if used, was also stopped 30 minutes before testing. Voltages were recordable in normal nonpremature children at 125 to 175 μV using these parameters.

Postoperatively, all the retinas were reattached and restudied every month for 3 months. One year after surgery, four of the five children with a retinal

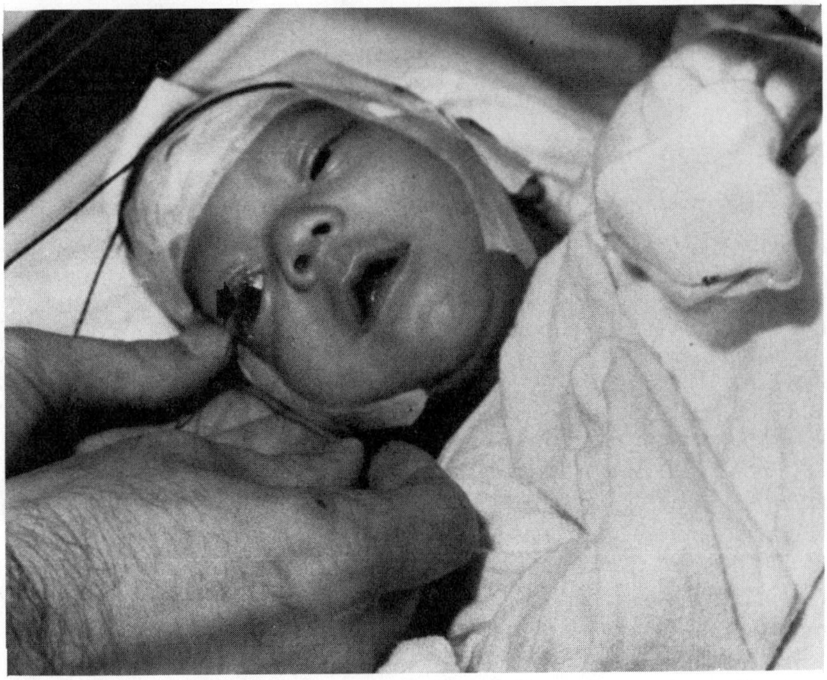

**FIG 11–10.**
This infant is being readied for an electroretinogram. After the skin has been cleansed, the ground electrode is placed on the forehead. A corneal contact lens *(arrow)* is used, and the reference electrode is placed at the temple.

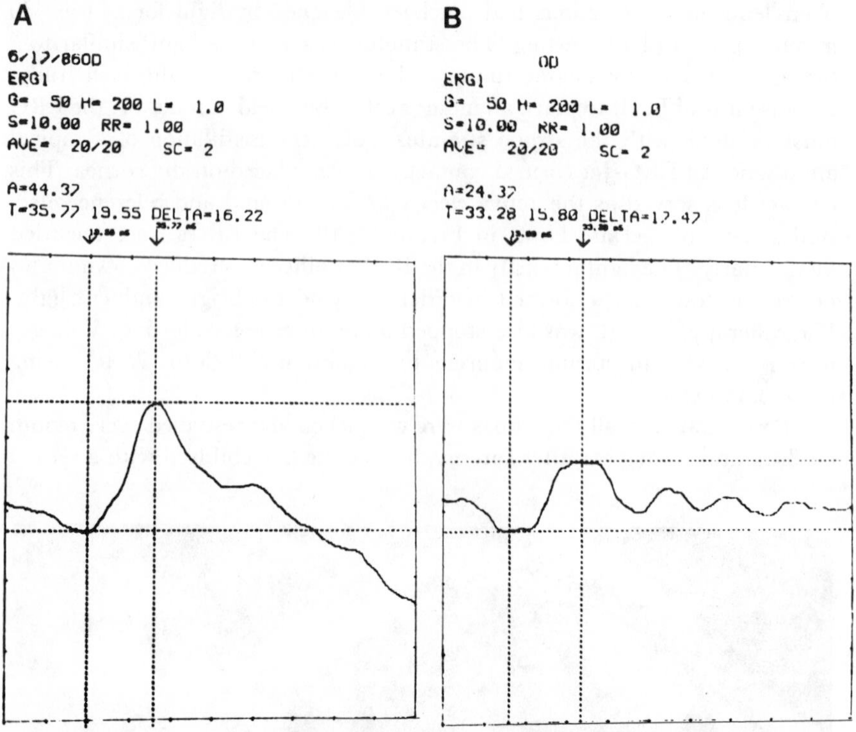


**FIG 11–11.**
A, this electroretinogram was taken in a 16-week-old premature infant girl with an extrafoveal detachment. **B**, after 2 weeks, the detahment progressed into the posterior pole and a reduction in the b wave was seen. The amplitude of the b wave has decreased. The a wave appears to be present in both studies, although it was difficult to obtain it in many cases.

detachment have been reevaluated by electrophysiological methods. Figure 11–11, A and B demonstrates such a case. This child was restudied 6 months after the buckle (No. 240 band) was cut (1 year after the buckling procedure had been performed) and demonstrated a reduced amplitude a and b wave in the ERG. Forty months after surgery, this child's visual acuity is 20/100. Preoperatively, the child's ERG demonstrated an absent a wave and a 50% reduction in the b wave.

The results showed that the ERG is extremely variable in these children. Each ERG must be compared to prior studies in the same individual. The a wave was decreased or absent in all eyes; however, in view of the prematurity of these children and the fact that the a wave can be difficult to elicit, this remains a phenomenon to be investigated. No significant abnormalities were found between the latencies observed in ROP vs. non-ROP infants. Eyes harboring a total detachment demonstrated an absent ERG.

As an extrafoveal detachment encroached upon the macula, the b wave amplitude began to decrease. Scleral buckling procedures were not performed until a significant decrease (usually 50%) was seen in the b wave. In view of the work described by Glass and coworkers,[9] dealing with high ambient light and the production of ROP, excessive light in nurseries may play a role in producing a retinal detachment in these infants by its toxic effects on the RPE. This may explain the difficulty in obtaining an a wave in this series.

Reappearance of an a wave was seen 3 months after successful surgery. Even 1 year after surgery, no difference could be seen between the 3-month and the 1-year readings. In the two eyes with a total detachment, a rudimentary b wave returned within 1 month. At one year, the a and b wave were present (Fig 11–12).

Several studies evaluating the ERG in patients with retinal detachments have been published.[10–13] Several authors have found that the b wave potential decreases as the area and the duration of detachment increase.[10, 11, 13]

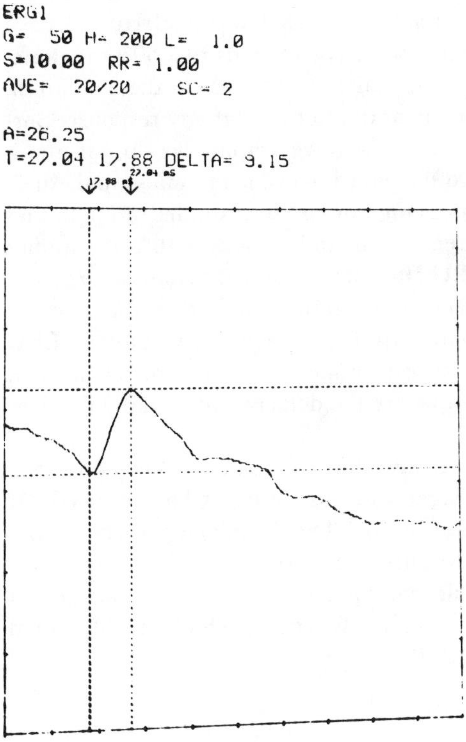


**FIG 11–12.**
Preoperatively, this child demonstrated a flat ERG with total detachment. The detachment was treated with a scleral buckle and drainage, and 1 year after surgery—6 months after the buckle was released—the ERG has a and b waves. Compared with controls at the same age, this ERG is abnormal.

Eyes with total retinal detachments will have a flat ERG.[14, 15] In most series, the ERG remained subnormal in spite of successful reattachment.[10, 11, 13] It is important to remember that any type of ERG (conventional or bright flash) is a mass response and does not give adequate information about the status of the macula. The above protocol uses a high-intensity flash to produce a small-amplitude, short-latency ERG with sharply peaked a and b waves. Variables that can adjust the height of the b wave, such as ambient room illumination, flash-to-eye distance, and flash intensity, were kept as uniform as possible. This can be especially difficult when dealing with premature infants in an ICU. An ICU can have anywhere from 35 to 90 ft-c of illumination. The lights were dimmed as much as possible in these settings. This factor could not be controlled, but an effort was made to decrease the lighting in the immediate testing area by 50%. Moreover, electrical shielding is not optimal in this setting. The children that were tested preoperatively in the ICU were tested postoperatively as much as possible in the ICU. Children tested preoperatively in the office were tested postoperatively in the office. The ambient light intensity in the office averaged 35 ft-c. A decreased a wave was possibly the initial electrophysiological response to a retinal detachment seen in these children; however, I cannot be sure because the a wave can be elusive in children.[8] Although Fuller and Hutton have noticed that a 50% reduction in the a wave corresponds to a 50% nonfunctional retina in adults,[16] this did not appear to be the case in these children. Children with a total retinal detachment did not exhibit any response. Surgery does improve the ERG; however, the wave amplitudes do not attain the initial amplitudes seen prior to macular involvement. Yinon and Auerbach noted that the ERG did not change in children studied prior to and after cataract surgery.[17] This current small study agrees with prior studies that demonstrated a subnormal ERG after successful reattachment surgery.[12] Work is needed using pattern electroretinography to further evaluate the macula in children pre- and postoperatively. A preoperative pattern ERG may be helpful in assessing the effects of a chronic detachment on the macula. The macula may be damaged even before the detachment actually involves macular tissue.

I use the b wave reduction as my indicator that the detachment is progressing to the point where a significant loss of cones has occurred. At this point, I intervene with a scleral buckle. The technique is certainly not free of problems because many factors are uncontrollable. Protocol flexibility must be maintained with these children; however, I do believe that the test is useful as a linear observation of the retinal function in children with retinal detachments secondary to active ROP.

## DISCUSSION

Machemer has theorized that the late stages of ROP develop as a result of several factors: contraction of the shunt area with retinal stretching, elevation of the retina by contraction of proliferative tissue, intravitreal tissue proliferation, and the anteroposterior location of the proliferative tissue.[18] The children who presented with stage 4a disease have all had intravitreal tissue proliferation with tissue-vitreous interaction. This interaction, coupled with the circumferential contraction of the shunt, served as the leading edge of the detachment. I also believe that there is a poor neurosensory-retinal pigment epithelial (RPE) adhesiveness, possibly caused by the immaturity of the pigment epithelium. This concept of a poor neurosensory-RPE bond strength is shared by other authors as contributing to the development of a traction detachment in these children.[19] A poor neurosensory-RPE bond will allow more and more retina to detach, often within a short time. If the shunt quiets down when the retina is detached, the picture may be a total detachment with pliable retina.

I have chosen the current surgical methodology for several reasons. Careful identification of the shunt region is important because this area needs to be well supported. The retina must be visualized with an indirect ophthalmoscope and the anterior retina treated with a cryoprobe. Because the sclera is very thin, extensive cryopexy is unnecessary. The production of a large iceball may stimulate further contraction of the shunt, which in turn increases the height of the shunt and further detaches the retina. For the retina to settle, support must be given to this shunt and the neovascularization halted. To this end, cryotherapy is applied to the avascular retina anterior to the shunt. The shunt should not receive cryotherapy as this may cause segmental contraction, as seen in Figure 11–6.

The published literature indicates that the rate of anatomical success in children with active ROP under 1 year of age varies between 50% and 100%. Koener described two cases of retinal detachments in two patients in which he placed donor sclera in an encircling episcleral fashion.[20] He reported anatomical attachment in one case, with improvement of vessel dragging. Yassur and coworkers treated two cases of retinal detachment with an invaginated lamellar strip of sclera.[21] They prefer a localized, equatorially placed buckle because this permits further growth of the globe. Also, it does not introduce a foreign substance such as solid silicone or a silicone sponge, which can theoretically become infected. They do not discuss the timing of the procedure, but feel that once a traction detachment has begun, no spontaneous regression is possible. Grunwald and coworkers describe three cases where only one eye received a scleral invagination procedure and one received a localized Lincoff sponge.[22] A third child received an equatorial encircling

Lincoff sponge. All three cases were reattached with one procedure. They remark on one fellow eye that had a shallow temporal detachment. It resolved spontaneously without therapy, but exhibited marked traction on the disc and macula.

McPherson et al. reported their extensive experience with the scleral buckling procedure in active ROP.[2, 23, 24] Her opinion is that when the macula is threatened or when the detachment involves the posterior pole, a scleral buckling procedure should be performed. This study reported on 101 eyes that underwent the scleral buckling procedure, including 35 eyes which had previously undergone cryopexy. Overall, McPherson et al. reported a 54% success rate in anatomically reattaching the retina despite macula dragging. Their follow-up ranged from 6 to 132 months. Snellen visual acuities have been recorded for 11 eyes, and six eyes have counting-fingers vision.

Bert and coworkers reported their experience with combined cryotherapy and scleral buckling in seven eyes of six premature children with an acute retinal detachment.[25] In their series, four cases had an identifiable peripheral break. They reported postoperative visual acuities ranging from 20/40 to 20/200 and a 100% reattachment rate. The infants in their series were younger than those reported here, and had a much longer follow-up period of up to 6 years. I have not seen any traction breaks as described by Bert and coworkers. However, I agree with Bert and coworkers that a detachment, once it has entered the posterior pole, should be repaired. Careful limitation of the number of cryo applications is also important. Excessive cryotherapy in terms of numbers of applications or maximal temperature can produce large folds, which may limit postoperative visual acuity (Fig 11–6). They cause segmental contracture of the shunt. A nasal fold may not have any consequences; a temporal fold, however, may ultimately involve the macula, producing a poor functional outcome. Excessive cryotherapy can also cause a more generalized contraction of the shunt, which may lead to retinal breaks. This may be a factor in causing the peripheral breaks seen after cryotherapy for stage 3 ROP.

Topilow and coworkers reported five successful outcomes in seven eyes.[19] Their surgical approach does not include drainage, but they do stress the need to relieve areas of vitreoretinal traction and placement of the buckle to adequately support these areas. In another chapter of this book, they describe their surgical approach, which does not greatly differ from mine. The principles of adequate cryopexy and appropriate buckle placement are also emphasized. They also state that extreme temperatures are not necessary to adequately treat these eyes. Attaining $-25°C$ will effectively ablate the avascular region.

At the American Academy of Ophthalmology meeting in Las Vegas in 1988, Topilow and Ackerman reported successful reattachment of the retina in 8 of 11 eyes that developed a tractional detachment after cryotherapy.[26] In their series, all the retinas reattached within 72 hours of scleral buckling with or without drainage. Although I have drained the detachments with a large amount of fluid, it may indeed not be necessary.

Tasman reported five successful attachments in six eyes. He prefers to operate on eyes that exhibit a tractional component as evidenced by peripheral cicatrization.[27] Baruch and coworkers reported only one case with successful reattachment of the retina.[28]

A separate question involves the use of a prophylactic buckle along with cryopexy. Hittner and coworkers reported an 81% success rate in preventing the development of a retinal detachment using both cryopexy and a scleral buckle.[29]

In summary, stages 4 through 5 respond to cryotherapy and scleral buckling. It is important not to overtreat the retina with cryopexy, as this may induce peripheral cicatricial changes that have a tendency to extend into the posterior pole. A detachment can be total (stage 5) and have a freely mobile funnel configuration. This may still respond to scleral buckling and drainage. This type of detachment appears to be unusual, and may represent resolution of the shunt after the retina has detached. Electroretinography demonstrates a flat ERG in patients with a total detachment, which reverts to a subnormal ERG after a scleral buckling procedure. A threatened macula may be diagnosed by involvement of the b wave. Further clinical and surgical correlations should help resolve questions about these eyes.

## REFERENCES

1. Ashton NW: Oxygen and the growth and development of retinal vessels. *Am J Ophthalmol* 1966; 62:412–435.
2. Patz A: The role of oxygen in retrolental fibroplasia. E Mead Johnson Award Address. *Pediatrics* 1957; 19:504–524.
3. Foos RY: Acute retrolental fibroplasia. *Graefes Arch Clin Exp Ophthalmol* 1975; 195:87–100.
4. Orellana J: Examination of the premature infant, in McPherson, Hittner, and Kretzer (eds): *Retinopathy of Prematurity: Current Concepts and Controversies.* Toronto: BC Decker Inc, 1986.
5. McPherson AR, Hittner HM, Kretzer FL: Treatment of acute retinopathy of prematurity by scleral buckling, in McPherson AR, Hittner HM, Kretzer FL (eds): *Retinopathy of Prematurity: Current Concepts and Controversies.* Toronto: BC Decker, 1986.
6. Hollyfield JG, Frederick JM, Rayborn ME: Neurotransmitter properties of the newborn human retina. *Invest Ophthalmol Vis Sci* 1983; 24:893–897.
7. Abramov I, Gordon J, Hendrickson A, et al: The retina of the newborn human infant, *Science* 1982; 217:265.

8. Zetterstrom B: The electroretinogram of the newborn infant. *Int Ophthalmol Clin* 1969; 9:1039–1049.
9. Glass P, Avery GB, Subramanian KNS, et al. Effect of bright light in the hospital nursery on the incidence of retinopathy of prematurity. *N Engl J Med* 1985; 313:401–404.
10. Rendahl I: The ERG in detachment of the retina. *Arch Ophthalmol* 1957; 57:566–576.
11. Stephens G and Safir A: The ERG as a prognostic aid in retinal detachment. *Arch Ophthalmol* 1958; 59:515–520.
12. Schmogen E: Die Prognostische Bedeutung des Elecktroretinenogramms bei Ablatio Retinae. *Klin Monatsbl Augenheilkd* 1957; 131:335–343.
13. Francois J and Verriest G: Les fonctions visuelles dans le décollement de la retinae. *Ann D'oculist* 1955; 188:97–162.
14. Karpe, G: The electroretinogram in detachment of the retina. *Acta Ophthalmol* 1948; 26:267.
15. Hamasaki DI, Machemer R, Norton EWD: Experimental retinal detachment in the owl monkey. VI. The ERG of the detached and reattached retina. *Graefes Arch Clin Exp Ophthalmol* 1969; 177:212–221.
16. Fuller DW and Hutton WL: *Presurgical Evaluation of Eyes with Opaque Media.* New York: Grune & Stratton.
17. Yinon U and Auerbach E: The electroretinogram of children deprived of pattern vision. *Invest Ophthalmol Vis Sci* 1974; 13:538–543.
18. Machemer R: Description and pathogenesis of late stages of retinopathy of prematurity. *Ophthalmology* 1985; 92:1000–1004.
19. Topilow HW, Ackerman AL, Wang FM: The treatment of advanced retinopathy of prematurity by cryotherapy and scleral buckling surgery. *Ophthalmology* 1985; 92:379–387.
20. Koerner FH: Retinopathy of prematurity: Natural course and management. *Methods Ophthalmol* 1978; 2:325–329.
21. Yassur Y, Grunwald E, Ben-Sira I: Surgical treatment of retrolental fibroplasia in infants. *Methods Ophthalmol* 1978; 2:333–334.
22. Grunwald E, Yassur Y, Ben-Sira I: Buckling procedures for retinal detachment caused by retrolental fibroplasia in premature babies. *Br J Ophthalmol* 1980; 64:98–101.
23. McPherson AR, Hittner HM: Scleral buckling in $2^1/_2$ to 11 month old premature infants with retinal detachment associated with acute retrolental fibroplasia. *Ophthalmology* 1979; 86:819–835.
24. McPherson AR, Hittner HM, Lemos R: Retinal detachment in young premature infants with acute retrolental fibroplasia: Thirty-two new cases. *Ophthalmology* 1982; 89:1160–1169.
25. Bert MD, Friedman MW, Ballard R: Combined cryosurgery and scleral buckling in acute proliferative retrolental fibroplasia. *J Pediatr Ophthalmol Strabismus* 1981; 18:9–12.
26. Topilow HW, Ackerman AL: Cryotherapy for Stage 3+ retinopathy of prematurity: Visual and Anatomic results. Presented at the American Academy of Ophthalmology Annual Meeting, Las Vegas, 1988.

27. Tasman W: Management of retinopathy of prematurity. *Ophthalmology* 1985; 92:995–999.
28. Baruch E, Bracha R, Godel V, et al: Buckling procedure in infant retrolental fibroplasia. *J Ocular Ther Surg* 1981; 1:65–66.
29. Hittner HM, McGee JK Jr, Kretzer FL: Anticipating traction and growth in severe retinopathy of prematurity. Presented at the American Academy of Ophthalmology Annual Meeting, Las Vegas, 1988.

Chapter 12

# Open-Sky Vitrectomy in Stage 5 Retinopathy of Prematurity

Juan Orellana, M.D.

## INTRODUCTION

Retinal detachments in retinopathy of prematurity (ROP) develop as a function of the arteriovenous shunt (AV) line. Continued contraction of a thickened napkin-ring shunt region that deposits collagenous tissue ultimately produces the characteristic leukocoria seen in end-stage ROP. The collagen deposition is responsible for the hazy white tissue seen behind the clear lens (Fig 12–1). Often, neovascularization continues, even though the retina has totally detached and has contracted into the center of the globe in a funnel configuration. This process may change an open funnel detachment into a closed funnel detachment by virtue of a continued shunt-vitreous interaction. Infants who have either been unsuccessfully treated for stage 3 ROP or who have had an unsuccessful scleral buckling procedure can present with leukocoria and a clinical picture of severe stage 5 ROP.

The surgical approach to these cases can be either through open-sky vitrectomy or through the anterior segment-pars plicata route, more commonly referred to as a closed vitrectomy procedure. The route chosen depends on the surgeon's preference. Tasman reported a 25% anatomical success rate using closed vitrectomy techniques.[1] Merritt et al. did not achieve any successes in their group of 12 cases.[2] Lightfoot and Irvine[3] reported a 60% success rate, while Machemer[4] reported a 58% success rate using a closed vitrectomy approach. In a series of more than 400 patients, Charles reported a 50% success rate.[5] Chong et al. reported a 43% success rate using the anterior segment approach.[6] In a follow-up report, Charles described a 46%

success rate in 586 cases of total retinal detachment.[7] Trese achieved 48% anatomical success with a 31% functional success in his series.[8]

In these children, I prefer not to approach vitreous work via the trans-ciliary body, pars plicata, or anterior segment route, as has been previously proposed by the aforementioned authors. Entry into the anterior segment through the cornea is associated with a distorted view of the surgical field caused mostly by the suturing of an infusion cannula at the corneoscleral limbus. This is a problem that can be overcome by using a two-hand dissection technique.[9] Before beginning surgery, the surgeon must consider the altered anatomy of the eye in this condition. The pars plana is often detached in these children, and the peripheral retina as well as the pars plana is rolled forward and into the vitreous cavity. This is caused by contraction of the shunt and stretching of the peripheral avascular retina. This shunt region becomes the leading edge of the detachment, leaving the vascularized retina behind and located much closer to the eye wall. Foos attributes the retinal foreshortening, posterior detachment, and funnel formation to this rolling of the peripheral retina.[10] Entry into the eye at the pars plana can contribute to the formation of multiple iatrogenic breaks, which are extremely difficult to close. Surgery for severe stage 5 ROP is not true vitreous surgery as we commonly refer to it. For the most part, this surgery requires slow, piecemeal dissection techniques and patience on the part of the surgeon.

I prefer to use the open-sky vitrectomy approach, the technique introduced by Schepens and Hirose. In this approach, the anatomy is readily observable during surgery. Dissection is easier and much safer than through the closed vitrectomy approach. The surgeon has much more control over the field.

## Materials and Methods

A retrospective review was conducted of children undergoing open-sky vitrectomy for ROP between 1984 and 1987. During this period, 25 infants (40 eyes) had lensectomy, membranectomy, and vitrectomy for a total retinal detachment in one or both eyes. All patients had a leukocoria and had been born prematurely. The gestational age at birth ranged from 27 to 31 weeks, and the series included 10 boys and 15 girls. At the time of surgery, some patients exhibited aspects of active and cicatricial disease. The follow-up period ranged from 24 to 48 months. In many cases, preoperative assessment included echography and more recently electrophysiology.

## Echography

In an eye with stage 5 ROP, there is frequently no view of the posterior pole. In these eyes, echography helps the surgeon decide the best approach to the funnel-shaped detachment, and determine whether the funnel detachment is open both anteriorly and posteriorly, closed anteriorly and posteriorly, or a combination of both. It always reveals the relationships between retrolental membranes and detached retina.

I prefer the Biophysic unit (Ophthascan "S"), a contact unit, which has a small and easily maneuverable probe. The unit is adjusted for sensitivity, near and far gain, and image position on the screen.

When an older child is examined, the probe is shown to the child. The physician may want to touch the child's hand with the probe to demonstrate that the test is painless. The patient can be seated upright or supine. If axial measurements are taken, it is preferable for the child to be seated. If necessary, the infant may be wrapped in a sheet or restrained in a papoose for examination.[11] The examination of a young infant is preferably scheduled at the child's mealtime: the parent can feed the hungry child while the test is being performed. Because the intraocular pressure will have been previously tested with a Tonopen or pneumotonometer, the anesthetic effects of the topical anesthetic should still be in effect. Without a topical anesthetic, the gel may burn the child's eye and prematurely end the echographic examination.

Funnel detachments in children with ROP can be described as open, partially open, or closed. The funnel's opening may lie in any quadrant and not necessarily in the midline. Such a funnel detachment may begin its course arising from the optic nerve and progressing anteriorly, with a bend occurring at the equator and ending in one of the quadrants. On a quick scan of the eye, the surgeon may erroneously decide that a funnel-shaped detachment is not present simply because the midline horizontal and vertical scans appear normal. The eye must be examined in at least three vertical and three horizontal planes and the information pooled to reconstruct a three-dimensional view of the globe. Figure 12–1 demonstrates such a case. Using an isolated scan in this case suggested an attached retina with membranes. Additional views of the globe were necessary to compose a complete picture, which differed greatly from the initial impression. Figures 12–2 (Plate 10) and 12–3 also demonstrate this point. In Figure 12–4 it appears that only a shallow detachment is present. However, other views (Fig 12–5) demonstrate that a hyaloid system is present and that there is significant intravitreal tissue proliferation. The scans should evaluate the size of the globe, the configuration of the detachment, the most anterior point at which retinal tissue will be found, and finally, the position of the retrolental membranes.[12] Although a closed funnel detachment does not necessarily correlate with a poor prognosis, it is essential to know that the funnel itself is closed. This knowledge will dictate to the surgeon where it is possible to dissect deeper, in cases with open funnels, and where the dissection must be kept in a shallow plane, in

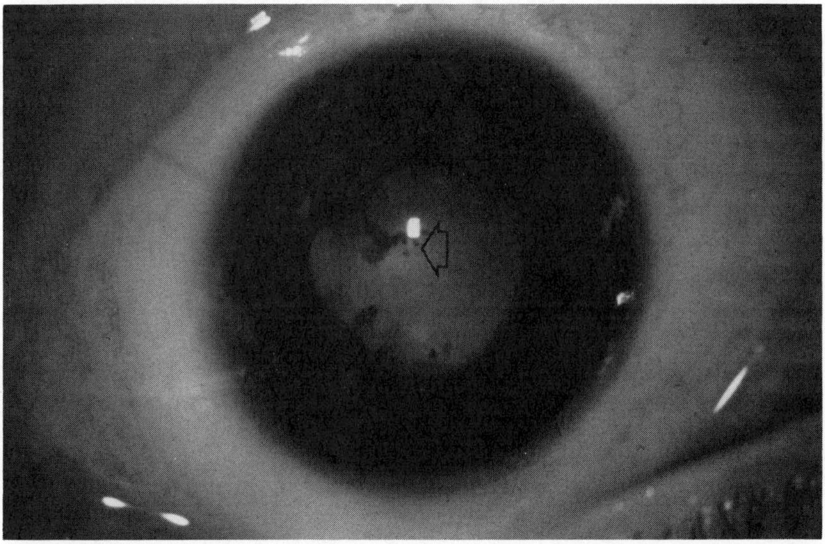

**FIG 12–1.**
**A**, deposition of collagen within the funnel produces the white retrolental tissue seen in severe stage 5 ROP *(arrow)*. When collagen deposition is heavy, the tissue is opaque. Frequently there is no view of the posterior pole.

cases with a closed funnel. During surgery, small hemorrhages can reduce visibility; thus, having a complete three-dimensional picture of the globe allows the surgeon to proceed safely.

It is imperative that the surgeon and not a technician perform the examination. A photograph of the scan is not a substitute for the surgeon's examination because the photograph does not convey the same information. The technician will not be performing the surgery, and may see several configurations on the scan that may not seem important enough to photograph or to tell the surgeon about. If surgery will not be performed within days of the examination, the test should be repeated before surgery in the operating room or in the physician's office. This will prevent iatrogenic complications at surgery. Investing a few moments to make certain the funnel is unchanged can make a difference between success and failure.

Over the last 4 years, I have evaluated 40 eyes by ultrasonography, and only 30 (75%) of these eyes have had funnels that were open in the midline. Of these 30 cases, 18 globes had funnel detachments open anteriorly. The remaining 12 demonstrated a closed anterior funnel. Ten globes had funnels that opened eccentrically. One third of the 40 cases (13 eyes) demonstrated a thickened choroid, which agrees with the findings reported by Shapiro and Stone.[13]

All of the cases in this series had a retinal detachment which was demonstrable by contact B-scan examination. In 90% of eyes, multiple low-amplitude echoes were seen, which corresponded to the retrolental membranes and epiretinal membranes situated in the anterior vitreous, behind the lens, and in front of the retinal mass. This is the tissue we readily see when examining the child with advanced ROP.

## Visual Evoked Potentials

An even more difficult technique to interpret is the visual evoked potential (VEP). Characteristically, the VEP is clinically useful in demonstrating an abnormal sensory system function, in documenting demyelinating disease, in defining the anatomical location of a disease process, and in objectively monitoring the patient over a period of time. VEPs were recorded in infants with severe stage 5 ROP using light emission diodes (LED) (Fig 12–6) and a Cadwell 5200 machine. This produced a pattern reversal evoked potential (PVEP). The active electrode was placed about 1 cm above the

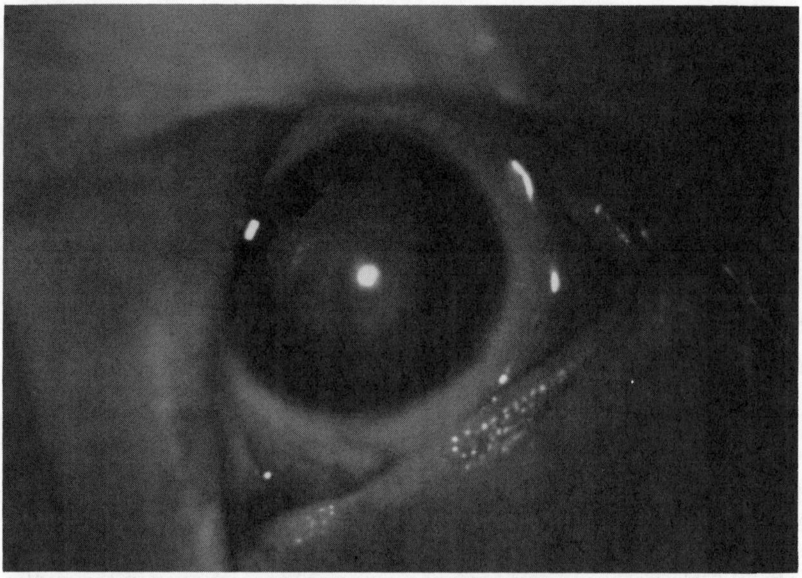

**FIG 12–2.**
Prominent retinal vessels in the detached retina *(arrow)* are easily seen through the clear crystalline lens. The center of this funnel has a moderately transparent membrane bridging the funnel opening. See also Plate 10.

inion. An inactive electrode was placed at the temples and the patient was grounded. The filters were set at 1 to 3 Hz low cutoff and 100 to 300 Hz high cutoff. Four trials were averaged to determine the latency. Each trial consisted of 100 sweep repetitions.

To date, 10 children (14 eyes) with stage 5 ROP were tested prior to open-sky vitrectomy. Testing revealed an absence of detectable waveforms in these children. Three months after surgery, five of these children with attached retinas were again tested, and there was no appreciable difference between pre- and postoperative test results. By visual assessment even 2 years after surgery, the optimal acuity was counting fingers, which would correlate with the poor PVEP results obtained again 2 years after surgery. Although the posterior pole was attached (zone 1 or zone 2 attachment), the VEP had been permanently altered. The PVEP appears to be more sensitive to hypoxia than is the ERG. In nine of the 14 eyes with attached retinas, postoperative ERGs returned, indicating that although the postoperative

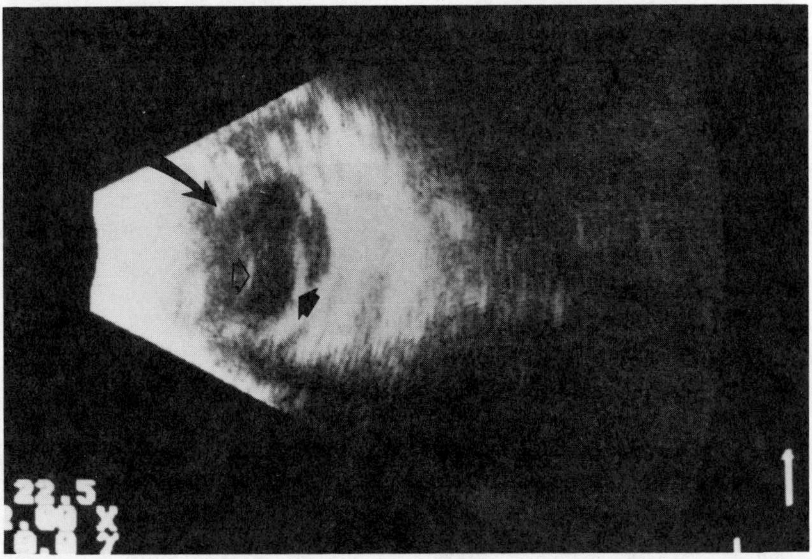

**FIG 12–3.**
Echography can be the most useful preoperative test in a child with severe stage 5 ROP and no view of the posterior pole. This study is a vertical midline section. It shows peripheral membranes *(white arrow)* and a bridging posterior membrane *(solid arrow)* in an eye with an attached retina. Reconstruction of the eye using other views demonstrated that the eye harbored a detachment with an open anterior and a closed posterior portion. The *curved arrow* demonstrates the peripheral scrolled retina and trough.

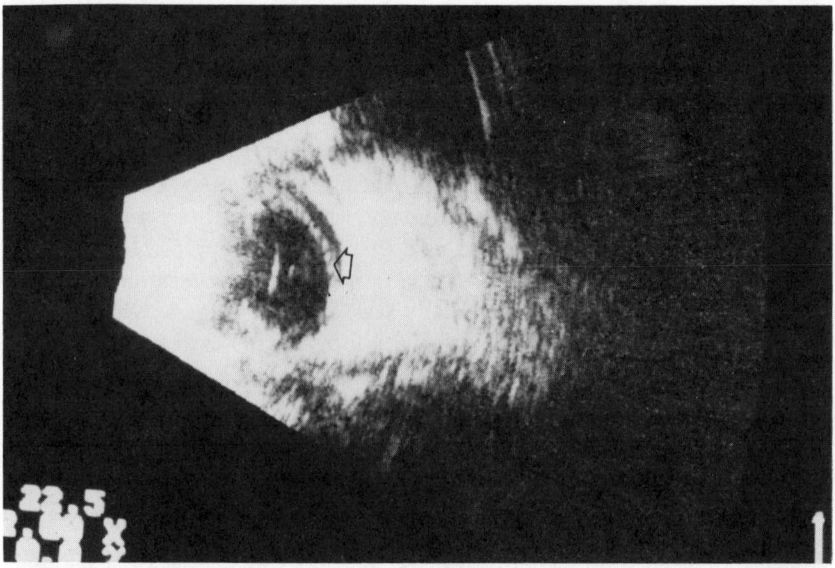

**FIG 12–4.**
This study suggests a shallow detachment *(open arrow)*. This section is a vertical-nasal view.

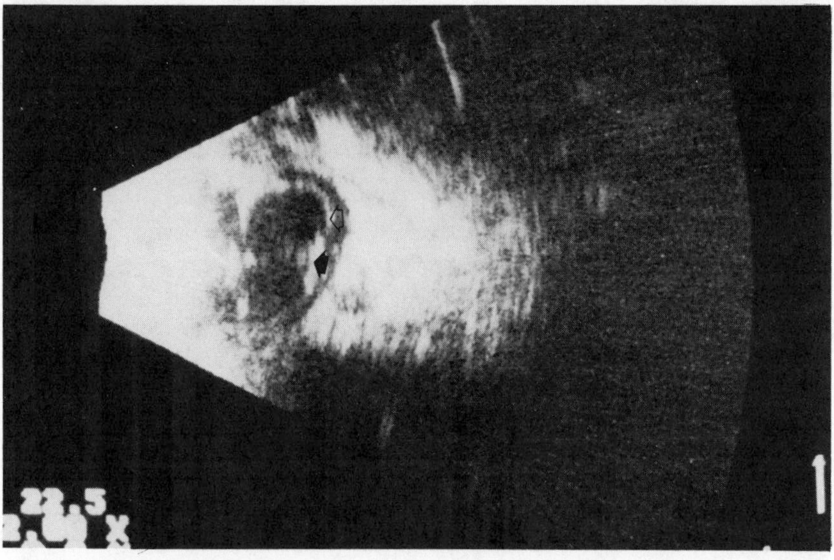

**FIG 12–5.**
In a vertical midline view of the same patient in Fig 12–3, there is indeed a retinal detachment *(open arrow)*. A central stalk corresponding to a persistent hyaloid system *(arrow)* and intravitreal proliferation can also be seen. Multiple views in different planes must be taken to adequately assess the position of the intraocular tissues.

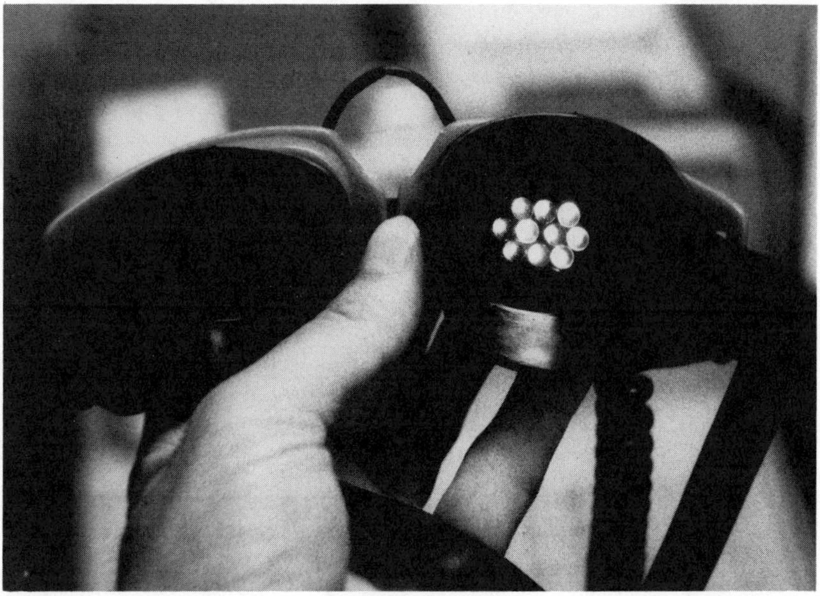

**FIG 12–6.**
These light emission diode (LED) goggles produce a pattern-reversal visual evoked response. The stimulus is intense, even through the eyelids. This enables the physician to test the infant without using a monitor and without being concerned about the infant's eye movements.

ERG was subnormal, some electrical activity was present. Prior to surgical intervention, the preoperative ERGs had been flat. The hypoxic damage to the retinal tissue at the posterior pole was too great to allow for a functional return of activity; thus the PVEP remained flat. This was true for all cases, whether the attachment was zone 1 or zone 2.

The surgical technique is as follows: The child is prepped and draped as for a scleral buckling procedure. A Flieringa ring or any type of scleral support is sewn into the episclera to keep the globe supported during surgery. I prefer a running silk suture because it holds the tissue well and is easy to see during the procedure. The cornea is measured and a corneal trephine is chosen that will leave at least 1.5 mm of healthy cornea on all sides. The corneal button is trephined and placed into fresh McCarey-Kaufman (M-K) medium. The routine principles of corneal surgery with regard to grafting techniques are adhered to during this procedure.

After the cornea has been removed and the marking sutures on the graft and host tissues are in place, the iris should be examined. Adhesions between the lens and iris should be lysed, and the vessels located near the pupillary border can be treated with underwater diathermy. Meticulous care paid to the iris vessels will help ensure good visualization throughout the surgery. It is important to avoid aggressive cautery of the iris vessels. A sphincterotomy is performed at the 12- and 6-o'clock meridians and permits good exposure of the lens. The lens is dried with a surgical spear and then removed in an intracapsular fashion (Fig 12–7). The removal is performed slowly to minimize any disruption of the tissues located behind the lens. Both the vitreous face and the retrolental membranes are now exposed. At this time, the surgeon refers back to the ultrasound pictures.

The surgeon must proceed depending on the configuration of the funnel. Is the funnel open both anteriorly and posteriorly, open only anteriorly, or only posteriorly? I grasp the membrane located over the opening of the funnel using a Kelman-McPherson forceps and open a small hole in the membrane with a Vannas scissors (Figs 12–8 and 12–9). Care must be taken to work carefully without producing traction on the peripheral trough. Excessive tugging will produce a dialysis of the peripheral retina, which will not be noticed until the trough dissection is complete. The membrane is removed piecemeal, with alternating dissection and tissue removal. The process is continued to the site of the original shunt, the leading edge of the detachment

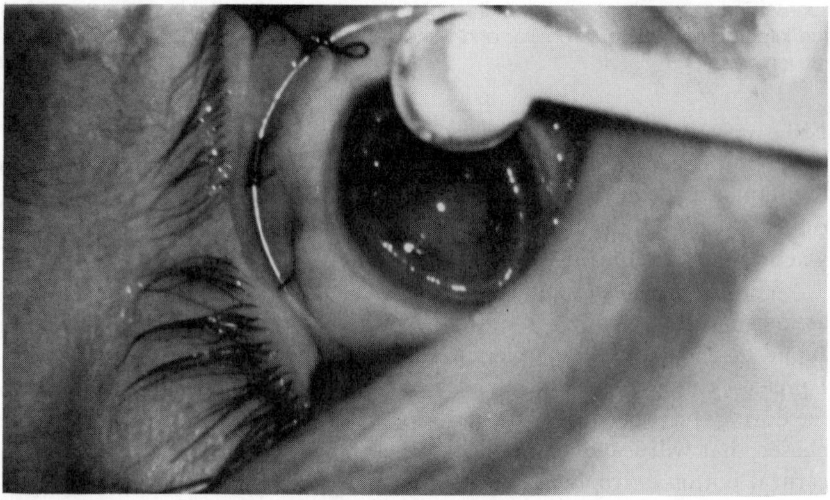

**FIG 12–7.**
After an iris sphincterotomy is made at the 6-o'clock and 12-o'clock meridians, the lens is removed in an intracapsular fashion. Lens extraction is easy, and with slow and gentle traction the surrounding tissue is not disturbed.

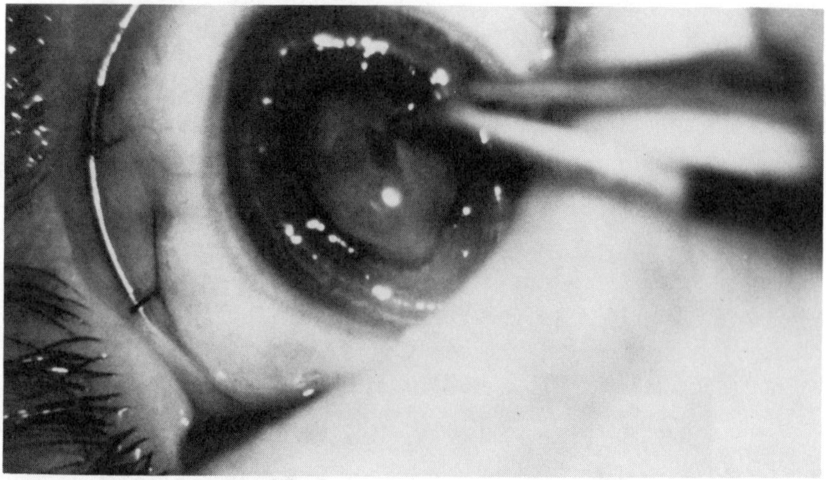

**FIG 12–8.**
Echography studies indicate that the funnel in this case opens in the midline. After the lens and vitreous face have been removed, the center membrane is incised and the dissection proceeds to the peripheral trough.

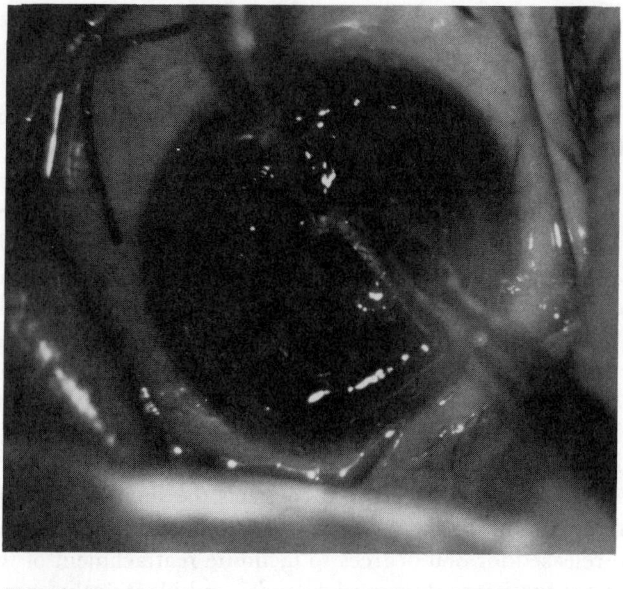

**FIG 12–9.**
The dissection continues as the surgeon opens the funnel. Once a small opening is made, the dissection becomes easier, as the surgeon obtains a clearer picture of the retinal detachment. The surgeon should consult echography studies because they may point out potential pitfalls.

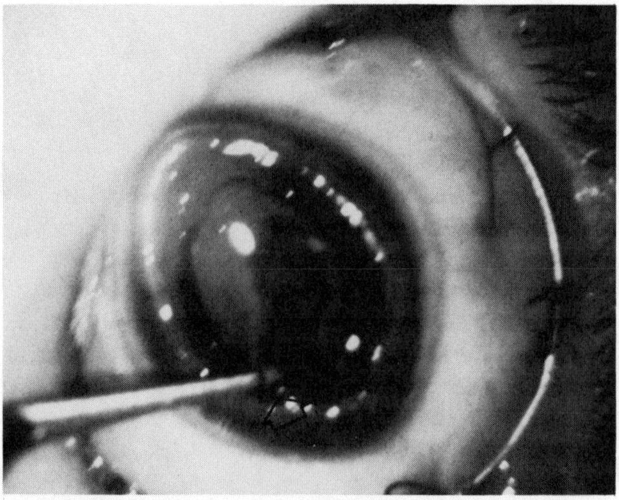

**FIG 12–10.**
The dissection has reached the leading edge of the detachment *(arrow)*. When the dissection has opened the entire funnel, attention should be paid to the peripheral trough. The iris should be gently elevated and the trough incised, allowing the retina to drop posteriorly.

(Fig 12–10). The epiretinal tissue is slowly removed to prevent excessive bleeding. Hemorrhage is unavoidable, but can be minimized by gentle tissue manipulation. After the superficial membranes have been removed, attention is paid to the funnel itself. If the funnel is moderately open, the dissection continues posteriorly in a blunt fashion. Sharp dissection must be avoided because it is easy to mistake retinal tissue for proliferative fibrovascular tissue. Healon is very useful as an adjunct to dissection. Injected into the funnel, it helps expand the funnel and isolate epiretinal membranes which must be removed. In eyes that harbor a tight funnel detachment, the same techniques are employed; however, the overall rate of tissue dissection and removal is even slower.

After the funnel has been opened, attention is shifted to the peripheral trough. The retina anterior to the shunt extends to the ora serrata and is located underneath a membrane that connects the shunt to the ora serrata. This membrane prohibits the retina from relaxing and dropping posteriorly. It must be released for 360 degrees to facilitate reattachment of the retina. I gently retract the iris with a surgical spear and identify the area with the most diaphanous membrane. I incise the membrane and continue with scissors, releasing as much as is safely possible. The more tissue is incised, the greater the amount of retinal mobilization. Traction on these peripheral tissues will also produce a disinsertion of the peripheral retina. The surgeon will notice that after the trough has been completely released, the plane of tissue will drop posteriorly. I do not ordinarily drain subretinal fluid in these cases. I have drained three eyes that were laden with cholesterol crystals. Reattachment of these retinas can take months in cases where longstanding detachments are present. Any center stalks that may represent remnants of the primary vitreous or hyaloid artery are carefully examined before further dissection is carried out. Tugging at these structures produces posterior tears which cannot be seen. I inject Healon into the cavity, which functions to control small bleeders in the perioperative and postoperative periods. The iris tissue is pulled gently away from the angle and the pupil is reconstructed using 10-0 Prolene. The cornea is resewn into place using either a running or interrupted 10-0 nylon suture (Fig 12–11).

To date, 19 of 40 eyes in 25 patients have been anatomically reattached. The visual acuities range from no light perception to counting fingers. Table 12–1 summarizes the postoperative visual acuities in this group of patients. The period of follow-up in these patients varies between 24 and 48 months. Although other cases have been added within the last two years, most do not have measurable visual acuity and have not been included in this series.

Ultrastructural and histopathological evaluation of the retrolental membranes in six of these eyes demonstrates a high connective tissue concentration (Figs 12–12 and 12–13; Plate 11). This increases the older the tissue. Foos reported that in 40 autopsy eyes, the pathogenesis of the retinal detachments was unique and represented progressive changes in the peripheral retina.[10] He stated that although the retina detaches, there is no tissue behind the lens or bridging across the vitreous cavity during the stage in which the peripheral retina had scrolled and the posterior vascularized retina had detached. Ultrastructural study of 37 retrolental membranes by Kretzer demonstrated vascularity of the membranes obtained from infants 4 to 5 months postnatally as well as the presence of actin.[12] Soong and coworkers demonstrated the presence of actin in retrolental membranes.[14] The actin filaments contained in the myofibroblast-like cells are the prime generators of the traction detachment in these children. Kretzer noted that a fibrillary matrix was present in infants 6 months postnatal and still represented a pliable retina that could be anatomically corrected.[12] Samples from infants 7 to 16 months old demonstrated multiple ghost vessels and a condensation of the fibrillary matrix. It correlated clinically with a decrease in the pliability of the retina during surgery. Older children (ages 2 through 6) demonstrated dense cables composed of the fibrillary matrix. The optimal time for surgical intervention appeared to be between the ages of 4 and 7 months, while the retinal tissue was still pliable and the membranes could still be easily dissected.

I cannot overemphasize the importance of echography in these cases. de Juan and coworkers have studied ultrasound examinations in these children and have found them helpful in determining the extent of ROP and associated malformations seen in these retinal detachments.[15] They have used ultrasound to accurately place their drainage sclerotomies for the hemorrhagic choroidal detachments that can be found in some eyes. They stated that the technique becomes more and more valuable as the examiner gains more experience.

Jabbour and coworkers also found echography a useful tool because it provided details about the retrolental membrane, the funnel, retinal folds, the hyaloid system, and retinoschisis.[16] McPherson et al. also emphasized

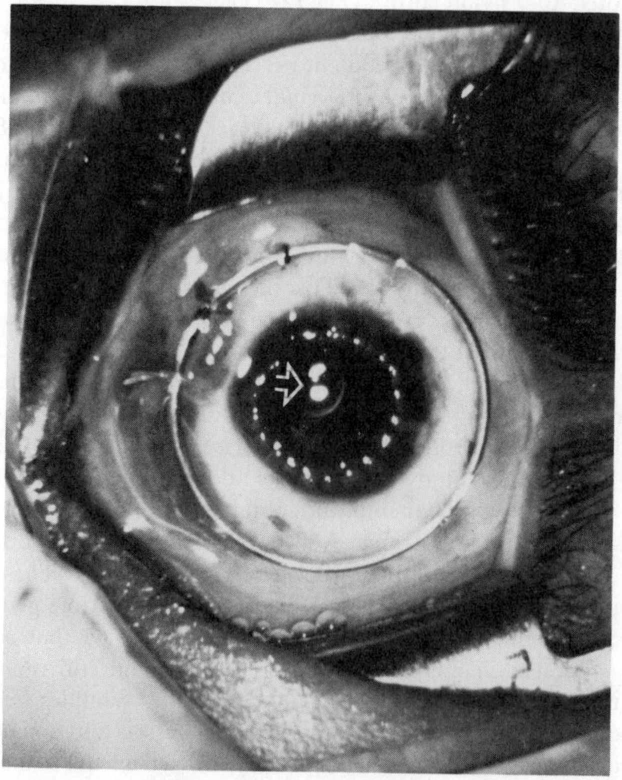

**FIG 12–11.**
The cornea has been resewn using interrupted 10-0 nylon sutures. There was excellent opening of the funnel during surgery. A small air bubble is present in the anterior chamber *(arrow)*.

**TABLE 12–1.**
Visual Results in Anatomically Reattached Retinas After Open-Sky Vitrectomy

| Patient # | Eye | Birth Weight (gm) | Gestational Age (wk) | Follow-up (mo) | Visual Acuity |
|---|---|---|---|---|---|
| 1 | OD | 780 | 28 | 24 | NLP |
| 2 | OD | 820 | 28 | 24 | LP |
| | OS | 820 | 28 | 26 | LP |
| 3 | OD | 800 | 29 | 28 | CF |
| | OS | 800 | 29 | 26 | HM |
| 4 | OD | 1,000 | 29 | 26 | HM |
| | OS | 1,000 | 29 | 28 | HM |
| 5 | OS | 1,100 | 28 | 29 | CF |
| 6 | OD | 830 | 29 | 29 | CF |
| 7 | OD | 820 | 29 | 30 | LP |
| | OS | 820 | 29 | 32 | LP |
| 8 | OD | 1,000 | 30 | 36 | HM |
| | OS | 1,000 | 30 | 37 | CF |
| 9 | OD | 800 | 30 | 40 | HM |
| | OS | 800 | 30 | 42 | LP |
| 10 | OS | 1,000 | 29 | 42 | LP |
| 11 | OS | 800 | 29 | 44 | HM |
| 12 | OD | 800 | 28 | 48 | HM |
| 13 | OD | 800 | 28 | 48 | LP |

*CF = count fingers; HM = hand movement; LP = light perception; NLP = no light perception; OD = right eye; OS = left eye.*

the value of preoperative echography. They pointed out that multiple scans must be obtained to fully elucidate the configuration of the detachment.[12] I feel that a careful study will tell the surgeon the data described by the above authors, but will also show whether the funnel is midline or shifted into another region. This information permits easier dissection in those cases where the retrolental plate and tissue are very dense.

Although the visual evoked potential can be performed using a strobe (flash) stimulation or the pattern reversal method, the latter is more consistent.[17] Evaluating children with VEPs has usually been mentioned as a means of assessing their visual acuity and providing an indirect measure of macular function. VEPs in newborn infants were first described in 1957 by Ellingson.[18] Using an LED type of stimulation is one way of generating pattern reversals with a greater luminance and a faster pattern reversal (Fig 12–6). The rapid rate of pattern reversal shortens the latency of P100 in pattern reversal evoked potentials (PVEP). In normal children, the P100 latency occurs approximately 10 ms earlier than the P100 elicited by the television monitor.

Retinal damage was implicated as a cause of the abnormal test results in this series. Sokol and Jones, and Moskowitz and Sokol, have found that

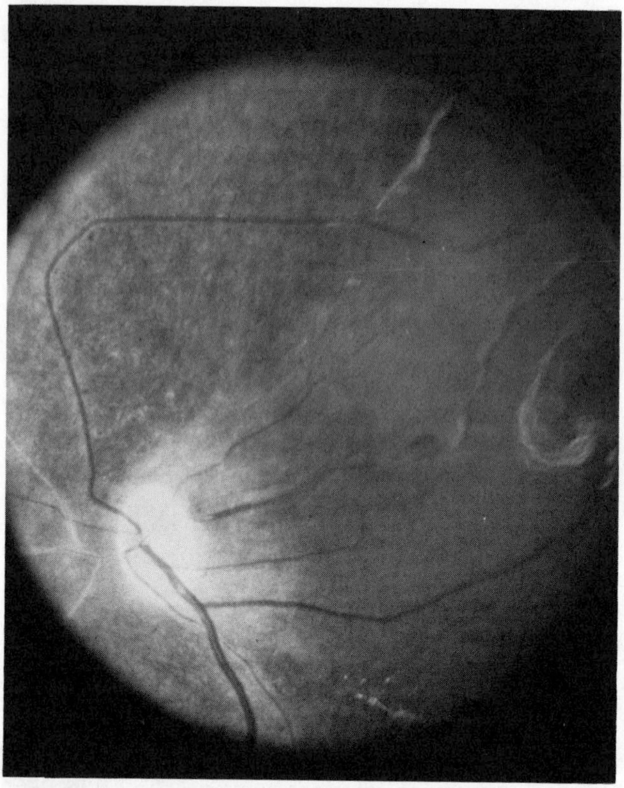

**FIG 12–12.**
One year after open-sky vitrectomy, this patient has zone 2 attachment. The child was 16 months old at the time of surgery. Visual acuity is counting fingers.

the latency of 30' checks reaches adult levels by 20 weeks, and smaller checks do not reach adult latency levels until the child is 5 or 6 years of age.[19, 20] We know that P1 can be obliterated by inattention to the stimulus by the subject. However, the LEDs placed directly over the infant's eyes make this highly unlikely (Fig 12–6). In our laboratory, P1 latencies range from 100 to 125 msec in normal eyes of children under the age of 15. Pattern visual evoked potentials under chloral hydrate sedation have been reported by Wright and coworkers.[21] They obtained reproducible PVEP waveforms under anesthesia. They felt it provided control of eye position, ensuring a testing of the central 12 degrees of the visual field, which is responsible for the majority of the PVEP.

In summary, although the retina can be anatomically attached after surgical repair of severe stage 5 ROP, electrophysiological testing demonstrated that only a moderate amount of electrical activity returned to the tissue. The macular region was apparently permanently damaged. Certainly, this is a very small sample, and a larger group of children must be tested to further evaluate retinal function after open-sky vitrectomy.

The visual results obtained in this series, however, underscore the fact that the parents must be told what to expect. The best visual acuity is counting fingers, and most acuities are light perception or hand motions. These remain low percentage cases which can fail at any point during the surgery. Even at the end of what may appear to be successful surgery, a small, unnoticed break or reproliferation will result in an adverse outcome within 2 weeks. Posterior dissection can cause small unoticed breaks which will cause failure. Eller and coworkers describe a 9% incidence of a persistent hyaloid artery in patients with ROP.[22] They believe it is the scaffold for further membrane growth in these eyes. With contraction, the persistent hyaloid artery may cause the posterior tight funnel configuration. Care must be taken when dissecting these membranes and the stalk, because excessive

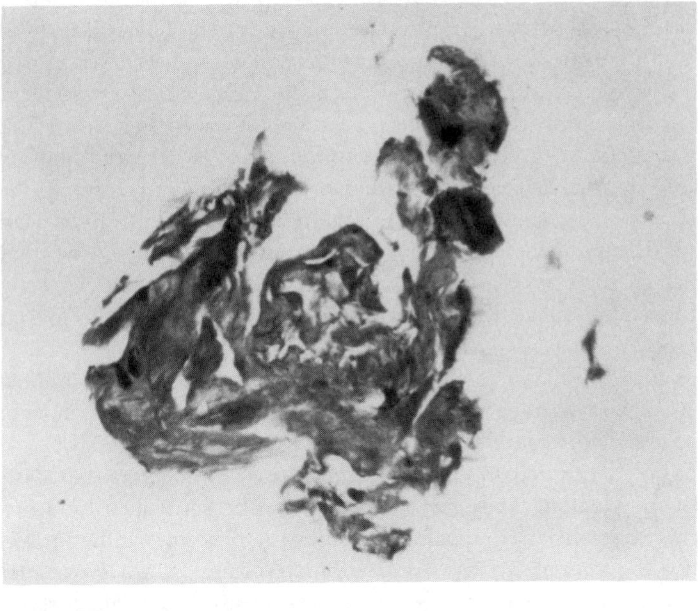

**FIG 12–13.**
Specimen taken from a 2-year-old child. The tissue, which was located behind the lens and bridging the funnel, demonstrates a large amount of minimally vascularized connective tissue. See also Plate 11. (Pathologic study performed by Alan H. Friedman, M.D.; Masson-trichrome; ×60.)

traction will produce breaks. This stalk should be trimmed; I find that its adherences to the surrounding tissue must be identified and released.

The anatomical success rate of 47.5% of this report compares favorably with the results of Charles (46%), Trese (48%), and de Juan (42%), using closed vitrectomy techniques.[7, 23, 24] McPherson et al. reported a 22% success rate in partially open funnel detachments, and an 11% success rate in closed funnel detachments using open-sky vitrectomy techniques.[12] Chong and co-workers reported a 57% anatomic success with open funnels and a 29% success rate with closed funnels.[16] Tasman reported a 37.5% success rate using open-sky vitrectomy techniques.[25] He felt that an elevated intraocular pressure and an opaque cornea are the two contraindications to surgery. The presence or absence of pupillary synechiae, a shallow anterior chamber, or a tight funnel anteriorly or posteriorly on ultrasound examination did not preclude a successful outcome. Several cases which demonstrated a tight funnel opened up quite nicely, especially if the patient was under 8 months of age. I agree that a flat anterior chamber is not a contraindication but should be taken into account as the surgeon trephines the cornea.

Certainly, it has been difficult to standardize what constitutes anatomic success in these children. de Juan et al. utilize the descriptions of retinopathy of prematurity as detailed by the Committee for the Classification of Retinopathy of Prematurity. The minimal amount of attached retina necessary to fulfill anatomic success is zone 1.[26] Of the 19 eyes that are reported as a success in this series, 5 were zone 1 successes. This includes one child with no light perception, 2 with light perception, and 2 with hand motions. The children with zone 2 successes all had counting fingers results. Still, for all the work that is expended on these children, I agree with other authors in lamenting the poor visual results. I try to have the children wear aphakic spectacles as soon as possible, although amblyopia is surely present in all cases. Even after successful surgery, the retina can take up to four months to reattach.

This surgery is associated with many technical pitfalls, most notably the problems of hemorrhage during surgery and iatrogenic tears. Hemorrhage can be controlled by underwater diathermy, although excessive diathermy can produce a tear. Tamponade of small surface bleeders can be accomplished with Healon, while large bleeders can be controlled by a thrombin drip. This must be used sparingly because it produces inflammation that can cause the surgery to fail. After sphincterotomy, the iris retracts under the host cornea and a fibrinous membrane develops over its surface. Heparinized balanced salt solution plus will help prevent this membrane from forming. Alternatively, the fibrous membrane can be stripped from the iris surface at the end of the procedure without adverse sequelae. During the dissection, I prefer to use the Kelman-McPherson IOL forceps to dissect because they grasp but do not tear the tissue. They have a long nose which allows them to be used for open-sky vitrectomy. A slow and steady dissection will eventually produce a retina that is freely mobile. Quick dissection will cause a retina break, which is almost impossible to repair. In this series, every eye that had an iatrogenic break failed and represented most of the initial attempts at open-sky vitrectomy. I am sure that small breaks cannot be averted and so I tamponade with Healon and air at the end of the procedure in the hope that this will keep the retina expanded and help close any small break.

In this series, I found that meticulous surgery correlated with a successful outcome. I made it a crucial part of the procedure to ensure that the peripheral trough was incised for 360 degrees, allowing the retina to drop posteriorly. I agree with other authors that release of the posterior pole membranes is important to the final outcome.[6, 24]

Reported complications included hypotony, iris-retina adhesions, corneal decompensation, cyclitic membranes, and ectropion uvea.[27] All the cases I have done have resulted in an intraocular pressure of less than 12, as tested by Tonopen or pneumotonometer. The lowest recorded intraocular pressure is 40. I have not had a problem with rubeosis or cyclitic membranes because I refrain from cautery as much as possible. Reproliferation certainly is the most devastating complication and may occur despite uneventful surgery.

Four weeks after surgery, the child is usually examined under anesthesia to ascertain whether or not the retina has begun to settle. Although it can take up to four months for the retina to settle, the sight of an open funnel will indicate that traction has been released. It will also indicate that reproliferation has not begun and that the detachment is settling. These are traction detachments, and settle when the forces keeping the retina elevated have been removed. Internal drainage is not necessary, and even external drainage is not advised. The sudden decompression of the subretinal space allows the retina to suddenly drop, and if the traction has not been completely released, a large retinal tear will result.

Time will tell if this heroic endeavor will pay dividends to the patient. The parents express joy that their children appear to ambulate and interact with their surroundings to a higher degree. It is possible that the children are simply getting older and becoming more accustomed to their handicap.

## REFERENCES

1. Tasman W: Late complications of retrolental fibroplasia. *Ophthalmology* 1979; 86:1724–1736.
2. Merritt JC, Lawson EE, Sprague DH, et al: Lensectomy-vitrectomy for stage 5 cicatricial retrolental fibroplasia. *Ophthalmic Surg* 1982; 13:300–306.

3. Lightfoot D, Irvine AR: Vitrectomy in infants and children with retinal detachments caused by cicatricial retrolental fibroplasia. *Am J Ophthalmol* 1982; 94:305–312.
4. Machemer R: Closed vitrectomy for severe retrolental fibroplasia in the infant. *Ophthalmology* 1983; 90:436–441.
5. Charles S: Vitrectomy for retrolental fibroplasia. Presented at American Academy of Ophthalmology Annual Meeting. Atlanta, Nov 12, 1984.
6. Chong LP, Machemer R, deJuan E: Vitrectomy for advanced stages of retinopathy of prematurity. *Am J Ophthalmol* 1986; 102:710–716.
7. Charles S: Vitrectomy with ciliary body entry for retrolental fibroplasia, in McPherson AR, Hittner HM, Kretzer F (eds): *Retinopathy of Prematurity: Current Concepts and Controversies.* Toronto, BC Decker, 1986, pp 225–234.
8. Trese MT: Surgical results of stage V retrolental fibroplasia and timing of surgical repair. *Ophthalmology* 1984; 91:461–466.
9. Trese MT: Two-hand dissection technique during closed vitrectomy for retinopathy of prematurity. *Am J Ophthalmol* 1986; 101:251–252.
10. Foos RV: Chronic retinopathy of prematurity. *Ophthalmology* 1985; 92:563–571.
11. Orellana J: Examination of the premature infant, in McPherson AR, Hittner HM, and Kretzer FL (eds): *Retinopathy of Prematurity: Current Concepts and Controversies.* Toronto: BC Decker Inc, 1986.
12. McPherson AR, Hittner HM, Moura RA, et al: Treatment of retrolental fibroplasia with open-sky vitrectomy, in McPherson AR, Hittner HM, Kretzer FL (eds): *Retinopathy of Prematurity: Current Concepts and Controversies.* Toronto, BC Decker Inc, 1986.
13. Shapiro DR, Stone RD: Ultrasonic characteristics of retinopathy of prematurity presenting with leukokoria. *Arch Ophthalmol* 1985; 103:1690–1692.
14. Soong HK, Eller AW, Hirose T, et al: In situ actin distribution in excised retrolental membranes in retinopathy of prematurity. *Arch Ophthalmol* 1985; 103:1553–1556.
15. de Juan E Jr, Shields S, Machemer R: The role of ultrasound in the management of retinopathy of prematurity. *Ophthalmology* 1988; 95:884–888.
16. Jabbour NM, Eller AE, Hirose T, et al: Stage 5 retinopathy of prematurity: prognostic value of morphologic findings. *Ophthalmology* 1987; 94:1640–1646.
17. Shahrohki F, Chiappa KH, Young RR: Pattern shift visual evoked responses: Two hundred patients with optic neuritis and/or multiple sclerosis. *Arch Neurol* 1978; 35:65–71.
18. Ellingson RJ: "Arousal" and evoked responses in the EEG of newborns. *Proc First Int Congr Neurol Sci* 1957; 3:57.
19. Sokol S, Jones K: Implicit time of pattern evoked potential in infants: An index of maturation of spatial vision. *Vision Res* 1979; 19:747–755.
20. Moskowitz A, Sokol S: Spatial and temporal interaction of pattern-evoked cortical potentials in human infants. *Vision Res* 1980; 20:699–707.
21. Wright KW, Eriksen J, Shors TJ, et al: Recording pattern visual evoked potentials under chloral hydrate sedation. *Arch Ophthalmol* 1986; 104:718–721.
22. Eller AW, Jabbour NM, Hirose T, et al: Retinopathy of prematurity: The association of a persistent hyaloid artery. *Ophthalmology* 1987; 94:444–448.

23. Trese MT: Visual results and prognostic factors of stage V retinopathy of prematurity. *Ophthalmology* 1986; 93:574–578.
24. de Juan E Jr, Machemer R: Retinopathy of prematurity: Surgical technique. *Retina* 7:63–69.
25. Tasman W, Barrone RN, Bolling J: Open sky vitrectomy for total retinal detachment in retinopathy of prematurity. *Ophthalmology* 1987; 94:449–452.
26. de Juan E Jr, Charles ST, Hirose T, et al: Surgery for stage 5 retinopathy of prematurity. *Arch Ophthalmol* 1987; 105:21.
27. Hirose T, Schepens CL: Complications in open-sky vitrectomy, in Freeman HM, Hirose T, Schepens CL (eds): *Vitreous Surgery and Advances in Fundus Diagnosis and Treatment.* New York, Appleton-Century-Crofts, 1977.

# Index

## S